Radiation Oncology and Radiation Biology

Joel Greenberger

Radiation Oncology and Radiation Biology

The Next 100 Years

Springer

Joel Greenberger
University of Pittsburgh
Pittsburgh, PA, USA

ISBN 978-3-031-66299-7 ISBN 978-3-031-66300-0 (eBook)
https://doi.org/10.1007/978-3-031-66300-0

This Springer imprint is published by the registered company Springer Nature Switzerland AG
The registered company address is: Gewerbestrasse 11, 6330 Cham, Switzerland

Concept of the Book

This book has two large sections: one describing the current status of the medical specialty of Radiation Oncology and predictions for the evolution of the specialty over the next decades.

The second section deals with the predictions for the future of Radiation Biology. This more comprehensive and detailed section will deal with two major categories: space travel and adaptation of humans to continuous, but sporadic galactic cosmic irradiation, and combined injury factors from multiple other physiological and medical consequences of long-term exposure to space irradiation. This section deals with the late effects of ionizing irradiation on humans, who have received therapeutic radiotherapy. Expanding use of high dose rate, small volume targeted stereotactic radiosurgery, and stereotactic ablative radiosurgery is expected to increase the numbers of long-term surviving patients. The medical, physiological, and radiobiological consequences of radiation late effect is described in detail. The current novel techniques of radiotherapy including FLASH irradiation, high LET particle irradiation, and novel strategies for a theranostics (combined radiographic diagnosis of metastatic deposits and delivery of therapeutic radiation) are described. The use of clinical radioisotopes in cancer therapy is described.

Prologue

This book has two large sections: one describing the current status of the medical specialty of Radiation Oncology and predictions for the evolution of the specialty over the next decades.

The second section deals with the predictions of the future of Radiation Biology. This more comprehensive and detailed section will deal with two major categories: space travel and adaptation of humans to continuous, but sporadic galactic cosmic irradiation, and combined injury factors from multiple other physiological and medical consequences of long-term exposure to space irradiation. This section deals with the late effects of ionizing irradiation on humans, who have received therapeutic radiotherapy. Expanding use of high dose rate, small volume targeted stereotactic radiosurgery, and stereotactic ablative radiosurgery is expected to increase the numbers of long-term surviving patients. The medical, physiological, and radiobiological consequences of radiation late effect is described in detail. The current novel techniques of radiotherapy including FLASH irradiation, high LET particle irradiation, and novel strategies for a Theranostics (combined radiographic diagnosis of metastatic deposits and delivery of therapeutic radiation) are described. The use of clinical radioisotopes in cancer therapy will be described. The section on Radiobiology also includes several chapters on radiation countermeasures, which are drugs that would be delivered to people after they had been exposed to unplanned ionizing irradiation from a nuclear reactor accident or a will full radiation terrorist or wartime event. These radiation countermeasures are being developed in an attempt to save lives, but also will provide much new information on the effects of ionizing radiation on the bone marrow, intestine, lungs, and other organs.

Acknowledgments

I am most grateful to my three mentors: William C. Moloney, M.D., my mentor at Harvard Medical School, who taught me the importance of being a physician first, and then a Radiation Oncologist, and above all, inspired me to keep research with animal models and basic science closely linked to patient care; Stuart Aaronson, M.D., my mentor at the National Institutes of Health in the Viral Carcinogenesis Program, who taught me the love for basic science research and importance of hard work; and Samuel Helman, M.D., Professor and Chairman of Radiation Oncology at the Joint Center for Radiation Therapy at Harvard Medical School, where I did my residency, and who taught me the importance of critical thinking in understanding patient outcomes. With respect to Radiation Oncology during residency and attending training, I am most grateful to Ralph R. Weichselbaum, M.D., Fellow Resident, and subsequent Chairman of Radiation Oncology at the University of Chicago, who emphasized the importance of being a physician-scientist. For the colleagues in my laboratory at Harvard Medical School, I am very grateful to Mary Ann Sakakeeny, who was my Head Laboratory Technician colleague, and who followed me to the University of Massachusetts through my years of Chairman of Radiation Oncology 1984–1993. At the University of Massachusetts, Thomas Jeffrey Fitzgerald, M.D., who ran the Clinical Department, and was a constant source of support in my laboratory. At the University of Pittsburgh during the years 1993–2022, when I was Chairman of the Department of Radiation Oncology, all faculty and staff at all levels and at all people at UPMC Cancer Center hospitals, who supported me in my role as chairman and supported my laboratory at the University of Pittsburgh from 1993 to the present I have maintained uninterrupted NIH funding for my laboratory. Many colleagues, helped my research including Michael Epperly, Ph.D., Amitava Mukherjee, Ph.D., Renee Fisher, Donna Shields, Wen Hou, and many Radiation Oncology residents, fellows, and medical students, who devoted research years working in my laboratory and allowed me to be their mentor. Colleagues in the Radiation Countermeasures Program at the National Institutes of Health, National Institute of Allergy and Infectious Diseases (NIAID), who have inspired me to continue working and contributing to develop radiation countermeasures include Andrea DiCarlo, Ph.D., Carmen Rios, Ph.D., Lanyn

Taliaferro, Ph.D., David Cassatt, Ph.D., and my colleagues at NASA, who have continued to update me on the importance of Space Radiation Biology; Jeffrey Jones, M.D., Carlos Montesinos, Ph.D.; Fathi Karouia, Ph.D. For continuous support in manuscript and book preparation, Susan Shimko. For moral support in book writing and preparation, Kees Gispen, my wife Catherine Greenberger, and children, Benjamin, Joshua, Emily, and Rachel. For love and guidance throughout my life, my parents Julius Paul and Freeda Greenberger and my trumpet teacher, Anthony Louis Pasquarelli.

Contents

About the Author

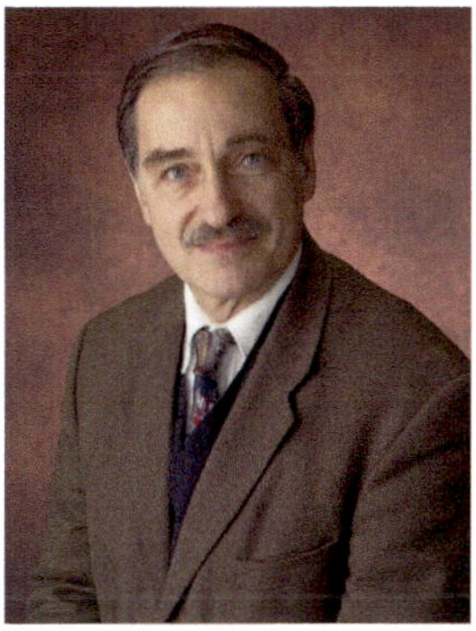

Joel S. Greenberger, MD, FACR, FACRO, FASTRO graduated from Taylor Allderdice High School in Pittsburgh, Pennsylvania in 1964, completed undergraduate education at Columbia University with a major in Music, and then attended Harvard Medical School graduating in 1971. He did a medical internship at Boston City Hospital, residency in Radiation Oncology at the Harvard Joint Center for Radiation Therapy, and was a Staff Associate at the National Cancer Institute focusing on research in retroviruses, animal models of cancer, and in in vitro techniques of studying Hematopoiesis and Leukemogenesis. His interest in Radiation Biology initiated with his mentor, William C. Moloney, MD, Chief of Hematology at Brigham and Women's Hospital in Boston, Massachusetts. Upon completion of his residency, he has practiced Radiation Oncology for over 50 years focusing on treatment of patients with Lung and Esophagus cancer.

He is a principal investigator managing an independent research program focused on discovery and development of radiation countermeasures and also lung cancer models. For the past 45 years, he has supervised over 30 postdoctoral fellows, junior faculty at the assistant professor level, and medical students. As a principal investigator, he has maintained uninterrupted NIH funding since 1977 and is a National and International manuscript reviewer in areas of radiation countermeasures, lung cancer, radiation biology, stem cell transplantation, and stem cell plasticity. He has been investigating the effects of irradiation on normal tissue responses and protecting and mitigating radiation acute and late effects on normal tissue. Support and inspiration for my career came from my beloved parents, Julius Paul and Freeda Greenberger, and my trumpet teacher, Anthony Louis Pasquarelli.

Chapter 1
Evolution of Radioresistance on Earth: From Single-Cell Organisms to Humans

Ionizing Irradiation in Our Everyday Lives

Since the first use of ionizing irradiation to treat cancer [1, 2], there has been a continual series of reports of individuals who appear to be sensitive [3] to irradiation and others and who seem to be resistant [4]. These reports led to the discovery of multiple disease states that are associated with sensitivity to radiotherapy. These include patients with Fanconi Anemia [5], Blooms Syndrome [6], Fragile XSyndrome, and Nijenmen Break Syndrome [7]. Analysis of the mechanism of radiation sensitivity led to the discovery of a series of genes and their products that are involved in the repair of DNA double-strand breaks [8]. Another mechanism of radiosensitivity of some cancer patients to the use of therapeutic radiation has been the knowledge and involvement of inflammatory mediators in the radiation response [9]. Patients who have a hyperactive induction of some inflammatory cytokines in response to unrelated inflammatory diseases have also shown radiosensitivity. These include patients with ulcerative colitis, Crohn's colitis, and other chronic conditions. Radiation oncology residents are taught to observe hyperactive response patterns in their patients and to appropriately dial back or reduce radiation dose, fraction size, or volume of tissue treated.

Variation in Radiation Resistance Among Humans: Where Did It Originate?

Radiation resistance of specific subpopulations of humans has been more difficult to categorize. Such observations would not even be possible in the absence of our current ability to precisely measure radiation dose. The first measurement devices included ionization chambers, then biologic assessment of radiation killing of cells

J. Greenberger, *Radiation Oncology and Radiation Biology*,
https://doi.org/10.1007/978-3-031-66300-0_1

in vitro [10, 11], and, most recently, the new development of precise physical measuring devices such as thermoluminescent dosimeters (TLD) [12], which are chips that can be placed in the radiation beam and convert physical elements to emit light that can be quantitated. Physical measurements of radiation dose, dose rate, and dose distribution within tissue-equivalent phantoms (3-dimensional structures that simulate the human body) have led to the precise calculation of radiation doses for therapeutic radiation. At the present time, it is established that some patients are radiosensitive and must be treated with extreme caution, while the majority of patients seem to respond in the same way when normal tissue side effects appear. Patients now receive fractionated irradiation—a dose of 1.8 to 2.0 Gy per day (180–200 rads). There is also information available on the radiation response of veterinary animals (pets and livestock). At the present time, veterinarians are subspecialized as oncologists, who are experts in the delivery of therapeutic irradiation to dogs, cats, and other domestic animals. Furthermore, there is evidence of the radiation sensitivity of other nondomesticated species from reports that have been derived largely from nuclear accidents, such as that in 1986 in Chernobyl, Ukraine [13], and in Fukushima, Japan, in 2011 [14]. Finally, there is a plethora of publications regarding the use of animals in irradiation research (mice, rats, dogs, nonhuman primates, ferrets, rabbits, and others) [15].

The radiation biology literature contains information on the radiation responsiveness of most taxonomic phyla from single-cell organisms, multicellular organisms, and nearly all categories in the plant and animal kingdoms. There are several ways in which the plant and animal kingdoms have been organized since the original system as defined by Linnaeus in 1758 [15]. The evolution of life on Earth has been estimated to have begun 4.0 to 3.5 billion years ago based on fossil evidence (Table 1.1), but how this estimate can ever be verified remains a mystery. We do have elegant descriptions of plant and animal taxonomy (Tables 1.2, 1.3, 1.4, and 1.5), and the radiation sensitivity of many of these species has been studied [16, 17, 21–27]. With regard to humans, the now routine use of ionizing irradiation to treat cancer patients and others with certain benign diseases has led to a vast concern for the effects of ionizing irradiation on not only the patient but also the environment. This concern has prompted a focus on ionizing irradiation safety and the multiple ways in which humans can be injured. The concern also relates to the future including how we will prepare for the radiation of space travel [28] and the discovery of countermeasures for unplanned radiation exposure.

The deployment of nuclear weapons first tested in the 1940s and first deployed in 1945, as nuclear fission bombs at Hiroshima and Nagasaki in World War II [29], first necessitated that physicians and scientists develop an approach to analyze, quantitate, and manage the effects of ionizing irradiation on humans. While the precise measurement of irradiation doses that were sustained by the Japanese survivors in 1945 was incomplete, there have been more precise studies of the second and third generations (children and grandchildren) of the survivors of the bombing. These data provided information on not only the late effects of irradiation but also the genetic changes and late sequelae of radiation exposure.

Table 1.1 Origin of life on Earth: importance of magnetosphere, water, and oxygen

Years ago									
Big Bang	Earth forms	Magnetosphere begins	Water forms	Life earliest fossils	Single cells	Oxygen	Photosynthesis	Eukaryotes (first mitochondria using oxygen 1.45)	Multicellular animals (poriferea-sponges 0.6)
43.8[a]	4.54 ± 1.4[a]	4.6[a]	4.4–4.0[a]	4.0[a]	4.0-3.5[a]	3.5[a]	3.0[a]	2.1[a]	1.6[a]

[a] Billion years ago

Table 1.2 Examples of taxonomic ranks

Taxonomic rank	Name	Measure of radioresistance
Domain	Eukaryotes	Wide variation
Leinstom	Animal	Wide variation
Phylum	Chondates	Wide variation
Subphylum	Vertebrates	Wide variation
Class	Mammalian	Wide variation
Order	Primates	Rhesus monkey LD50/30 = 8 Gy Cynomolgou monkey LD50/30 = 8.5 Gy
Family	Hominidae	Not known
Genus	Homo	Not known
Species	Homo sapian (human)	LD50/30, 4.5 Gy

Table 1.3 Time-based evolution of classification of plant and animal kingdom members (Carl Linnaeus, 1758)

Nucleated single cells	When appeared	Radiation resistance available data
1. Prokaryotes	4.0–3.5[a]	Not known [16]
2. Eukaryotes (yeast)	2.0–1.45[a]	Wide variation [17]
3. Porifera-sponges (multicellular organisms)	0.7[a]	Not known
4. Coelenterates	0.5[a]	Not known
5. Platyhelminthes (flatworm)	0.5[a]	*C. elegans* [18]
6. Nematoda (roundworm)	0.4[a]	Not known
7. Annelida (segmented worm)	0.54[a]	Not known
8. Mollusca (octopus/squid)	0.54[a]	*Crepitula fornicada* [19] Snails [20]
9. Echinoderms (starfish)	0.54[a]	Not known
10. Arthropoda (insects, spiders)	0.54–0.48[a]	*Drosophila melanogaster* [21] Cockroach Ants
11. Vertebrates Chondrichthyes (sharks) Osteoichtes (fish)	0.518[a] 0.395[a] 0.410[a]	Shark Zebrafish [22]

[a] Billions of years ago

Table 1.4 Radioresistance of vertebrates is age dependent and has wide variation

	Examples
Amphibians	Frogs
Reptiles	Lizard
Birds	Parrot
Mammals	Dogs
Cartilaginous fish	Shark
Bony fish	Zebrafish
Eel	Lamprey

Table 1.5 Radioresistance of invertebrates: examples that have been incompletely studied

Phylum	Examples by phylum (Linnaeus, 1758)
Platyhelminthes	Flatworm
Nematoda	Roundworm
Annelida	Segmented worm
Anthropoda— Crustacean Insecti Labiatan	Spider Crab wasp Centipede
Porifera	Sponge
Echinodermata	Starfish
Cnidaria	Coral
Mollusca	Octopus

How did humans arrive at their current state of biological responsiveness to ionizing irradiation? To begin to answer this question, we must evaluate the history of the solar system and the origins of life on Earth.

There is an emerging consensus in the scientific community that water arrived around 4.4–4.0 billions of years ago on the planet Earth long after its initial formation at 4.5 billion years ago [30] (Table 1.1). Water perhaps arrived by the contact of the developing planet with an asteroid bringing frozen water to the planet some time approximately 4.4–4.0 billion years ago [30]. Astronomers continue to evaluate the potential capacity of planets in other solar systems to support life, by detection of water. To astrobiologists, water means life. If water arrived on the developing planet Earth at some point in time and led to the creation of oceans, where life originated, then the chemistry of the origin of life began 4.0 billion years ago. The data suggest that in biochemistry, several elements combined must have included carbon, oxygen, and nitrogen, and these formed nucleic acids. Most likely, the chemical reactions necessary for the creation of single-cell organisms must have first been nucleic acids. Where did the lipids and proteins come from? This question is unanswered. Many theories have been suggested as to how DNA was formed and how initial transcription to RNA in translation to proteins became the foundation necessary in a sequence that is required for creating the first single-cell organisms. The most primitive organisms, prokaryotes, are thought to be cells without nuclei (Table 1.1). The other single-cell organisms called archeobacteria are also now thought to be the origin of the mitochondria 1.45 billion years ago. The two organisms combined to form Eukaryotes (Table 1.1). The mitochondria-free prokaryotes and then mitochondria containing more complex single-cell organisms, eukaryotes, were believed to be the first examples of "life" on Earth (Table 1.1). What were the conditions during the creation of the first single-cell organisms? To answer this question, one must know the relative time of development of the magnetosphere [31] or "radiation shield" that surrounds the planet Earth and the time of the first detectable presence of water (Table 1.1).

Unlike other planets in the solar system, the Earth contains an iron core. Scientists continue to describe the Earth as a "young planet" in which the core is molten but also displays a condition in which there is rotation of the core containing iron. This rotation of the Earth produces gravity on the planet's surface. If the planet formed as expected from the expulsion of solid objects from the sun, there was an interval during which the iron core was established, gravity on the surface of the planet was established, and the magnetosphere formed (Table 1.1). Key questions, which deal with space irradiation, are how adaptations to ionizing irradiation occurred in developing organisms and whether further adaptation would be affected by gravity. The development of life on Earth over billions of years did so in the presence of irradiation and gravity. So, if and when humans leave the planet, they must adapt to a setting in which these dimensions will be different: less gravity and more irradiation. In space, there will be different forms of radiation to which organisms on Earth have not been required to adapt. The adaptation must occur to facilitate space travel [28].

It is now established that there are several layers of "protective" magnetic shielding on the planet, which led to the direction of any radioactive solar particles directed to the planet's surface now redirected to the poles. When did the magnetosphere [31] form and for how many millions of years did it exist before the origins of the first life on the planet? These questions cannot be answered at the present time. Other questions include whether life formed on Earth from the chemistry of DNA before the magnetosphere directed radioactive particles to the poles or in the presence of the magnetosphere. Was there a second asteroid which hit the water-containing planet and which brought life or building blocks of life with it? To answer these questions, we only have available evidence from the current state of life on the planet. If the polar regions are indeed the focus of direction of radioactive particles from sources outside the Earth [31], which include: (1) Galactic Cosmic irradiation—which are charged ions from Supernova from other solar systems and (2) protons from solar proton events—sunspots, then the radiation levels at the poles would be expected to be higher. Meteorites collected from the poles of the planet demonstrate high concentrations of different materials, which include both "collected" and "directed" ionized particles, which are unique in the polar regions [31]. The discoveries lead to more questions. Radiation levels at the poles would be expected to be higher. So, how does this concentration of charged particles relate to the decreased temperature and polar ice formation in these areas? Would not life develop more slowly in these areas and would surviving organisms be more radiation resistant due to their evolution in a region of higher background levels of radiation? The taxonomy of the plant and animal kingdom fails to support such a theory (Table 1.3) unless new fossil evidence is yet to be discovered. Many more questions are associated with the astrophysics of planet formation and its linkage to the developing biology of life.

Origins of Life and Associated Radiation Resistance

Measurement of irradiation on Earth has proven that higher altitude elevation above the planet's surface is associated with higher radiation levels [32, 33]. In the United States, the highest habitable areas such as Leadville, Colorado (Table 1.6) display increased radiation levels compared to levels at sea level. There are data to support the hypothesis that there is no threshold for radiation-induced cancer in humans [34–37]. This means that even modestly increased radiation levels will cause more cancer and other late radiation effects. Is there a higher incidence of cancer and other late effects of irradiation occurring in lifelong residents of Leadville, Colorado [33] (Table 1.6)? If so, then the increased relative radiation doses that are measured in humans, who spend a significant amount of time at commercial airline altitudes of around 35,000 ft. above sea level, which are much higher than that on the planet's surface, should be at increased risk. Do pilots and other frequent fliers have a higher incidence of cancer and other late effects of radiation exposure [34, 35]? All data collection has confounding variables since humans are complex in genetics and lifestyle, but the analysis is useful. Radiation levels outside the protective magnetosphere (Van-Allen Belt of the magnetosphere, which provides a shield of the planet's surface from ionizing irradiation) are higher. Much of the information on the cumulative radiation dose that is sustained by humans, who are outside the magnetosphere, comes from the data collected on the International Space Station, space shuttle programs, and the lunar orbiting and landing missions [35]. Long-term follow-up of astronauts has led to the accumulation of data that are still being analyzed. Did the single-cell organisms that constitute the origins of life (both plant and animal) evolve in an environment where there was a protective magnetosphere that minimized ionizing irradiation exposure from outside the Earth (Tables 1.7 and 1.8)?

Table 1.6 Examples of estimated radiation dose rates from natural background sources at different locations on Earth

Natural background source	Amargosa Valley, NV	Leadville, CO Effective dose rate ($mSv\ y^{-1}$)	State of Colorado	State of Nevada
Cosmic radiation	0.33	0.85	0.50	0.39
Terrestrial radiation	0.47	0.97	0.49	0.22
Radon and its decay products	0.52	3.44	3.01	1.66
Total (±1 SD)	1.32 ± 0.12	5.26 ± 1.08	3.86 ± 2.18	2.27 ± 0.81

Moeller DW, Sun L-SC (2006) Comparison of natural background dose rates for residents of the Amargosa Valley, NV, to those in Leadville, CO, and the states of Colorado and Nevada. Health Phys 91(4): 338–353

Table 1.7 Mean shell length (in μm) of metamorphosed Crepidula fornicata larvae irradiated to each x-ray dose

X-ray dose (Rad)					
Shell length[a]	Control	500	1000	2000	5000
Mean	976.7	889.2	910.6	960.7	751.8
S.D.	±181.8	±129.2	±140.6	±144.7	±145.7
Number measured	39	41	45	39	4

[a] Metamorphosed individuals in groups surviving 21 days after each irradiation dose were measured for shell length as described in the methods. Results are presented as the mean ± standard deviation (S.D.) for the number of animals in each group tested

Table 1.8 Growth rates of Crepidula Fornicata larvae as a function of x-irradiation dose

Experiment	0 rad (μm/day)	5000 (μm/day)	10,000 (μm/day)	20,000 (μm/day)
#1	47.3	33.0	18.5	12.0
#2	51.5	41.4	17.2	8.4
#3	53.6	35.7	16.4	12.6

[a] Results are presented as the rate of growth in μm/day after daily measurement of the growth of at least 40 animals per group in each of three experiments. The growth rate was calculated as the slope of the line relating shell length to larval age for each group. Results are presented as mean for each group

The magnetosphere does not protect the planet's surface from all radiation and doses that are sustained, are measurable, and still significant. Radiation that is emitted from the core of the Earth from radioactive decay of isotopes that have been there since the formation of thc planet also contributes to the exposure levels during the origins of life and today [36, 37]. The existing radioactive elements in the core of the planet include radium, uranium, and from radium, the evolution of radon gas. Some geographic areas of Earth have greater emission of radiation from the planet's core, and these levels are predictably higher in geographic areas where there has been significant coal mining and drilling deep beneath the planet's surface, where more radon is released [36, 37]. Do miners and people, who live in these high radiation areas, have a higher incidence of radiation-induced late effects including cancer [37]. There are observations from current measurements in these geographic areas.

We have data from radiation biology experiments that are being carried out with multiple species of plants and animals. There is one very interesting observation from all of these studies. The size and complexity of an organism do not directly relate to its radiosensitivity (Tables 1.2, 1.3, 1.4, and 1.5). Furthermore, within each taxonomic category (both plants and animals), there are multiple possible explanations for the relative state of radiation responsiveness of each species. Single-cell organisms including bacteria, amoeba, paramecia, and both phytoplankton and zooplankton all have been studied for responsiveness to ionizing irradiation. In the single-cell organism, radiation responsiveness is measured by individual cell survival and its proliferative capacity. With bacteria taxa, the difference between the responsiveness to radiation of two taxons has been documented [38]. These studies led to genetic analysis of the genes on the bacterial single chromosome and to the discovery of gene products that determine the capacity of each bacterium to survive irradiation. The discovery of single- and double-strand breaks in DNA, and their repair by specific enzymes, is part of the repair capacity. Data on the molecular biology of DNA repair has provided the tools by which to compare the radiation responsiveness of many organisms including single cellular species, from the first multicellular organisms and all species up to and including humans.

There are different levels of responsiveness of bacterial taxa to irradiation. Some bacteria are more radiosensitive than others. The clonogenic assay was developed for medical analysis of bacterial infections [38]. Bacteria are plated into semisolid agar gel-containing nutrients, including sugars, amino acids, and lipids, and bacteria form colonies, which then can be quantitated. These assays were first developed to detect bacterial growth in humans with suspected infections by culturing urine, blood, sputum, and other sources of suspected infection. Clonogenic assays for bacteria allowed measurement of radiation dose–response curves. Different bacteria are relatively sensitive or resistant when this assay is carried out. What is the mechanism of bacterial resistance to radiation and why are some bacterial taxa more resistant? The answer is associated with the genes in the bacterial chromosome. Several categories of genes responsible for radiation resistance include those associated with the repair of DNA strand breaks and genes that produce factors that neutralize ionizing irradiation effects. Ionizing irradiation produces reactive oxygen species (ROS). X-rays (gamma rays) produce their damaging effect in bacteria that is prominently indirect and starts with the creation of reactive oxygen species. Ionizing irradiation first hits water and oxygen within the bacteria and produces reactive oxygen species that bind to DNA and cause strand breaks [8, 10, 11, 29]. Other forms of irradiation such as charged nuclear particles (protons or electrons) or charged elemental nuclei (alpha particles—helium nuclei) directly damage the DNA without the need for the intermediate step of production of ROS [39]. Irradiation from protons and high linear energy transfer particles is very relevant to both clinical radiotherapy and space irradiation since both situations involve human exposure. Bacteria rapidly repair DNA strand breaks due to their rapid proliferative capacity [38, 40, 41].

Natural Selection and Radioresistance

Thus, there is expected to be a rapid natural selection of those variants that are more radiation resistant. The best evidence of this phenomenon is the discovery of *Deinococcus radiodurans* [38, 40, 41]. Experiments were carried out to deliver huge doses of irradiation to sterilize meat products. These delivery systems irradiated meat and sought to increase the capacity of these irradiated food products to withstand prolonged storage. The logic here was to kill bacteria, which even in small quantities could proliferate and destroy the stability of the food product. There was a discovery of the evolution of a bacterial species with great radiation resistance and capacity to withstand the huge radiation doses in that experiment. *Deinococcus radiodurans* was analyzed and found to contain a string of DNA repair genes and antioxidant genes [38]. The discovery of *D. radiodurans* confirmed the capacity of organisms to develop resistance to ionizing irradiation. Multicellular organisms were more complex and led to the discovery that different cell phenotypes had different capacities to withstand radiation damage. The evolution of species in those plants and animals and the discovery of differentiation capacity of stem cells in each organism led to the discovery of the relative radiation resistance of different cell phenotypes [42].

A dramatic discovery was that of the organism's capacity for indirect irradiation effects on radiation responsiveness. Radiation damages nuclear DNA and also mitochondrial DNA if mitochondria arose from the evolution of archaea bacteria fusion with single-cell organisms billions of years ago, but this was only the first step in the evolution of the response to ionizing irradiation (Table 1.1). Cellular death is not the only result of radiation damage, there is the phenomenon of radiation-induced cellular change without death. Radiation induces a change in growth and development [19, 43]. The response and repair process can lead to the production of injured but not killed cells, which produce cytokines and other communication molecules that arrive via the circulation to other cells within a multicellular organism. Indirect irradiation effects have been the major source of radiation responsiveness in complex multicellular organisms and prominently in humans. Do indirect effects explain the radiosensitivity and radiation resistance of some humans? The current answer to this question is probably: "in some cases." Individual resistance to irradiation is thought to be a complex responsiveness of both individual cell DNA repair capacity and also the degree to which indirect effects are induced in an individual. Production of inflammatory cytokines by irradiated cells includes those that are associated with other inflammatory diseases such as response to heat, chemical toxins, infectious agents, and reactions to foreign elements including drugs. Inflammatory cytokines are released into the circulation (blood and lymphatic system) and can produce cell death at distant sites. Irradiation responsiveness is complex in the capacity of an individual to stand the direct effects on DNA and indirect effects are an individual matter. Another point to be made is that the "complexity" of the species studied does not necessarily relate to its radiation responsiveness (Tables 1.2 and 1.3). The taxonomy of Linnaeus [15] was not the only methodology used. Looking at the taxonomic listing of complex organisms starting from the first multicellular animals to humans indicates that the complexity, size, and position in the evolutionary tree do not correlate with radiation response (Table 1.3). As will be shown in this book, the response to ionizing irradiation is not simply reliant on DNA damage and repair but involves organ-specific and indirect effects that make organisms vulnerable to damage and death. It must be tempting to conclude that species that survived for millions of years are radioresistant: crocodiles, insects, and bony fish, but the conclusion is unfounded given the multiple other variables. Ionizing irradiation was not the only stimulant of speciation [34]. This book will also address many of these issues and suggest ways in which scientists and physicians can approach explanations and treatments [35].

Evolutionary Changes Compared to Rapid Pace of Natural Selection

The evolutionary process takes hundreds or thousands of generations to select a species change [16, 44] as documented in the fossil record [20]. In contrast, intervention for selective breeding can create faster selection [45] or does it [20]? Can rapid environmental changes induce evolution to occur faster or are there changes in animals, not a new species, but rather a selection of traits in behavior [46]?

Specific Experimental Models of Irradiation Biology in Both Invertebrates and Vertebrates

There have been several informative approaches toward understanding the effect of radiation on whole organisms. The gastropod larvae experiments with X-rays show the resilience of these invertebrates to radiation (Fig. 1.1) [47, 48] at relatively high doses, but there is growth delay and abnormal metamorphosis.

The experiments with low-dose continuous irradiation delivered to mice show that vertebrates (mice) resist low-dose irradiation consistent with radioisotope fallout that produces genetic effects (Fig. 1.2).

DNA damage and mutations are well established for their carcinogenic effects. Several key markers of DNA damage and DNA damage responses in mice exposed to low-dose-rate radiation revealed few genotoxic effects associated with low-dose-rate radiation. We studied low-dose-rate radiation using a variable low-dose rate irradiator consisting of flood phantoms filled with ^{125}Iodine-containing buffer [47, 48]. Mice were exposed to 0.0002 cGy/min (~400-fold background radiation) continuously over 5 weeks. Base lesions, micronuclei, homologous recombination (HR; using fluorescent yellow direct repeat mice), and transcript levels for several radiation-sensitive genes showed little change in the levels of the DNA nucleobase damage products hypoxanthine, 8-oxo-7, 8-dihydroguanine, 1,N^6-ethenoadenine, or 3,N^4-ethenocytosine above background levels under low-dose rate conditions. The micronucleus assay revealed no evidence that low-dose-rate radiation-induced DNA fragmentation, and there was no evidence of double-strand break-induced HR. Low-dose rate radiation did not induce *Cdkn 1a, Gadd45a, Mdm2, Atm,* or *Dbd2.* Importantly, the same total dose, when delivered acutely, did induce micronuclei and transcriptional response. Lowering the dose rate suppresses the potentially deleterious impact of radiation.

Remaining Issues of Controversy at All Levels

The controversy over the mechanism of the origins of life on Earth remains active in many disciplines of basic science. The discipline of taxonomy, which all forms of life ranging from single-cell organisms such as bacteria to the complexity of mammals including humans, remains the basis for discussion of different forms of life on Earth. Taxonomy is the discipline in which animal and plant kingdoms are organized based on levels of complexity. The first taxonomy of Linnaeus, 1758 has given way to other forms of organization of the complexity of life based on several

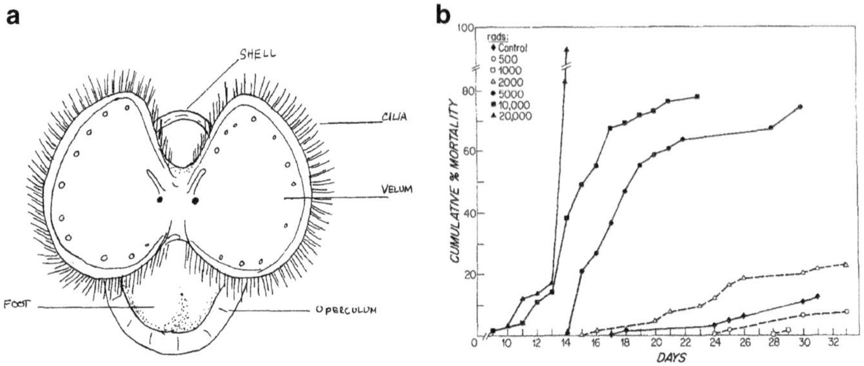

Fig. 1.1 (**a**) Schematic drawing of *Crepidula fornicate* prior to metamorphosis, showing the velum (↑) (Magnification, X95) [19]. (**b**) Effect of X-irradiation on mortality of *Crepidula fornicata* larvae. Groups of larvae were irradiated as described in the methods to each of 6 doses of irradiation and observed closely over 33 days for the number of dead animals. Results are presented as the cumulative percent mortality for at least 50 animals per group for unirradiated controls (♦) or after irradiation to: (&), 20,000 rad; (■). 10,000 rad; C•J. 5000 rad; (6), 2000 rad; (□), I,000 rad; or (0), 500 rad. (**c**) Effect of X-ray dose on shell length at 8–9 days after irradiation (results of single experiment). The group of animals described in Fig. 1.1b was measured at 8–9 days after irradiation for shell length as described in the methods. Results are presented as the mean ± SEM for at least 30 individuals measured per X-ray or control group. (**d**) Effect of X-ray dose on shell length at 10 days after irradiation, results of pooled data from three replicates. The data for each irradiated or control group are presented as described in the legend to Fig. 1.1c for each of 3 separate experiments designated by symbols: ▲, ●, and Δ, respectively. The grand mean (○) for pooled data is plotted with SEM of the pooled 3 experiments. (**e**) Effect of time after X-irradiation on shell length. Groups of 60 animals were irradiated to each indicated dose or left unirradiated. The shell length was measured four times over 20 days for animals in each group and plotted as the mean ± SEM for each group. Results are for: (♦), unirradiated controls; or animals irradiated to (▲), 20,000 rad; (■), 10,000 rad; (●), 5000 rad; (Δ), 2000 rad; (□), 500 rad (↑) indicates time of X-irradiation. (**f**) Effect of irradiation on biomass as a function of shell length. Biomass determinations were made as described in the methods for groups of control unirradiated or X-irradiated C. *fornicata* larva sorted according to shell length at 9 days after irradiation. Animals with a shell length within each 10 μ,m range were studied as a group and the mean shell length for that group shown on the abcissa and the mean biomass shown on the ordinate. Results are for animals irradiated to: (**A**), 20,000: (**Ill**), 10,000, or (e), 5000 rad. Two unirradiated control groups were also studied. Those controls from the identical hatch used in the experiment are presented as(♦) and those in a separate experiment shown as(◊). Results are the mean biomass for at least 30 animals per point. (**g**) Effect of X-irradiation on metamorphosis of *C. fornicuta* larvae. Groups of unirradiated control or irradiated larvae were observed daily for metamorphosis as described in the methods. Results are presented as the cumulative percent of larva that had metamorphosed to juveniles (as indicated by loss of the velum) for unirradiated controls, (♦); or irradiated animals receiving, (e), 5000 rad; (Li), 2000 rad;(□), I,000 rad; or (0). 500 rad. (**h**) Effect of X-irradiation on metamorphosis of *Crepidula fornicata* larvae. Metamorphosis of larval gastropods is signaled by loss of the velum, the ciliated organ used for swimming, respiration, and feeding. Groups of unirradiated control or irradiated larvae were observed daily for metamorphosis. Results are presented as the percent of larvae that had metamorphosed to juveniles (as indicated by loss of the velum) for controls (♦); or animals receiving: (0), 5000 rad; (6), 2000 rad;(□), 1000 rad; or (◊), 500 rad. From Greenberger JS, Pechenik J, Gould L, et al. X-ray irradiation effects on growth and metamorphosis of gastropod larvae (Crepidula fornicate): A model for environmental radiation teratogenesis. *Arch Environ Contam Toxicol.* 1986;15(2): 227–234. PMID: 3707206

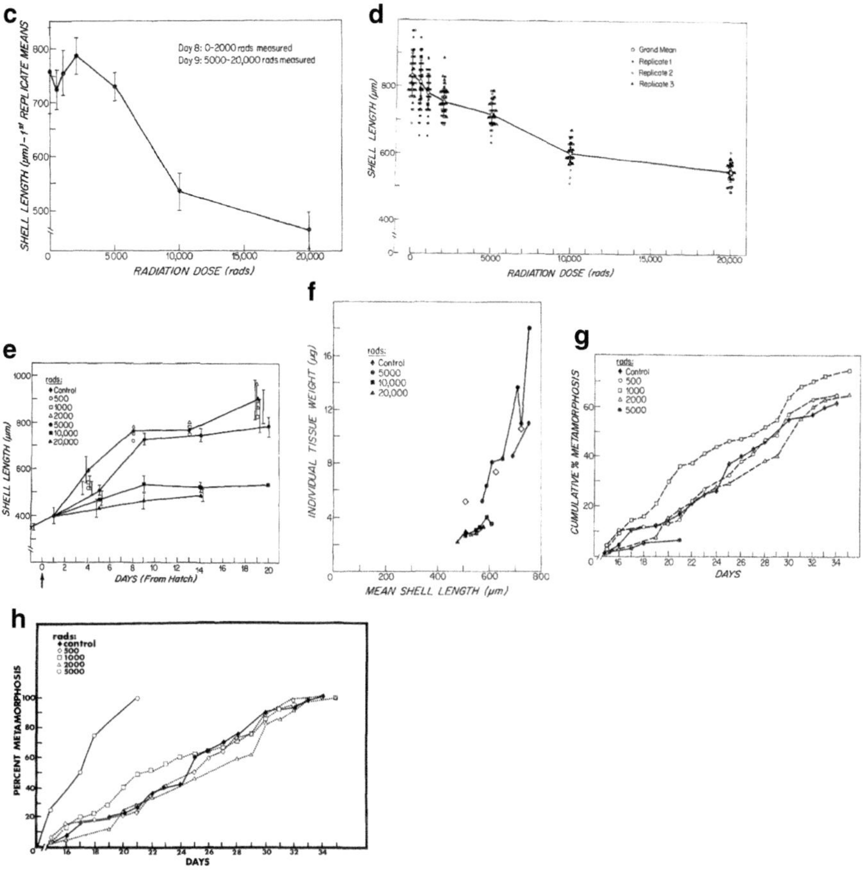

Fig. 1.1 (continued)

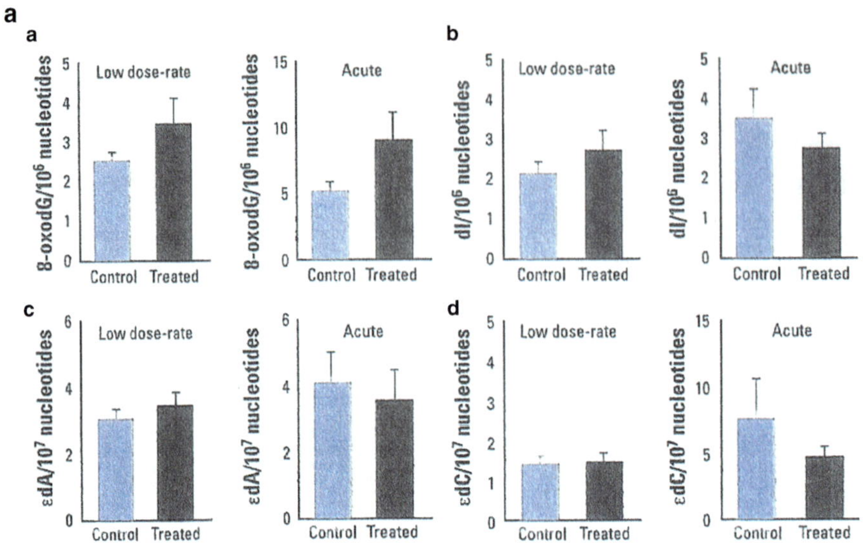

Fig. 1.2 (**a**) Exposure to 10.5 Gy acute (7.1 cGy/min) and chronic irradiation (0.0002 cGy/min) does not change steady-state base lesion levels. Effects of chronic, lowdose-rate and acute irradiation on DNA base lesion levels of (*A*) 8-oxodG, (*B*) dI, (*C*) εdA, and (*D*) εdC were measured by LC-MS/MS in splenic DNA. Data represent mean ± SE for $n = 6$ and were analyzed by Student t-test. (**b**) Representative image of a PCE-containing micronuclei (MN-PCE; arrowheads) and of a normal RBC (arrow) isolated from bone marrow; bar = 20 μm (*A*). Low-dose rate (0.0002 cGy/min) irradiation (*B*) does not induce micronuclei in PCEs, whereas acute (7.1 cGy/min) irradiation (*C*) does. Data (mean ± SE) are representative of two independent experiments; percent MN-PCE was calculated from >2000 scored PCE per sample. $^*p < 0.05$ using unpaired two-tailed Student t-test. (**c**) FYDR mice carry a recombination substrate (*A*) that results in expression of *Eyfp* upon recombination repair. The *Eyfp* signal can be detected by in situ imaging. The frequency of *Eyfp*$^+$ cells increased with age [(*B*) 4-week-old (young) mouse; (*C*) 24-week-old (old) mouse]. Chronic, low-doserate (0,0002 cGy/min; *D*, *F*) and acute (7.1 cGy/min; *E*, *G*) irradiation do not affect HR frequency in the pancreas; $^+$, positive. Chronic irradiation does not affect *Eyfp* expression in FYDR control mouse (*H*). Values are mean ± SE; statistical analysis was performed using two-tailed Mann-Whitney U test. (**d**) Effects of chronic, low-dose rate (0.0002 cGy/min; *A*, *B*) and acute (7.1 cGy/min; *C*, *D*) ionizing radiation on gene expression in WGCs. Gene expression changes were compared between control and treated groups after irradiation (*A*, *C*) and in irradiated animals before and after irradiation (*B*, *D*). Data (mean ± SE) are representative of two independent experiments. $^*p < 0.05$ using unpaired two-tailed Student t-test (*A*, *C*) and paired two-tailed Student's t-test (*B*, *D*). From Olipitz W, Wiktor-Brown D, Shuga J, et al. Integrated molecular analysis indicates undetectable DNA damage in mice after continuous irradiation at −400-fold natural background radiation. *Environ Health Perspect.* 2012;120(8): 1130–1136. PMID: 22538203; PMC3440074

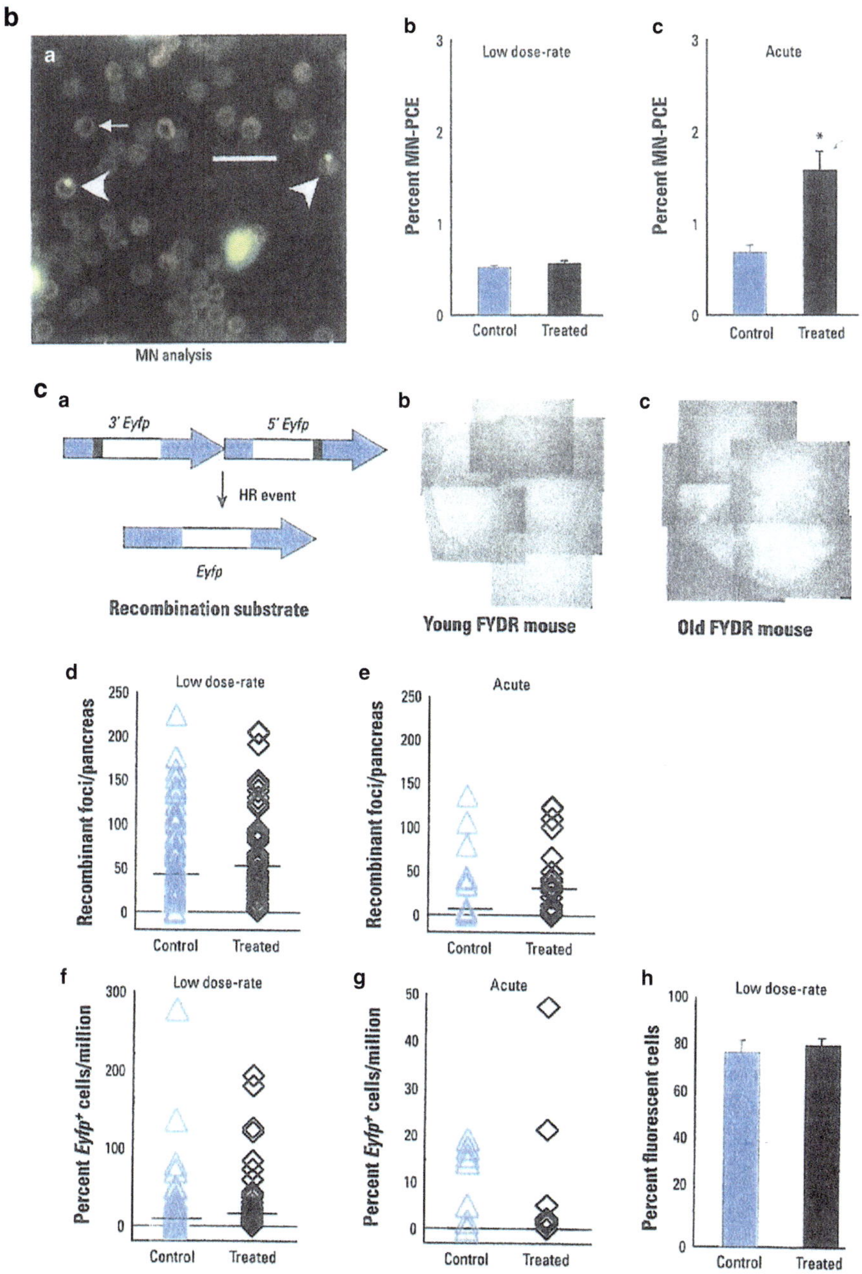

Fig. 1.2 (continued)

d

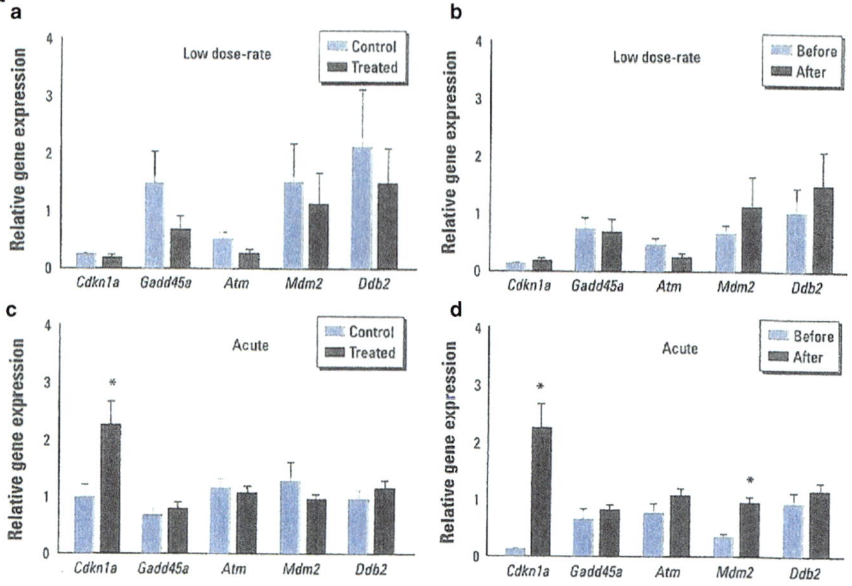

Fig. 1.2 (continued)

different parameters [27]. Linnaeus first described complexity based on criteria of multicellularity, formation of organs, asexual or sexual reproduction, and other structural factors. Other forms of taxonomy have organized the different forms of life using other parameters. Taxonomic classifications are closely related to the fossil record. It is clearly not possible to conclude that one type of animal or plant appeared in the planet's history before another unless there is fossil evidence to support this hypothesis.

Going back to the origins of the planet, the current concept is that there was a "Big Bang" event leading to the formation of our solar system and potentially the entire galaxy. After this event occurred in which the elements of gravity, energy, and matter produced the sun (our star), there followed the expulsion from this star of planets including Earth, and expulsion from some of these planets of other objects, which orbited each planet, including our single moon. From this point in the disciplines of physics, astrophysics, and astrochemistry, there is only conjecture and hypothesis. The major events leading to our "unique" planet include information on the magnetosphere [31]. [The magnetic field around the Earth is highly relevant to the topic of radiation biology since charged particles from supernovae and solar protons are transported to the polar regions of the planet, and this filtration device significantly limits the amount of radiation from these forms of particles that get to the planet surface; the arrival of water [30] on the planet and the creation of the first elements of life; namely, nucleic acids, which led to deoxyribonucleic acid (DNA) and ribonucleic acid (RNA).] The sequence of these events is probable but cannot be proven. The Earth has an iron-containing core, and this iron core has created the magnetosphere, which serves as a radiation-protective shield around the planet. The current hypothesis is that water arrived on the planet sometime later, potentially delivered by a meteor, which led to the formation of oceans and continents. Laboratory experiments in recent years have attempted to create conditions for the elimination of elements to form nucleic acids, and some of these experiments have been successful. However, the translation of this successful chemistry experiment to the formation of the first single-cell organisms remains speculative. Given the current taxonomic classifications of the elements of the animal kingdom, which form the basis for all biology, it is instructive to view these categories with respect to how they have impacted radiation biology.

Single-Cell Organisms and Evolution

These data are in fact estimates. As shown in Table 1.1, a suggested timeline for the detection of the first single-cell organism is speculative but shown relative to the origin of the planet and the evolution of other animal categories. The taxonomic classification, which is popular, but not the only one is shown in Table 1.2 and is related to some of the complexity but not 100% logical in the explanation of the differences between the different orders, classes, further specification of genus and species. There is no taxonomic classification that relates the complexity of animals or plants to their radiation resistance or radiosensitivity. How the different categories of plants and animals evolved is all speculative but must relate to the fossil record. Radiocarbon dating and the more recent uranium-thorium dating techniques have allowed a more precise evaluation of the age of a fossil. The first single-cell organisms suggested coming in billions of years ago when such cells first appeared.

The numbers in terms of billions of years reflect not only evolution of more complex animals and plants but also the fact that during these billions of years irradiation from the solar system and beyond was hitting the planet Earth, after filtration by the magnetosphere, such that all of these changes in complexity of animals and plants were occurring under the influence of low-level irradiation. In addition, the core of the planet Earth is still "young," and radiation-emitting isotopes such as radium and radon continue to deliver radiation from the center of the planet to the surface. Thus, the evolution of life occurred on Earth with radiation coming not only from outside the planet through the magnetosphere but also from the inside of the Earth's core, which still has active radiation emissions.

The phenomenon of the speciation role has been a subject of intense research [44]. The evolution of a new species has suggested that major genetic changes led to differentiation, such that a new animal or plant could have evolved. There is no direct evidence that recognizing irradiation can produce or influence speciation, but since these changes over billions of years on the Earth's surface and in the oceans took place with constant influence of both internal and external radiation sources, one must consider that irradiation did have a role in the evolution of life on Earth.

In discussing whether one group of animals or plants is radiosensitive or radioresistant, there is the phenomenon of identification by forms of asexual or sexual reproduction. With simple organisms including bacteria [16], yeast [30], Platyhelminthes (flatworms) [23], Echinoderms (sea urchin) [24], Arthropoda (insects) [21], amphibians (frog) [25], reptiles (crocodile) [26], and bony fish (zebrafish) [22], as well as mammals (laboratory mice), there is a clear phenomenon that early stages in reproduction arise to organisms that are different in the response to ionizing irradiation compared to the adults. Zebrafish may be relatively radioresistant compared to other animals if one looks at the dose-response of the adults. However, Zebrafish embryos are much more radiosensitive. The same holds for embryogenesis, and age applies to laboratory mice [44] and humans. Exposure to ionizing irradiation of early gestation embryos leads to spontaneous abortion and embryonic death at much lower radiation doses compared to mid-gestation and late gestation embryos. These data must be taken into account when comparing the radiation resistance of adults of each lifeform.

How Did Radioresistance Evolve?

The data on radiation resistance have come from decades of research with specific experimental models. While there is much information on irradiation of examples in the plant kingdom, this book will focus on the animal kingdom as the overall goal/mission of the book is to provide information relative to humans. However, the same type of experiments have been carried out with members of the plant kingdom and have led to confirmation of the results with members of the animal kingdom. General principles apply with respect to ionizing irradiation effects on plants and animals, namely, (1) higher radiation doses produce more lethality; (2) low continuous or sporadic radiation produces mutations in DNA, which can lead to physical and reproductive abnormalities; and (3) the type of irradiation/quality of irradiation (charged particles or atoms, protons, neutrons, electrons, or gamma rays—X-rays) lead to different effects on each experimental model. Much of the information in basic radiation biology has been obtained from the study of specific models. Bacteria contain cytoplasmic circles of DNA called plasmids, and even though these are the simplest single-cell organisms, the interaction of plasmids with the single chromosome in bacteria has been a subject of intense investigation. Bacteria are known as prokaryotes due to the presence of a nucleus, but the absence of mitochondria, which are the cell cytoplasm organelles responsible for oxidative metabolism. An accepted principle in taxonomy and in basic biology is the eukaryote difference from prokaryotes. The current accepted theory is that at some point in the evolution of life, single-cell organisms engulfed archeobacteria with the creation of mitochondria. These cell cytoplasmic organelles have a reproductive cycle similar to the nucleus and have provided the energy supply for oxidative metabolism. Yeast is the most primitive known eukaryote in this regard.

Both bacteria and yeast have been studied intensively with respect to gene sequencing and the discovery of many DNA repair genes and the equally complete study of the effects of ionizing irradiation on inducing mutations in each of these genes. Two primary strains of yeast have been intensely studied for the effects of irradiation-inducing mutations. A range of genetic controls of the ionizing radiation response have been discovered in both Ceravace and Pompe strains of yeast [17]. Banks of mutants of these single-cell organisms have served as the basis for the study of complementary genes in more complex organisms and humans. A large list of genes found in yeast is associated with ionizing irradiation as well as ultraviolet irradiation damage and repair. Many of these have analogs in more complex organisms including humans. Studies in bacteria and yeast have provided a foundation for basic radiobiology.

The taxonomy has led to the concept of phyla, which are major categories of organisms. Three phyla have been organized based on the anatomic complexity of these worms. Platyhelminthes-flatworms have generated a plethora of data on one subspecies, the *C. elegans*. The phylum Nematoda (roundworms) and the phylum Annelida (segmented worms) have been the subject of less intense study, but there are data published on the ionizing radiation response of several examples in these phyla. Studies with *C. elegans* have been intense, and there are many publications describing ionizing irradiation effects on this organism. The most dramatic study was that published by Doctrow et al. [18]. showing that these worms had a significant response to ionizing irradiation, which could be altered by adding an antioxidant MnSOD mimetic small molecule to the medium in which the worms were growing. Genes for radiation recognition and repair were discovered in these animals and correlated with similar data from bacteria and yeast.

Studies on the larvae and embryos of representative animals in each of these phyla have been based on other taxonomic categories. The phylum Mollusca, which includes many shellfish, octopus, squid, and others, has led to confirmation that the embryos are radiosensitive and much more easily studied with respect to the effect of radiation protectors than are the adults. One such study with shellfish embryos of *Crepidula fornicata* (Fig. 1.1) led to information that antioxidant drugs added to the water in which these embryos were expanding had the same effects as on flatworms and yeast. Thus, these studies with more complex organisms (according to the taxonomic classification) confirmed the uniform aspects of DNA damage and protection by specific categories of drugs with respect to ionizing irradiation. Other phyla including Echinoderms have been studied less intensively with respect to radiation biology. All of these categories represent invertebrate animals or those without vertebral bodies and a spinal cord or notochord. The category of vertebrates, which includes cartilaginous fish like sharks and rays, (chondryichtses) as well as bony fish (osteoithyces), provides the information on ionizing irradiation effects that have been consistent up to mammals and humans. The spinal cord of vertebrates facilitate studies of both the central nervous system (brain and spinal cord) compared to peripheral nerves. Peripheral nerve effects of irradiation can be studied in mollusks, most prominently, the squid species in which squid axons have been studied for movement of mitochondria in the nucleus down to the motor endplate in which nerves innovate muscles. So, the presence of a spinal cord is not necessary to study peripheral nerves. However, the interaction between the peripheral nervous system and the central nervous system has only been possible with examples of vertebrates. The phylum Arthropoda (insects) has led to much more complexity in the taxonomic categories and has reflected the effects of irradiation on valuable sexual reproductive capacity including effects of irradiation on sperm production, ova, larva, embryogenesis, and all complex organs of insects. The irradiation resistance of insects has been known for decades. Cockroaches have been shown to resist very high doses of ionizing irradiation. However, studies on their embryos also reflect a radiosensitivity that is seen in many other organisms with respect to age and radiation response.

In the insect realm, a great body of data on radiation biology has been obtained by the study of *Drosophila melanogaster* (fruit flies). The first experiments on radiation-induced mutations were carried out in fruit fly embryos [21]. A large number of fruit fly mutants were available for study of the effects of irradiation on many aspects of teratogenesis, inducing mutations that lead to abnormalities in structure, anatomy, and function. There are fruit fly subcategories that show the effects of irradiation on energy production, mitochondrial function, and many other aspects of energy metabolism. Progressing along the evolutionary tree as defined by the Linnean Taxonomy, one comes to the order and class of mammals. There have been many studies done on amphibians, the frog egg studies, but not nearly the degree of complexity of the studies that have been carried out with genetic inbred strains of mice. Some studies have been carried out on different strains of rats with respect to radiation effects, but the majority of these studies have been carried out in mice. Mouse genetic variations, which are associated with radiosensitivity in certain inbred strains, have led to the identification of many DNA repair pathways, oxidative stress response pathways, and age-related metabolic pathways, which have confirmed many of the genetic studies on bacteria, yeast, *C. elegans*, and fruit flies.

Some of the elegant experiments, which have been carried out with bacteria, yeast, *C. elegans*, Drosophila, zebrafish, and mice are the products of innovation and wisdom of specific groups of scientists, who chose to study these organisms. Generations of scientists have continued to focus on these examples of radiation-responsive organisms at large because the data have led to much historical information that can guide current research. However, with respect to the complexity of ionizing irradiation as it relates to the topics in this book including: Radiation Oncology for Use of Radiation to Treat Patients; the development of drugs to mitigate damage from radiation terrorism or environmental radiation exposure; and the adaptation of humans to space irradiation one must appreciate the overwhelming value of data that has been obtained with experimental mouse models.

Vertebrate Evolution and Radioresistance

To summarize the information up to this point, there are several useful conclusions: (1) The evolution of radioresistance on Earth is based upon studies related to the taxonomy or classification of animal species [27]. Much of this information has been obtained from taxonomy, which is the classification of animals based on their complexity. There are several systems of taxonomy available. Confirmation of the time sequence of appearance of these different categories of animals must be confirmed by the fossil record, which is continuously being updated with more sophisticated techniques of dating the age of fossils and including expansion of the science literature. (2) The radioresistance of an adult organism taxonomic category is not related to the radiosensitivity of embryos with respect to cell death, mutations, and teratogenesis. (3) Select animal systems have been chosen for decades of study, and these have generated the data, which supports a unified theory of DNA damage as one mechanism of response to ionizing irradiation. Studies with bacteria, yeast, *C. elegans*, flatworms, *Drosophila melanogaster* (fruit flies), zebrafish, and laboratory rodents have provided the basis for unifying theories of radiobiology. (4) As it relates to human exposure to ionizing irradiation, some of the principles of basic radiobiology may apply, but not all. The complexity of humans and the ionizing irradiation response is not unique, but it is certainly a response that goes far beyond DNA damage and repair as originally defined in single-cell organisms. Embryos are usually radiosensitive, perhaps, because all early-life cycles including larvae are similar "Ontogeny Recapitulates Phylogeny," was the quote from Ernst Haeckel (1834–1919) [27]. How does all of this information relate to the radiobiology of humans, the use of radiation to treat cancer, and the concern for ionizing irradiation exposure from weapons, nuclear power plant disasters, and the continuing challenge of how humans can survive in space without the radioprotective magnetosphere? Finally, if ionizing irradiation is dangerous and is to be avoided, why do we use it to treat cancer?

References

1. Kemikler G. History of brachytherapy. Turkish Journal of Oncology. 2019;34(Supp 1):1–10. https://doi.org/10.5505/tjo.2019.1.
2. Gianfaldoni S, Gianfaldoni R, Wollina U, et al. An overview on radiotherapy: from its history to its current applications in dermatology. Open Access Maced J Med Sci. 2017;5(4):521–5. https://doi.org/10.3889/oamjms.2017.122.
3. El-Nachef L, Al-Choboq J, Restier-Verlet J, et al. Human radiosensitivity and radiosusceptibility: what are the differences? Int J Mol Sci. 2021;22(13):7158. https://doi.org/10.3390/ijms22137158.
4. Foray N, Gourguignon M, Hamada N. Individual response to ionizing radiation. Mutat Res Rev Mutat Res. 2016;7770(Pt B):369–86. https://doi.org/10.1016/j.mrrev.2016.09.001.

5. Walden H, Deans AJ. The Fanconi anemia DNA repair pathway: structural and functional insights into a complex disorder. Annu Rev Biophys. 2014;43:257–78. https://doi.org/10.1146/annurev-biophys-051013-022737.
6. Keller C, Keller KR, Shew SB, et al. Growth deficiency and malnutrition in bloom syndrome. J Pediatr. 1999;134(4):479. https://doi.org/10.1016/s0022-3476(99)70206-4.
7. Digweed M, Sperling K. Nijmegen breakage syndrome: clinical manifestation of defective response to DNA double-strand breaks. DNA Repair (Amst). 2004;3(8–9):1207–17. https://doi.org/10.1016/j.dnarep.2004.03.004.
8. Kaina B. A genome-wide screening for DNA repair genes: much more players than hitherto known. Signal Transduct Target Ther. 2020;5(1):204. https://doi.org/10.1038/s41392-020-00314-4.
9. Epperly MW, Travis EL, Sikora C, et al. Manganese superoxide dismutase (MnSOD) plasmid/liposome pulmonary radioprotective gene therapy: modulation of irradiation-induced mRNA for IL-1, TNF-α, and TGF-β correlates with delay of organizing alveolitis/fibrosis. Biol Blood Marrow Transplant. 1999;5(4):204–14. https://doi.org/10.1053/bbmt.1999.v5.pm10465100.
10. Elkind MM, Sutton H. Radiation response of mammalian cells grown in culture. I. Repair of x-ray damage in surviving Chinese hamster cells. Radiat Res. 1960;13:556–93.
11. Puck TT, Markus PI. Action of x-rays on mammalian cells. J Exp Med. 1956;103(5):653–66. https://doi.org/10.1084/jem.103.5.653.
12. Tochilin E, Goldstein N, Miller WG. Beryllium oxide as a thermoluminescent dosimeter. Health Phys. 1969;16(1):1–7. https://doi.org/10.1097/00004032-196901000-00001.
13. McCall C. Chernobyl disaster 30 years on: lessons not learned. Lancet. 2016;387(10029):1707–8. https://doi.org/10.1016/S0140-6736(16)30304-X.
14. Hasegawa A, Ohira T, Maeda M, et al. Emergency responses and health consequences after the Fukushima accident. Evacuation and relocation Clin Oncol (R Coll Radiol). 2016;28(4):237–44. https://doi.org/10.1016/j.clon.2016.01.002.
15. Steyskal GC. Trend curves of the rate of species description in zoology. Science. 1965;149(3686):880–2. https://doi.org/10.1126/science.149.3686.880.
16. Confalonieri F, Sommer S. Bacterial and archaeal resistance to ionizing irradiation. J Phys Conf Ser. 2011;261:012005.
17. Bennett CB, Lewis LK, Karthikeyan G, et al. Genes required for ionizing radiation resistance in yeast. Nat Genet. 2001;29(4):426–34. https://doi.org/10.1038/ng778.
18. Srinivasan V, Doctrow S, Singh VK, et al. Evaluation of EUK-189, a synthetic superoxide dismutase/catalase mimetic as a radiation countermeasure. Immunopharmacol Immunotoxicol. 2008;30(2):271–90. https://doi.org/10.1080/08923970801925331.
19. Greenberger JS, Pechenik J, Gould L, et al. X-irradiation effects on growth and metamorphosis of gastropod larvae (Crepidula fornicate): a model for environmental radiation teratogenesis. Arch Environ Contam Toxicol. 1986;15(2):227–34. https://doi.org/10.1007/BF01059971.
20. Stankowski S, Zagrdozka ZB, Garlovsky MD, et al. The genetic basis of a recent transition to live-bearing in marine snails. Science. 2024;383(6678):114–9. https://doi.org/10.1126/science.adi2982.
21. Paithankar JG, Deeksha K, Patil RK. Gamma radiation tolerance in different life stages of the fruit fly drosophila melanogaster. Int J Radiat Biol. 2017;93(4):440–8. https://doi.org/10.1080/09553002.2016.1266056.
22. Kamstra JH, Hurem S, Martin LM, et al. Ionizing radiation induces transgenerational effects of DNA methylation in zebrafish. Sci Rep. 2018;8(1):15373. https://doi.org/10.1038/s41598-018-33817-w.
23. Sakashita T, Takanami T, Yanase S, et al. Radiation biology of Caenorhabditis elegans: germ cell response, aging, and behavior. J Radiat Res. 2020;51(2):107–21. https://doi.org/10.1269/jrr.09100.
24. Zeitz L, Ferguson R, Garfinkel E. Radiation-induced effects on DNA synthesis in developing sea urchin eggs. Radiat Res. 1968;34(1):200–8.

25. Masui Y. Effects of ionizing radiation on meiotic maturation of frog oocytes: I. In vivo studies. J Embryol Exp Morphol. 1973;29(1):87–104.
26. Wood MD, Beresford NA, Semenov DV, et al. Radionuclide transfer to reptiles. Radiat Environ Biophys. 2010;49(4):509–30. https://doi.org/10.1007/s00411-010-0321-1.
27. Levit GS, Hossfeld U. Ernst Haeckel in the history of biology. Curr Biol. 2019;29(24):R1276–84. https://doi.org/10.1016/j.cub.2019.10.064.
28. Montesinos CA, Khalid R, Cristea O, et al. Space radiation protection countermeasures in microgravity and planetary exploration—a review for special issue on space life science in life. Life. 2021;11(8):829. https://doi.org/10.3390/life11080829.
29. Putnam FW. The atomic bomb casualty commission in retrospect. Proc Natl Acad Sci USA. 1998;95(10):5426–31. https://doi.org/10.1073/pnas.95.10.5426.
30. Piani L. Earth's water may have been inherited form material similar to enstatite chondrite meteorites. Science. 2020;369(6507):1110–3. https://doi.org/10.1126/science.aba1948.
31. Davies CJ, Constable CG. Rapid geomagnetic changes inferred from earth observations and numerical situations. Nat Commun. 2020;11(1):3371. https://doi.org/10.1038/s41467-020-16888-0.
32. Anamika K, Malik RMP. Assessment of radiological impacts of natural radionuclides and radon exhalation rate measured in the soil samples of Himalayan foothills of Uttarakhand. India: J Radioanalytical Nuclear Chemistry; 2019. https://doi.org/10.1007/s10967-019-06876-0.
33. Moeller DW, Sun L-SC. Comparison of natural background dose rates for residents of the Amargosa Valley, NV, to those in Leadville, CO, and the states of Colorado and Nevada. Health Phys. 2006;91(4):338–53. https://doi.org/10.1097/01.HP.0000218426.41326.6d.
34. Scheibler C, Toprani SM, Mordukhovich I, et al. Cancer risks from cosmic radiation exposure in flight: a review. Front Public Health. 2022;10:947068. https://doi.org/10.3389/fpubh.2022.947068.
35. Reynolds R, Little MP, Day S, et al. Cancer incidence and mortality in the USA astronaut corps, 1959-2017. Occup Environ Med. 2021;78(12):869–75. https://doi.org/10.1136/oemed-2020-107143.
36. Chandra K, Proshad R, Chandra Dey H, et al. A review on radionuclide pollution in global soils with environmental and health hazards evaluation. Environ Geochem Health. 2023;45(12):9245–66. https://doi.org/10.1007/s10653-023-01725-2.
37. Alif SM, Sim MR, Ho C, et al. Cancer and mortality in coal mine workers: a systematic review and meta-analysis. Occup Environ Med. 2022;79(5):347–57. https://doi.org/10.1136/oemed-2021-107498.
38. Battista JR. Against all odds: the survival strategies of Deinococcus radiodurans. Ann Rev Microbiol. 1997;51:203–24. https://doi.org/10.1146/annurev.micro.51.1.203.
39. Greenberger JS, Kagan VE, Pearce L, et al. Modulation of redox signal transduction pathways in the treatment of cancer. Antioxid Redox Signal. 2001;3(3):347–59. https://doi.org/10.1089/15230860152409004.
40. Slade D, Lindner AB, Paul G, et al. Recombination and replication in DNA repair of heavily irradiated Deinococcus radiodurans. Cell. 2009;136(6):1044–55. https://doi.org/10.1016/j.cell.2009.01.018.
41. Zahradka K, Slade D, Bailone A, et al. Reassembly of shattered chromosomes in Deinococcus radiodurans. Nature. 2006;443(7111):569–73. https://doi.org/10.1038/nature05160.
42. Berhane H, Epperly MW, Goff J, et al. Radiobiologic differences between bone marrow stromal and hematopoietic progenitor cell lines from Fanconi anemia (Fancd2−/−) mice. Radiat Res. 2014;181(1):76–89. https://doi.org/10.1667/RR13405.1.
43. Epperly MW, Smith T, Zhang X, et al. Modulation of in utero total body irradiation induced newborn mouse growth retardation by maternal manganese superoxide dismutase-plasmid liposome (MnSOD-PL) gene therapy. Gene Ther. 2010;18(6):579–83. https://doi.org/10.1038/gt.2010.178.
44. Shapiro BJ, Leducq J-B, Mallet J. What is speciation? PLoS Genet. 2016;12(3):e1005860. https://doi.org/10.1371/journal.pgen.1005860.

45. Perri A, Widga C, Lawler D, et al. New evidence of the earliest domestic dogs in the Americas. Am Antiq. 2019;84(1):68–87. https://doi.org/10.1017/anq.2018.74.
46. Dutrow EV, Serpell JA, Ostrander EA. Domestic dog lineages reveal genetic drivers of behavioral diversification. Cell. 2022;185(25):4737–55. https://doi.org/10.1016/j.cell.2022.11.003.
47. Olipitz W, Wiktor-Brown D, Shuga J, et al. Integrated molecular analysis indicates undetectable DNA damage in mice after continuous irradiation at ~400-fold natural background radiation. Environ Health Perspect. 2012;120(8):1130–6. https://doi.org/10.1289/ehp.1104294.
48. Nayak T, Sengupta I, Dhal PK. A new era of radiation resistance bacteria in bioremediation and production of bioactive compounds with therapeutic potential and other aspects: an in-perspective review. J Environ Radioact. 2021;237:106696. https://doi.org/10.1016/j.jenvrad.2021.106696.

Chapter 2
Adaptation to Low-Dose-Rate Background Irradiation: Continuous Radiation Exposure Based on Geographic Location on Earth Relative to Other Sources/Hazards of Radiation

As the communication of new information increases, there is greater awareness of the potential dangers of ionizing irradiation. Many research projects that have been in existence for decades continue (Table 2.1). While the majority of nuclear power stations in the world are safe and well maintained, most Americans think about the disaster at Chernobyl in Ukraine in 1986 and the Fukushima Dai-Chi disaster in Japan in 2011. The historical events involving ionizing irradiation exposure are now many in number (Table 2.2). While people are concerned about the cost of energy and the efficiency of nuclear power stations, they are also quick to jump on promises that other sources of energy including hydroelectric, wind turbine power, and solar collection of energy in novel new batteries will replace the need for nuclear power stations. There is also the continuing threat of terrorism using a fission bomb and awareness of changes in global climate. People are aware of the effects of controlling climate change/global warming and other threats to the environment. Not all people may associate climate change with the loss of or change in the protective shield (magnetosphere) over the planet. This chapter deals with the reality of radiation levels in a variety of situations. The difficulty in making accurate measurements of radiation exposure is apparent [1–8], as is the importance of the radiobiologic effect (RBE) of different forms of irradiation, such as X-rays, protons, galactic cosmic irradiation, and neutrons.

As described in Chap. 1, the evolution of radiation resistance and radiation protector genes in organisms on the planet Earth going back over two billion years ago indicates that organisms were "aware" of ionizing irradiation and were selected for genes, the expression of which facilitated the repair of ionizing irradiation-induced DNA double-strand breaks. In the modern era, the techniques for measuring irradiation have dominated the concern for environmental safety [7, 8]. Badge dosimeters on hospital personnel and radiation workers have led to policies that have generated estimates of what a "safe" level of radiation exposure is and the development of radiation safety offices in all hospitals and medical facilities where X-ray machines are located. For radiation workers, in the nuclear power industry and in the production facilities that

J. Greenberger, *Radiation Oncology and Radiation Biology*, https://doi.org/10.1007/978-3-031-66300-0_2

Table 2.1 Current research on outcomes continue. Radiation exposure levels from historical experience: Challenges in data retrieval

Event (start of collected data)
Manhattan project uranium workers: 1940s
Plutonium production plant, Wyoming, USA: 1940s
Hiroshima survivors: 1945
Nagasaki survivors: 1945
Marshallese islanders: 1950s Fallout survival
Chernobyl survivors: 1986
Fukushima survivors: 2011

Table 2.2 Radiation exposure levels for humans in different locations

Category	Radiation quality
General population	X-rays, radon
Living at high altitudes	Leadville, Colorado
Radium workers	X-ray, radon
Uranium miners	Radon, gamma rays
Airline pilots	X-rays
Space shuttle Mission	GCR, proton, gamma rays
International Space Station (resident)	GCR, proton, X-rays
Lunar Mission (apollo)	Charged particles, protons, neutrons, gamma rays
Mars Mission planned 180 + 500 + 180 days	Charged particles, protons, neutrons, gamma rays
Hiroshima/Nagasaki survivors of atomic bombs	Gamma ray, neutrons
Marshallese Islands Fallout exposure from thermonuclear fusion bombs.	B-irradiation, gamma radiation
Bone marrow transplantation recipients	X-ray

produce weapon-grade plutonium, there is great concern for measuring exposure levels. Badge dosimetry continues to be the mainstay of measurements for the general population [8]. Using currently available radiation measuring devices including badge/film dosimetry, ionization chambers, and thermolescent dosimeters gives available data on radiation levels that are sustained by people.

Individuals, who work in radiation environments [9–13] or who live at high altitudes (Example: Leadville, CO) which is 2 miles above sea level, airline pilots, and people, or specific geographic locations [11] may be at greater risk of radiation effects. People who have been veterans of the space shuttle mission or residents in the International Space Station or even airline pilots who experience sources of irradiation from the atmosphere (or outside the Earth) including galactic cosmic irradiation, solar proton events, and gamma rays [14, 15] represent one source of data quantitating the effects of radiation exposure to humans. The higher the altitude above Earth, including location outside the protective Magnetosphere, the higher these radiation levels would be expected to be (Table 2.2). The other source of radiation is from the radon and isotopic conversion from radium in the Earth's core. As individuals mine the Earth deeper for uranium, coal, and other mineral excavation, exposure from this internal "inside the Earth" source of radiation increases. Relative levels are shown in Table 2.1. To compare these radiation dose levels sustained with other unplanned radiation exposure, such as a radiation terrorist event, a nuclear reactor accident, or a radioisotope "spill," these same measuring devices are used to detect the increased levels of radiation exposure [16]. Since there is measurable ionizing radiation everywhere, both originating from outside the Earth and from the Earth's core, there is a concern about what constitutes a "safe level" of exposure [7]. Is there a safe level [17]?

To measure levels of radiation exposure and relate such data to human biology, one must be aware of the continuing controversy over the "threshold" of radiation effects [17]. Acute radiation effects are those associated with clinical presentations of symptoms and signs of radiation exposure. Late radiation effects are those that occur after any acute exposure is long past and the body is producing a latent reaction to the radiation exposure. Animal models have provided valuable data (Table 2.3). Late effects in humans are seen routinely in clinical radiotherapy patients who have completed a course of radiation (Table 2.4). While they may experience some skin redness during the irradiation, for example, to treat breast cancer, the tissue returns to a normal state after completion of irradiation. There is a latent period in which the patient experiences no symptoms, and there is no visible sign of irradiation. After this latent period, some patients will experience late effects such as thickening of the skin or fibrosis. The question of late effects is one of the continuing challenges for radiation biology. A later chapter will present

Table 2.3 Experimental animal radiation exposure: results

Experimental model	Animal species	Cumulative dose	Outcome
Low-dose rate	Mice	600X background	Little effect
Total body irradiation (TBI)	Mice	Wide range	Hematopoietic death, gastrointestinal (GI) death
Partial body irradiation (PBI)	Mice	Higher dose	Survival at higher dose
Whole abdomen irradiation (WAI)	Mice	Higher dose	GI death
Thoracic irradiation	Mice	20–21 Gy	Pneumonitis, late fibrosis
TBI	Rhesus macaque monkey	8–9 Gy	Pneumonitis, late fibrosis
Thoracic irradiation	Rhesus macaque monkey	10–15 Gy	Pneumonitis, late fibrosis
TBI	Miniature swine	Wide range	Hematopoietic death
TBI	New Zealand white rabbit	Wide range	GI death
TBI 3–5 rad/day X 2 years	Out-bred beagle dogs	2.19–3.65 Gy Gamma ray Co^{60} gamma ray	Leukemia, aplastic anemia, radioaccommodation

Table 2.4 Known acute and late effects of ionizing irradiation on humans

Acute effects	**Syndrome**	**Outcome**	**Exposure dose**
Total body irradiation	Bone marrow failure	LD50/30	3–4 Gy
Total body irradiation	Gastrointestinal syndrome	LD50/10	10–15 Gy
Total body irradiation	CNS syndrome	Seizures and death	>30 Gy
Thoracic irradiation	Pneumonitis	Lung failure	>20 Gy
Radioactive fallout	Skin burns	Radiation dermatitis	>20 Gy
Late effects	**Syndrome**	**Outcome**	**Exposure dose**
Thoracic irradiation	Radiation-induced pulmonary fibrosis	Lung failure	Volume dependent 6–24 mos.
Kidney failure	Renal fibrosis, renal failure	Radiation nephritis	>13 Gy 6–24 mos.
Liver damage	Radiation hepatitis and fibrosis	Liver failure	Volume dependent 6–24 mos.
Skin fibrosis, muscle fibrosis	Skin variation and fibrosis	Scarring	Volume and dose dependent 6–24 mos.
Sterility Female Male	Ovarian failure Azo spermia	Ovarian failure Testicular failure	>10 Gy >10 Gy
Neurocognitive loss (hypocampus dependent)	Neurocognitive failure	Memory and brain function	50 Gy 12–24 mos.
Eye	Cataracts	Cataracts	1 + years

Table 2.5 Deleterious effects of irradiation in one instance and therapeutic effects in another

Radioisotope	Hazard	Therapeutic use
Radioiodine I131	Thyroid cancer induction	Radioablation for thyroid cancer
Strontium 90, strontium 89	Fallout	Treatment of bone (Sofigo) metastasis of prostate cancer
Transuranium compounds Antibody-labeled radioisotope	Cancer induction	Theranostics
Ultrahigh dose rate irradiation	Fission or fusion bomb—Death, H-ARS, GI-ARS	FLASH irradiation treatment of cancer
Low-dose rate irradiation	Cancer induction	Brachytherapy for head and neck or gynecologic cancer

details on what is known about late effects; however, there is a phenomenon that is associated with the "threshold" that has been observed in experimental animals and in human radiotherapy patients with respect to late effects. One great dilemma is the paradox that ionizing irradiation is both deleterious and in some cases therapeutic (Table 2.5).

The concept of radiation late effects is difficult to understand. As shown in Fig. 2.1, with continual radiation exposure including background levels of irradiation, for example, from radon in the basement of houses, cells repair radiation damage such that there is a balance. The level of radiation-induced DNA double-strand breaks is balanced by the continual repair of these double-strand breaks. As shown in Fig. 2.1, the "threshold" level for detecting any effects of irradiation is not reached until the amount of radiation sustained exceeds that threshold. Then, the repair mechanisms are overburdened, and there will be some evidence of irradiation exposure. This evidence is termed the "acute effects." For example, in a clinical radiation therapy patient, who is receiving 4 weeks of fractionated irradiation for breast cancer, there may be no detectable changes in the tissue for the first 2 weeks (10 treatments), but during the third week, the skin may become red, there may be some skin shedding—desquamation, and then by the fourth or fifth week, there may be some skin breakdown and ulceration.

How do clinical effects of radiation relate to radiation biology? After the DNA repair capacity of irradiated cells is exhausted, as are antioxidant stores in cells this would be an example of going over the threshold for acute effects (Fig. 2.1). One of the controversies about "threshold" [17, 18] is that some radiation biologists and radiation oncologists believe that any radiation exposure, which is still within the "balance" of neutralization by DNA repair and antioxidant stores, proves that there is a threshold below, which there are no biological effects. However, emerging evidence indicates that there is an accumulation of damage, which may not be

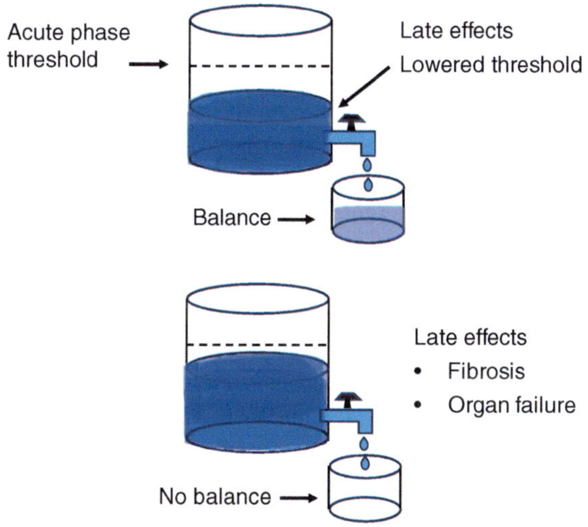

Fig. 2.1 The lowered threshold for radiation late effects. The cylinders in this figure represent the accumulation of radiation damage, which is in blue. There is a balance in the top part of the figure indicating that the dotted line is the threshold for acute effects. There is compensation for damage occurring and the drops coming out of the faucet represent management-reduction of the level of accumulated damage in blue. There is a balance here, and there are no acute effects. In contrast, in the lower panel, there is accumulation of an increased amount of damage indicated in blue, and the repair of the damage or the compensation-release coming through the faucet is ineffective to prevent the rising level of the blue to reach the threshold. Thus, exceding the dotted line would result in late effects of irradiation

detectable during the acute phase, and, in fact, changes the threshold. The evidence from clinical radiotherapy patients provides strong support for the hypothesis that the threshold can change over time. Cells in culture and tissues "remember" a previous radiation exposure, and there is a continuing presence of this memory. While there may be no clinical evidence of "memory" of the previous irradiation with respect to lack of symptoms and lack of signs in the tissue or in the organism, the patient or experimental animal that is exposed to irradiation again at some later time will often reveal evidence of the prior exposure and "late effects" may then occur after much lower levels of exposure for this second treatment course or second irradiation exposure (Fig. 2.1).

What is the mechanism of this "memory" of prior irradiation? At present, the answer to this question is unknown. One hypothesis is that a slowly proliferating group of cells is stable in the tissues after the first radiation course, and it is only after a second radiation exposure that these cells are pushed to go through a cell division, and during that division the cells die. Another hypothesis is that some types of cells within tissues such as endothelial cells (cells that line blood vessels) "remember" the radiation damage and are continually producing proteins that accumulate within the cells. There may be induction of inflammatory mediators that cause a late tissue reaction. The components of a "scar" formation are one example of a late reaction. As with late effects of thermal burn, the scar components, such as collagen, may not produce any visible effect or clinical symptoms until the scar appears. If the experimental animal or patient receives no further radiotherapy at the previously irradiated site, there may be no evidence of prior irradiation. However, a second irradiation exposure to the same anatomic site accelerates the accumulation of such proteins in cells and can push the tissue to generate the pathways associated with late effects. Figure 2.1 shows the hypothesized change in the threshold. The threshold for acute effects is still there, but there is a second threshold now, which is much lower for the induction of the late effects. This represents a hypothesis as to the mechanism of irradiation effects and is supported by evidence from clinical radiotherapy treatment courses and also from data in experimental animals.

Given the concept of "threshold" and that tissues can "remember" prior radiation exposure, there are several new questions.

Will a person who has a prior increased level of background radiation exposure, such as living at high altitude or having been an airline pilot or astronaut in a space shuttle mission, who then receives at some later date a course of clinical radiotherapy have a different outcome? Would such a person be at greater risk for symptoms and side effects of therapeutic irradiation? While some data are available on this subject, evidence suggests the continuous level of exposure in the first course of exposure that is below the threshold level, and it is being continually repaired that person would not be at greater risk of side effects of clinical radiotherapy.

What about second level of exposure, such as that in a nuclear power plant accident or in a radiation terrorist event releasing X-rays or radioisotopes? There is no evidence to support this hypothesis, but airline pilots who have received clinical radiotherapy have not been reported to be at greater risk for side effects at some later date [14, 15]. What about a person who has lived at a high altitude for his/her entire life and then becomes an astronaut and is involved in a space mission outside the radioprotective magnetosphere? The hypothesis regarding a threshold would follow here as well. If the person has experienced a high background level of irradiation for decades and shows no symptoms or signs, it would be expected that irradiation repair and neutralization of radiation effects by antioxidant stores have kept all tissues and organs below the threshold. Therefore, any subsequent radiation exposure, for example, from a space mission would not lead to any greater susceptibility to side effects. This conclusion is also a hypothesis.

There are other issues associated with the analysis of threshold effects of ionizing irradiation. Are radiosensitive animal models and people with expression of genes that are associated with radiosensitivity more susceptible to late effects? In the case of patients, many individuals do not know that they harbor genes for radiosensitivity. Only at later time when they are exposed to ionizing irradiation for therapeutic treatment of cancer, do they show a heightened radiosensitivity compared to the general population. Then, analysis of genotype may occur, and the patient may be found to have Fanconi anemia, Bloom's syndrome, or another genotype associated with radiosensitivity. This phenomenon will be described in a later chapter in this book.

In all the considerations for levels of radiation exposure and what constitutes a hazard or unsafe condition, there are basic principles which apply to every one of these situations. The basic principles of response to radiation involves volume treated, total dose, fraction size in the case of multiple sequential exposures, and, overall, the relative biologic effect (RBE) of the radiation. In basic radiobiology, it is well known that high linear energy transfer (LET) particle produce more DNA strand breaks and more damage than do X-rays and gamma rays. In clinical radiotherapy, the RBE of the radiation source is controlled by radiation oncologists and physicists delivering the treatment. However, when one analyzes the RBE of other situations including nuclear reactor accidents and in space irradiation, it is not so easy to determine the RBE of the exposure.

There is a fifth basic principle of radiation biology, which also applies but is rarely considered: that of dose rate. Clinical radiation oncology linear accelerators and treatment delivery devices are well calibrated for the level of irradiation produced per minute, and the dose rate is well known. Experimenting with low dose rate produces very few detectable effects [19]. In contrast, continuous radiation exposure is clearly deleterious and causes cancer if the dose per day is above the threshold [20]. However, in the case of unplanned radiation exposures such as a nuclear reactor accident or radiation terrorist event, the dose rate must be reconstructed from historical information. For example, the dose rate of irradiation in the survivors of the Hiroshima and Nagasaki atomic bomb events was calculated years later based on known information about nuclear fission reactions and the location of individuals from the hypocenter of the detonation. It was a very high dose rate, and, thus, any measurements that would be carried out by using current badge dosimetry, thermoluminescent dosimeters, or ionization chambers could not give information on the dose rate unless this was measured in real time. With respect to space irradiation and radiation dose sustained by astronauts, the same dilemma would apply.

Measuring devices produce data on cumulative radiation exposure, and the sporadic nature of a supernovae producing galactic cosmic irradiation would not be indicated on the dosimeter. This would have to be measured in real time. Furthermore, galactic cosmic radiation (GCR) could be associated with production of a different spectrum of high LET ions from a supernovae event [21]. Thus, the spectrum of ionized particles iron, silicone, and carbon may differ, and the RBE of each would be different as measured by current radiobiology techniques. Measurement of GCR and solar protons on Earth yield very low levels because the protective "magnetosphere" funnels these charged particles to the polar regions. Not so, during space travel or on the surface of Mars [21]. All of these uncertainties produce a situation in which it is very difficult to give definitive answers. With the understanding that there is uncertainty in data collection and many levels of hypotheses with respect to RBE, we can now approach available information on each of the sources of radiation in the environment.

General Population and Radiation Workers Are Concerned About Environmental Radiation Exposure

People in the United States are very concerned about exposure to ionizing irradiation. The best example of this concern is the rising focus on radon-gas measurements in the basements of houses that are being considered for sale [1, 2]. Most real estate agents, particularly in geographic areas where there has been a history of coal mining or deep excavation, have radon test centers close and available. Levels of radon detected in basement can result in changes in the purchase and sale agreements for homes. Fans and other gas mobilization devices are installed in basements to vent levels of radon. Radon is a natural decay product of radium in the Earth's core. Prior to the availability of sensitive radiation detection devices to measure radon, home sales did not include a "radon-test" [1, 2].

Another example of the concern of people for radiation levels is the policy of most hospitals concerning notification of patients and their families that they must be aware of radiation levels [3] that are associated with conventional X-rays [7]. Most emergency rooms and outpatient facilities have the equipment for routine chest X-rays, pelvic X-rays, and despite significant innovations to decrease radiation exposure, such as the use of image intensifiers and strict guidelines for using lead shielded aprons to cover critical areas during diagnostic examinations, people are still concerned about radiation levels. Policies in hospitals have changed in the last 50 years. Cancer patients with gynecologic malignancies (endometrial, vulvovaginal, or cervix cancer or head and neck cancer) frequently received intracavitary and/or interstitial radioisotope implants (radium or cesium) as part of their therapy [5]. The radiation delivery systems prior to the 1980 s was "low dose rate" applicators in which an applicator was placed in the cervix in the operating room, then patients taken to the floor, and radiation oncologists and radiation physicists accompanied by a radiation safety officer would later place ionizing irradiation sources into the device [4]. Patients would then lie in bed for 50 plus hours, while low dose rate irradiation was emitted from the sources and delivered the therapeutic doses to the structures including the residual cancer, regional lymph nodes and associated tissues felt to be at risk for local recurrence. The concern for low dose rate irradiation, and its recent change in the 1990s to the use of high dose rate (HDR) applicators was a necessary event. HDR deliverery of different isotopes are afterloaded after the patient is brought to the department. These isotopes such as iridium 192 are housed in department of Radiation Oncology. The patient is treated, the isotope removed and the patient returned to their bed. Several HDR treatments are repeated instead of one continuous LDR treatment. The entire paradigm of treatment has changed.

There was controversy among gynecologic oncologists initially that the HDR delivered using Iridium 192 sources that were placed into the apparatus in the protected basement environment of a Radiation Oncology Department and would result in a decreased local control of cervical and endometrial cancer compared to the low dose rate [5, 6]. However, therapeutic outcomes were shown to be the same with low-dose rate or the newer HDR delivery devices [5]. Thus, the medical controversy has been largely resolved. However, a major factor that pushed the change in policy was the concern for patients, their families, and house staff entering the patient's room over their own unintended radiation exposure. Hospital personnel including those that changed bedding, managed laundry, delivered food trays, and delivered or removed equipment from hospital rooms were concerned about their levels of exposure.

The Radiation Safety Offices in hospitals and medical centers have structured a program for the analysis of radiation exposure by creating policies that separate categories of levels of exposure. There is separation of the monitored exposure levels for radiation workers, from patients, and from the general population. The concept of "as low as reasonably acceptable" (ALARA) [7] led radiation safety officers to create a program of regular and in some cases mandatory measurement of radiation exposure for all people in the hospital environment, who routinely have contact with radiation-emitting sources. Badge dosimetry is a policy used in most hospitals and clinics. Workers will wear a dosimeter badge, either one or several that are placed in several locations on their body. The badge is usually placed on a laboratory or clinical white-coat, but for those individuals working closely with radiation sources on a routine basis (cardiologists carrying out cardiac catherization fluoroscopic procedures, and other physicians such as thoracic surgeons or neurosurgeons, who have fluoroscopic C-ARM X-ray units in the operating room) are asked to wear dosimeters on their hands (finger badge) and also other anatomic locations. Many hospital radiation safety offices monitor the dosimetry on a quarterly basis and change badges for everyone routinely. The levels that are measured then lead the Radiation Safety Office to alert individuals if they have reached ALARA-1, 2, or 3 levels. Individuals, who have reached high levels of exposure as detected by badge dosimeters, are often asked to carry out fewer procedures, limit their exposure, and in some cases have been asked to cease their proximity to fluoroscopic or radioisotope sources for several months. The badge data as interpreted by radiobiologists have not been reported. This topic will be discussed in a later chapter.

Public Awareness of the Estimated Radiation Exposure from Air Travel and Known Historical Space Missions

With all of the concern for radiation exposure, it is useful to review the data, which actually support of the hypothesis that increased radiation exposure leads to increased risk. Airline pilots, current astronauts, and shuttle missions or International Space Station workers have been studied [14, 15]. How is exposure measured and what are the risks? Much of the data leading to the concern for radiation exposure levels come from animal experiments that were carried out as far back as the 1940s. Experimental animal studies have been well documented (Table 2.3), and new models continue to be reported [22–24].

When radiation workers in the 1940s including those working on development of the atomic bomb and in the plutonium manufacturing facility (Tables 2.1 and 2.2) began to increase their levels of exposure, certainly during the "Manhattan Project" for the development of the atomic bomb, there were routine measurements of exposure with the Manhattan Project. The purification of Uranium 235, there followed a development of breeder factories to produce Plutonium239. At this time, there were clear cases of injury from radiation exposure of workers. The high levels of exposure are recorded for radiation workers in some cases. Cautionary measures were installed.

The recent nuclear reactor accidents at Chernobyl in 1986 and Fukushima in 1911 further emphasized the needs to prepare for unplanned radiation level release into the environment. There are two major current industries to consider: (1) Breeder reactors that produce plutonium for weapons [9] and (2) nuclear power stations that contain plutonium fuel rods that are regulated by insertion of graphite rods [10]. Recently, there has been the creation of the Radiation Injury Treatment Network (RITN) [16]. The RITN organization and others created systems, whereby exposed individuals could be triaged to hospital facilities that are appropriate and skilled for handling radiation injuries, particularly injuries to those individuals who had radioisotope contamination on or inside the body (nuclear reactor accident, nuclear weapons preparation, or test facilities). RITN Network hospitals have now been organized to handle casualties from high-dose exposure. After the 9/11 terrorist events, which involved airplane crashes in Washington, DC, New York City, and rural Pennsylvania, there was heightened concern for all forms of terrorism including radiation terrorism. There followed the creation of the Center for Medical Countermeasures Against Radiation (CMCR)—this Consortium, which was organized and funded by the National Institutes of Allergies and Infectious Diseases (NIAID) and other organizations. The federal government organized and funded research through NIAID for the development of radiation countermeasures that could be administered to people after radiation exposure.

Historical Radiation Exposure Levels and Medical Outcomes

The heightened concern about radiation exposure has filtered through to the general population and enhanced the concern for continuous low-level exposure including that from radon gas levels in home basements. A useful body of data has come from the study of miners, who had relatively higher levels of exposure to radon gas emitted from the Earth's core. Uranium miners [11] in the United States and other countries cooperated for the collection of data on the level of exposure to miners and their subsequent possible increased incidence of cancer and other medical conditions that could be associated with chronic radiation exposure mostly from radon [11]. There are two ways to interpret this published data. A significant fact is that many of those miners, who were also cigarette smokers, revealed a significant increase in the incidence of lung cancer [11]. However, the data on radiation exposure alone, in the absence of documented cigarette smoking, were more complicated to decipher. Given the sophisticated and improved measuring devices for levels of exposure, all of these datasets there are published have increased the level of anxiety within the general population with respect to radiation exposure.

Does the available information support the hypothesis that increased levels of exposure do lead to an increased incidence of late effects including cancer? From basic radiobiology experiments with animal models, late effects of radiation exposure do include cancer, accelerated aging, and neurocognitive deficits, but the time course of exposure and radiation quality must be included in the analysis. Are the observed late effects clearly caused by or associated with increased levels of exposure to ionizing irradiation to humans? There is no clear answer.

Animal Irradiation Exposure Experiments: Lessons Learned and Cautions for Interpretation

The question about relating radiation cumulative dose to late effects cannot be answered definitively because of the continuing controversy about the "threshold" levels of radiation exposure with respect to each detectable medical condition. What is the "threshold" controversy? One group of scientists have concluded that there is a threshold below which radiation exposure cannot be associated with any detectable changes in cells in culture or in experimental animals or in humans. Another group of scientists insists that there is no threshold and that every level of increased radiation exposure above background levels (coming from radon leaking from the Earth's core) leads to a detectable and possibly deleterious outcome. What has changed regarding this controversy? There is an understanding that there are two elements at work in such a model [17]: (1) the sensitivity of the measuring device and (2) the capacity of the model system to repair or neutralize any detectable change during the exposure and during the measurement. Chronic low-dose radiation is cumulative [19], but every organism (species) has an adaptation response including DNA repair. Radiation late effects including bone marrow failure and cancer are definitely dose dependent, but at much higher cumulative doses [20]. The threshold relates to biological effects and must take into account both issues of adaptation and DNA repair. Thus, as radiation dose is sustained, it is also neutralized (Fig. 2.1). Background radiation levels cannot be translated to sensitive enough biological effects. Devices for measurement of physical effects of radiation are accurate and include: Ionization chambers [18], and thermoluminescent dosimeters [18], but the biological effects of radiation are dynamic and are continually being repaired in real time. While dosimeters accumulate data, they report the sum of exposures over a particular time. This fact alone applies to the detection of levels of space radiation [21]. Given the existence of repair gene products in cells, the controversy about thresholds continues.

Radiation Exposure from Long-Planned Space Missions

We can now detect MILLI REMS of irradiation in badge dosimeters (1000th of an REM or radiation equivalent man) [7, 8]. We can now make measurements that might not have been possible without these highly sensitive dosimeters. The concept of REM is important because it takes into account the quality of the radiation (whether photon, proton, neutron, or high linear energy transfer LET-ionized particles, such as products from galactic cosmic radiation (GCR) helium nuclei, alpha particles, or carbon nuclei). The ability to measure radiation exposure levels in MILLIREM allows radiation safety offices in hospitals to deploy a metric by which to measure radiation and translate the data into an estimate of the increased risk of each individual to exposure level, but badges accumulate the data from 3 month intervals. Astronauts will also need real-time measurements of time-related fluxes [21]. Another controversy is whether the reported exposure level can be translated to increased risk that is realistic and relevant. While this controversy leads to continued debate these badge dosimeters are still used, and reports are delivered to each individual hospital worker who turns in a badge for evaluation.

Are there people living in some high-altitude levels who are at greater risk of injury from radiation?

Comparisons between ultraviolet (UV) irradiation (sun exposure) and ionizing irradiation continue to be recorded, although the mechanism of injury by these two forms of irradiation is entirely different. UV exposure is uniform to exposed areas and is measured by an entirely different metric [18]. The mechanism of ultraviolet (UV) irradiation-induced DNA strand breaks is by creation of cyclobutane-dimers, and its repair is very different from that caused by ionizing irradiation, namely, the local (angstrom sized) deposition of ionizing irradiation energy in localized areas (purine and pyrimidine base) of elements of DNA. However, UV irradiation measurements, which predominantly are made on the skin, do record exposure levels and have led to sound data showing that people living at high altitudes with higher levels of UV exposure do have a greater incidence of skin cancer [18]. UV irradiation penetrates through superficial tissues (several millimeters depth at most), whereas ionizing irradiation from gamma rays or X-ray photons dependent on the energy of the photons can transmit to the entire body and produce energy deep deposition within tissues. Protons, electrons, neutrons, and charged high LET particles penetrate even deeper.

Comparisons of ionizing irradiation sources (photons from X-rays or gamma rays) can be compared with UV irradiation, but with human exposure levels, these data are much less robust with respect to ionizing irradiation. One of the highest geographic elevations in the United States is that in Leadville, Colorado. Analysis of the data on cancer incidence and other late effects associated with ionizing irradiation in that location is complicated by the role of other variables: smoking history, genetic predisposition to cancer, and the presence in residents of other comorbid background diseases [12, 13]. The physical environment, where more robust data can be collected and interpreted is that with airline pilots, frequent flier passengers, and other personnel, who have spent a significant time at high altitudes [14, 15]. Most commercial airline altitudes are around 30,000–35,000 feet above sea level and are now known to be associated with a definite increase in level of exposure to ionizing irradiation [15]. These data have been published. Multiple attempts to correlate the cumulative level of radiation exposure at this altitude with incidence of late effects does lead to the same confounding variables, but more data are available. It can be concluded that there is a detectable increase in ionizing irradiation-induced effects in humans, who spend a significant amount of time in commercial airline travel. The controversy with interpretation of the data is whether it is "significant" with respect to effects on human health.

Higher levels of radiation exposure are present in individuals, who have spent time in the International Space Station or in the former Space Shuttle Program. These data are also published, but here the issue is the number of individuals in the study (Table 2.1) [18]. While there are potentially hundreds of thousands of airline passengers or airline employees studied, the numbers with respect to radiation exposure for these other groups are much less. How can all these data be translated into useful information that can be applied to the two areas of discussion in this book, namely, space irradiation and measurement of casualties from a willful (terrorist) or clandestine radiation terrorist event or nuclear reactor accident? For the planned Mars Mission, NASA has calculated the radiation exposure. There is controversy over when there will be a mission to Mars, but the data from robot dosimeters suggest that there will be 1.0 Gy cumulative dose from a planned 860-day mission [21].

Radiation Exposure Levels in Victims of Nuclear Accident, Military Exposure, and Experiments to Simulate Military Missions

All victims of unplanned radiation exposure are closely observed for decades (Table 2.1). One recommended answer to these questions is as follows: (1) Continue to make measurements and record data; (2) use of artificial intelligence (AI) algorithms may be useful in analyzing this data and should be considered; and (3) if analysis of data leads to the conclusion that levels of exposure are significantly associated with deleterious medical outcomes, then what radiation countermeasures can be safely delivered to individuals with a documented higher exposure level and higher risk of experiencing a deleterious outcomes?

The information from animal experiments will be used to predict outcome of radiation exposure to humans. The National Institutes of Health (NIH) had a "low dose rate" program for decades [19], and the results of such experiments are very interesting. Some animal experimental models have been designed to measure the effects of low dose rate. A particularly interesting technique was that used by Olipitz et al. [19], placing mice in an environment in which 600 times background irradiation was delivered by radioisotope liquid in a tray under the animal living cages. Measurements of single strand and double DNA strand breaks and other measures of radiation damage led to detectable, but insignificant changes from LDR exposure in this model. Analysis of the data from this study included recommendation for restriction of conclusions to the level of irradiation delivered by each of multiple gamma ray energies associated with the radioiodine degradation. In contrast, the data from other pioneering studies by Seed et al. [20] from the 1980 at Argonne National Laboratories showed that outbred beagle dogs, which had been placed in a room with continuous exposure to Cobalt 60 gamma ray irradiation over 2 years at 3–5 Roentgens in air daily (a dose roughly equivalent to 3–5 rads or Centigray irradiation), showed three significant and different categories of response. These studies in dogs showed that 1/3 of animals died from continuous exposure, over a two-year period due to bone marrow failure. The animals received 3–5 roentgens in air, and death was from drop in blood counts leading to anemia, leukopenia, thrombocytopenia, and overall bone marrow failure. This exposure level was roughly associated with daily 3–5 rad, Centigray total body dose, and these animals died of aplastic anemia that was manifested by progressively reduced peripheral blood cell counts leading to subsequent death. A second 1/3rd of the animals developed cancer, primarilymyeloid leukemia or erythroleukemia. The third cohort of 1/3rd of dogs survived. An interesting observation from these studies was the third group of animals showed "radio-accommodation" [20].

Adaptation of the animals that accommodated to continuous irradiation exposure showed that white blood cell counts dropped and then over time returned to normal levels. Although these animals showed signs of accelerated aging (graying of hair), they survived with the return of blood counts to the preirradiation normal range. Follow-up studies by Seed et al. [20] showed that these dogs with radio-accommodation displayed increased blood serum levels of colony-stimulating factor-1 (CSF-1 also called macrophage (M) M-CSF). These data may be very useful for understanding how to deal with individual human responses to irradiation. This topic will be discussed in the later chapters of this book.

Incomplete Data Collection Does Not Allow Precise Planning at This Stage

The conclusions from all of the available data indicate that space irradiation (including the moon habitat missions and the Mars Mission and beyond) must prepare to address radiation exposure levels. This will be a significant concern because the data on humans exposed to irradiation from first Earth—orbiting space vehicles, the moon landing, the International Space Station, and the shuttle program have provided enough evidence and enough follow-up data on these cohorts of individuals to show that the available early biomarkers of radiation exposure do lead to measurable medical events [21]. The most dominant of these is cataract formation in astronauts that has been observed and is detectable at earlier ages than that in the general population [14, 15].

While there is much less information with respect to airline travel and with humans living at high altitudes on the planet surface and including miners and other individuals working at depths in the Earth, where radon exposure level is higher, all the data needs to be collected and continually updated as we move forward. Confounding variables for analysis of data are the genetic outbred nature of humans, history of comorbid disease, medication history, and other medical conditions that may be additive or synergistic with radiation effects in an analysis of late effects of irradiation. What is helpful is the plethora of data on animal model systems that provide information on what to measure, whether it be incidence of cancer, neurocognitive deficits, neurological deficits, cataracts, bone loss, and other conditions (Table 2.3). A later chapter in this book on analysis of the data from irradiated nonhuman primates (NHP), mainly from Rhesus Macaque monkeys at the Wake Forest NHP Center, may prove to be very helpful to understand the magnitude of irradiation-induced deleterious medical events, and how these late effects of radiation exposure can be measured in humans.

At the present time, there are multiple examples of how the same radiation delivery techniques or exposure can be either hazardous or therapeutic depending on how the radiation is delivered and under what circumstances. Many of these examples seem contradictory, confusing, and inconsistent. Explanation of each will be provided in future chapters in an attempt to provide some clarity.

References

1. Reddy A, Conde C, Peterson C, et al. Residential radon exposure and cancer. Oncol Rev. 2022;16(1):558. https://doi.org/10.4081/oncol.2022.558.
2. National Radon Program Services, Kansas State University, 2323 Anderson Avenue, Suite 300, Manhattan, KS 66502.
3. Frane N, Bitterman A. Radiation safety and protection. In: StatPearls [Internet]. Treasure Island, FL: StatPearls Publishing; 2024, January 2023. Bookshelf ID: NBK557499.
4. Koh WJ, Abu-rustum NR, Bean S, et al. Uterine neoplasms, version 1,2018, NCCN clinical practice guidelines in oncology. J Natl Compr Cancer Netw. 2018;16(2):170–99. https://doi.org/10.6004/jnccn.2018.0006.
5. Andring LM, Corrigan KL, Rooney M, et al. Patient reported outcomes for women undergoing definitive chemoradiation for gynecologic cancer: a prospective clinical trial. Pract Radiat Oncol. 2023;13(6):e538–46. https://doi.org/10.1016/j.prro.2023.07.004.
6. Song J, Alyamani N, Bhattacharya G, et al. The impact of high-dose-rate brachytherapy: measuring clinical outcomes in the primary treatment of cervical cancer. Adv Radiat Oncol. 2020;5(3):419–25. https://doi.org/10.1016/j.adro.2020.02.003.
7. ALARA—As low as reasonably achievable. Radiation and Your Health, CDC Center for Disease Control and Prevention, May 17, 2002.
8. Pardue LA, Goldstein N, Wollan EO. Photographic film as a pocket radiation dosimeter. At Energy Biophys Biol Med. 1948;1(5):169.
9. Waltar AE, Reynolds AB. Fast breeder reactors. New York, NY: Pergamon Press. ISBN 978-0-08-025983-3. Archived https://web.archive.org/web/20140105044948/; http://books.google.com/books?id=4m6o1jMcIIIC from the original on 5 January 2014. Retrieved 4 June, 2016
10. Park ES, Moon K, Kim HN, et al. Radiation exposure and cancer mortality among nuclear power plant workers: a meta-analysis. J Prev Med Public Health. 2010;43(2):185–92. https://doi.org/10.3961/jpmph.2010.43.2.185.
11. Wagoner JK, Archer VE, Lundin FE, et al. Radiation as the cause of lung cancer among uranium miners. N Engl J Med. 1965;273:181–8. https://doi.org/10.1056/NEJM196507222730402.
12. Iannacone MR, Youlden DR, Baade PD, et al. Melanoma incidence trends and survival in adolescents and young adults in Queensland, Australia. Int J Cancer. 2015;136(3):603–9. https://doi.org/10.1002/ijc.28956.
13. Moeller DW, Sun L-SC. Comparison of natural background dose rates for residents of the Amargosa Valley, NV, to those in Leadville, CO, and the states of Colorado and Nevada. Health Phys. 2006;91(4):338–53. https://doi.org/10.1097/01.HPH.0000218426.41326.6d.
14. Reynolds R, Little MP, Day S, et al. Cancer incidence and mortality in the USA astronaut corps, 1959-2017. Occup Environ Med. 2021;78(12):869–75. https://doi.org/10.1136/oemed-2020-107143.
15. Scheibler C, Toprani SM, Mordukhovich I, et al. Cancer risks from cosmic radiation exposure in flight: a review. Front Public Health. 2022;10:947068. https://doi.org/10.3389/fpubh.2022.947068.
16. Case C Jr. 10 years of preparedness by the radiation injury treatment network. Curr Hematol Malig Rep. 2017;12(1):39–43. https://doi.org/10.1007/s11899-017-0360-7.

17. Little MP, Wakeford R, Tawn EJ, et al. Risks associated with low doses and low dose rates of ionizing radiation: why linearity may be (almost) the best we can do. Radiology. 2009;251(1):6–12. https://doi.org/10.1148/radiol.2511081686.
18. Seco J, Clasie B, Partridge M. Review on the characteristics of radiation detectors for dosimetry and imaging. Phys Med Biol. 2014;59(20):R303–47. https://doi.org/10.1088/0031-9155/59/20/R303.
19. Olipitz W, Wiktor-Brown D, Shuga J, et al. Integrated molecular analysis indicates undetectable DNA damage in mice after continuous irradiation at −400-fold natural background radiation. Environ Health Perspect. 2012;120(8):1130–6. https://doi.org/10.1289/ehp.1104294.
20. Seed T, Fritz TE, Tolle DV, et al. Survival patterns and hemopathological responses of dogs under continuous gamma irradiation. 1983. https://doi.org/10.1007/978-94-009-6048-0_9.
21. Hassler DM, Zeitlin C, Wimmer-Schweingruber RF, et al. Mars' surface radiation environment measured with the Mars science laboratory's curiosity rover. Science. 2014;343(6169):1244797. https://doi.org/10.1126/science.1244797.
22. Arhelger RB, Smith PN, Walker BL, et al. Influence of local abdominal radiation on response of rabbits to nephrotoxic serum. Am J Pathol. 1961;39(6):631–42.
23. King GL. Characterization of radiation-induced emesis in the ferret. Radiat Res. 1988;114(3):599–612.
24. Moroni M, Coolbaugh TV, Lombardini E, et al. Hematopoietic radiation syndrome in the Gottingen minipig. Radiat Res. 2011;176(1):89–101. https://doi.org/10.1667/rr2481.1.

Chapter 3
Genetic Mediators of Radiation Sensitivity and Radiation Resistance

There are two major disconnects in our understanding of ionizing irradiation. First is that the origin of species, which describes the evolution of life on planet Earth over the billions of years of adaptation. Organisms, speciation (origin of new species) [1–3], occured under conditions of a magnetosphere [4], which provided the protection of the surface of the planet from the majority of deleterious high-energy charged particles from galactic cosmic irradiation and solar proton events. The second disconnect is that we use irradiation to treat cancer and doses are prescribed by physicians who have a very different understanding of radiation safety.

There is an assumption that human beings can live in space outside the protective magnetosphere-if specific modifications in their radiation adaptation and radiation countermeasures administration can be organized and facilitated. This assumption must be addressed for safety with respect to astronauts and will be a challenge [4].

Ther must be an understanding of radiation dose and the importance of the relative biological effect (RBE) of different qualities of ionizing irradiation. Clinical radiation oncologists, are physicians who spend their lives treating patients with cancer, and are accustomed to understanding what a high dose of irradiation is compared to a low dose [5, 6]. However, these clinicians, who receive basic training in radiation biology during their residency programs, have their understanding of what a high dose of irradiation is. Therefore, when one sees data on measurements of space irradiation, from the Curiosity Mission to Mars experiments, and others in which ionization chambers and radiation detector devices were placed on the spacecraft and robotic landers on the surface of Mars, the doses reported seem low. The reported doses did not take into account the RBE and when interpreted by physicians, who are accustomed to clinical radiotherapy doses, the information appears to suggest that the radiation levels are "low" and that a mission to Mars would be safe. This information does not take into account the facts that the RBE of galactic cosmic irradiation, which are charged ions, which have not reached the Earth's surface for billions of years, because of the magnetosphere, is foreign to humans so human adaptaion to it cannot

J. Greenberger, *Radiation Oncology and Radiation Biology*,
https://doi.org/10.1007/978-3-031-66300-0_3

be assumed to be safe. The RBE must be factored into a measurement of radiation dose to be able to understand what is safe and what is not safe for humans.

This chapter will address the issue of understanding that the evolution of life on Earth, occurred during constant exposure to radiation levels that were filtered to create a "background radiation" to which all life forms adapted over billions of years. In his book *Origin of Species*, Charles Darwin established the principle of natural selection [1–3]. Organisms evolved under conditions in which those having a proliferative advantage in the current environment would survive, whereas those that had difficulty adapting would not. The natural selection process can understandably be slower with respect to organisms that have a long lifespan compared to those with rapid proliferation. Furthermore, the process of natural selection would necessarily take into account all of the environmental factors at play during the selection process. While this chapter deals with ionizing irradiation, the constant level of this variable over billions of years would be one factor to consider under conditions in which organisms would be evolving with changes in climate temperature, rainfall, volcanic activity, the availability of food supplies With more complex organisms predator to prey relationships and atmospheric conditions including relative availability of oxygen and decreased amounts of toxins in the atmosphere are factors that affect natural selection.

Evolution Under Constant Radiation

Each of multiple factors was occurring on planet Earth during the evolution of single-celled organisms to multicellular zooplankton and phytoplankton all within the ocean environment. Once, the migration of amphibians to land occurred for part of their life cycle the environmental factors on land also came into play, as well as, those in the ocean. Evolution led to reptiles that did not require return to the ocean for part of their life cycle nor did the evolution of mammals. Within the order Mammalia, there were three categories ranging from monotremes (egg-laying mammals that nursed their young—such as the duckbill platypus); then to marsupials, such as the Kangaroo, in which the step of the egg laying was bypassed to live birth, but in which newborns were totally dependent on physical contact with the mother for some time; and finally to placentals, in which gestation occurred in the female for much longer times until birth.

Mammalian Subtypes: Placentals

The evolution of the placenta cannot be minimized with respect to the robust survival capacity of this subdivision of mammals [7, 8]. The fact that the female could nurture and harbor within the body, the developing embryo until a late stage was only possible because of the powerful capacity of the placenta. The placenta functions as both an immunological organ and a physiological organ. The developing embryo is protected from infection and toxic influences by the immunological system in the placenta. Most importantly, the placenta functioned as liver and kidney processing metabolized nutrients from the mother's circulation to the developing embryo. The process of evolution and the importance of "survival of the fit" natural selection were slower under conditions in which a gestation inside the mother would occur for periods of 21 days for the mouse compared to 2 years for the elephant, and generations of natural selection would naturally take hundreds or thousands of years for a newly adapted creature to evolve. This time frame is in stark contrast to the rapid adaptation possible with single-cell bacteria that have a doubling time of 4 h [9]. The role of the environment in natural selection can be seen dramatically observed by this comparison of time of life cycle More complex species were selected for radiation repair and resistant genes as yeast [7, 8], flatworms [10], and insects [11]. These genes have been preserved during evolution [12].

The environment for bacteria in cell culture is precisely controlled by ambient oxygen and other volatile gasses, as well as, nutrients and other constituents in the medium, whether this be a laboratory culture tube or the ocean. Changes in the environment result in the selection of a resistant/adapted variant very quickly. For example, adding an antibiotic to the culture medium of bacteria and increasing the concentration of this antibiotic can result in the selection of antibiotic-resistant bacteria after periods as short as several weeks. A selected variant survives with complete resistance to that particular antibiotic. Contrast this evolutionary simplicity to the environment mammals such as the wooly mammoth, and the mastodon compared to the modern elephant. The gestation time of 2 years in the environment of a terrestrial mammal may change including levels of atmospheric oxygen, nutrients including availability of plants, food supply, and predators. So in contrast to bacteria it would take thousands of years of natural selection to evolve resistant mammals. In the case of these two predecessors of the modern elephant, the failure to adapt led to extinction.

Radiation in the Environment

What many scientists and evolutionary biologists often forget is that all of these changes on Earth for both the bacteria and the mammoth/mastodon/elephant occurred under conditions of ionizing irradiation at "background levels" [13]. These background levels included soil-based internal radiation emission from the natural decay of radium and radon, but also the external background radiation coming from those sources that penetrated the magnetosphere. What is also forgotten in this process is that there was the absence of significant galactic cosmic irradiation—charged particle and solar proton events—proton irradiation in the evolutionary process. X-irradiation from external sources including solar proton events that are proceeded by X-rays and other X-rays penetrating the magnetosphere levels was relatively constant as was the internal production of gamma rays from radioisotope decay from the Earth's core. While these events may seem trivial given the huge impact of other stresses that lead to adaptation and "survival of the fit," the fact becomes increasingly important as we leave the magnetosphere and astronauts in their space vehicle travel for extended times in the absence of the protective magnetosphere [4]. Furthermore, as will be described later in this book regarding space irradiation, adaptation to these new forms of irradiation with RBE that is incompletely understood will be required of the astronauts, who are also experiencing the conditions of weightlessness and other environmental stresses.

The evolution of life on Earth including the evolution of the molecular mechanisms of ionizing irradiation resistance and repair, occurred under conditions of minimal if any influence of solar proton events (proton irradiation) and galactic cosmic irradiation (radiation radioactive charged particles including iron, silicon, carbon, and others that were largely filtered by the magnetosphere). It must be understood that all discussions in this chapter; as well as, future chapters on the mechanism of ionizing irradiation damage repair and radiation resistance; as well as, the development of radiation countermeasures, radioprotective and radiation mitigator drugs, have been studied under conditions of the currently available organisms and animal models. All models have evolved in an environment with minimal or no influence of the RBE of galactic charged particles and protons.

The radiobiology response of humans to each of these forms of irradiation must be interpreted given the current conditions of background environmental irradiation on Earth.

Adaptation to Constant Radiation in the Environment

The recent scientific literature describes the hypothesized molecular mechanism of the appearance of the first nucleic acids and evolution and the creation of new species in plants and animals [1–3]. More difficult to explain is the molecular biologic basis for the evolution of major taxonomic categories that occurred over billions of years [2]. In the animal kingdom, it is well established from fossil evidence that life began in the oceans with the evolution of single-cell bacteria leading to multicellular zooplankton, then leading up to the class coelenterates, echinoderms, mollusks, then to vertebrates including cartilaginous fish, and finally, Osteichthyes (bonyfish). While natural selection is an established principle of the origin of species, it is unclear how this phenomenon applies to the origin of the major subgroups (classes) of the phyla. Evidence for the timing of genetic evolutionary steps is constantly being updated by new discoveries of fossils and evolutionary models [2] that bridge the gaps between the major taxonomic categories. The evolution of amphibians requires an understanding of what led oceanic species to evolve and migrate to land for reproduction. Next is the evolution of reptiles and then mammals, which is a consistent focus of paleontology. Here, there is an abundance of fossil evidence and new dating technologies in addition to radiocarbon dating. Recent evidence for the separation of theropod dinosaurs from the ancestral precursors of modern birds has also been in the literature. Evolutionary pressures led to natural selection and the generation of new taxonomic categories; however, this fact does not explain why some species of plants and animals persisted over billions of years, while others became extinct? For example, the persistence of crocodilians in the reptile taxonomic class of the animal kingdom and ferns in the plant kingdom are a continuing subject of curiosity.

As one reflects on the diversity of animal and plant species and their evolutionary history, the question remains as to how these events occurred over billions of years in an atmosphere on Earth that was exposed continually to multiple forms of ionizing irradiation, but not all forms. Evolution must have occurred with the biological consideration of survival in an irradiated environment. Even with the magnetosphere [4] protecting the Earth from solar proton events and galactic cosmic irradiation, and filtering out much of the X-rays reaching the Earth's surface, there must have been an evolutionary pressure overlaying all of these taxonomic changes that involved adaptation to ionizing irradiation. This adaptation was continual leading up to the evolution of non-human primates and humans.

The current scientific literature on the biology of cell division has led to astonishing conclusions regarding the conserved evidence of adaptation to ionizing irradiation. Cell death is caused by irradiation-induced breaks in double-stranded nuclear DNA [14–16]. There are over 1000 DNA double-strand breaks that occur with every mammalian cell division [14]. These breaks are repaired by a group of intranuclear enzymes called endogenous DNA repair enzymes that have been conserved during the billion years of the origin of life on Earth.

Over millenia, the process of DNA repair has also been involved in the creation of new species and involves gene mutations that must have given these mutants a survival advantage that has persisted during evolution [11]. Other mutations that were conserved have resulted in either a sensitivity to ionizing irradiation or radioresistance, which did not lead to a selective advantage in evolution, but which have persisted with respect to humans, who have these specific genes in their genome. Studies of individuals with these genes have provided insight into radiation biology, as well as, the evolution of species.

How these mutations affect the specialty of Clinical Medicine, which uses radiation to treat cancer, termed Radiation Oncology, and the current responses of some humans to irradiation is also relevant and very compelling.

Fanconi Anemia, Bloom's Syndrome, Nijmegen Break Syndrome, Ataxia-Telangiectasia, and Radiosensitivity

There are patients with genetic mechanisms of DNA repair deficiency [17–27].

Several genetic changes that cause radiosensitivity of humans were first discovered by the observation of select Radiation Oncology patients, who were receiving therapeutic irradiation. Analysis of their cells in culture led to the discovery of genes, which when mutated (altered) lead to the production of either absent or altered proteins that result in decreased DNA repair. There followed an analysis of the similarity of these gene mutations in those genes in other species, revealing that in some cases, these genetic mutations are also present in primitive taxa, including bacteria and yeast [12]. The fact that these mutations have persisted during evolutions and still occur in humans and are persistent provides evidence that they were and are non-lethal. Many mutations arise during embryogenesis and in experimental systems in which mutations are induced and are fatal resulting in gestational or embryonic death and some produce perinatal death of newborn animals. Lethal mutations are difficult to analyze due to the lack of ability to study both developability and with multiple future generations of animals. However, some mutations or genetic disorders, which are non-lethal, but are associated with radiosensitivity have been elucidated in great detail [18].

Fanconi Anemia was first described in children, who had several physical attributes associated with low red blood cell counts (anemia) [19, 20]. These children displayed short stature, sometimes the absence of thumbs, and had other physical abnormalities [19]. Anemia was associated with the sensitivity of the cells to DNA cross-linking agents, such as mitomycin-C, and a test of cells from FA patients for mitomycin-C sensitivity became a diagnostic criterion for this disorder [20]. Children with FA presented with rapid and often fatal anemia, and many died in the first decade of life [19]. In the 1980s, bone marrow transplantation became widely available to FA patients and resulted in the normalization of hematopoiesis and correction of the anemia in many; although, the toxicity of drugs to prepare patients for transplant of donor marrow was itself often fatal [20] in early clinical trials. The development of less toxic preparatory drugs such as Fludarabine made successful marrow transplants a realistic therapeutic option [20]. However, as will be described in future chapters of this book, the correction of the anemia in patients, who survived successful marrow transplants, uncovered other clinical problems from the FA genetic defects that were associated with mutations in the FA genes. The most serious of these other sequelae of FA is the sensitivity of these patients to the induction of cancer in multiple organs primarily in those of the aerodigestive system [5, 6, 28].

FA has been widely studied in part attributable to the multiple pathways leading to the phenotype of anemia [18]. To date, there have been over 23 genes involved in FA, which have been discovered [18], and which are mutated either singly or in combinations and lead to the clinical syndrome of FA. The genes that are altered in the diagnostic category of FA include those that produce a scaffold of proteins along DNA double-strand breaks within the cell nucleus (Fig. 3.1). The scaffold is located at the site, where DNA double-strand breaks occur—either at baseline conditions (1000 per cells division) or after exposure of cells to toxin including ionizing irradiation, the scaffold allows the attachment of DNA repair enzymes to repair DNA [14]. When the scaffold is defective, DNA repair cannot occur. Fanconi Anemia has been a subject of intense interest, not only because of the complexity of the genotype but also because of the phenotypic alterations/sequelae that occur during the process of effective DNA repair. Many, but not all, FA patients display a prominent sensitivity to irradiation.

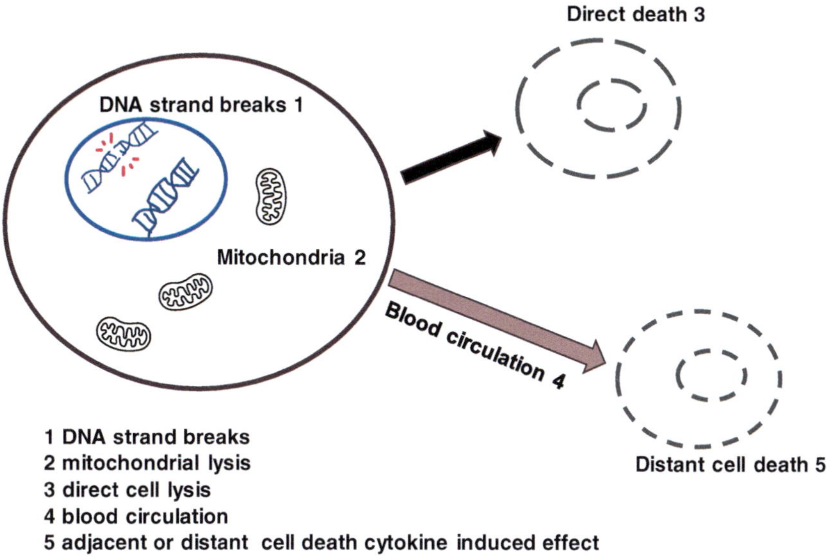

Fig. 3.1 Mechanisms of radiation-induced cell death. The figure demonstrates a cell nucleus (green), mitochondria (purple), and the methods by which radiation can induce cell death. These also represent targets for the generation of radiation protectors and radiation mitigators, as will be described in a future chapter. DNA strand breaks, mitochondrial lysis from transported messengers from the nucleus to the mitochondria including: p53, p21, BAX, and the differentiation of the direct effects, which cause cell lysis of the cell that is hit by irradiation, as well as, indirect effects, which affect cells that are either adjacent to the irradiated cell or distant and affected by inflammatory cytokines through the circulation

Why only some FA patients are radiosensitive and why only some display clinical features of short stature, absent thumbs, and other features remains a subject of investigation. Many older patients in their 30 s, 40 s, and 50 s have presented with cancer and the need for chemotherapy including the use of drugs that kill cancer cells by inducing DNA strand crosslinking [16] and clinical radiotherapy. Why such patients are found to have FA late in life and why only they are genotyped is attributable to their sensitivity to DNA-crosslinking drugs such as Cis-Platinum or Mitomycin-C, or radiation. There are reports of sensitivity to even low dose fractions of ionizing irradiation that have led to a diagnosis of FA by genotyping their peripheral blood cell. These studies of the complex mechanism of radiosensitivity in these patients are very enlightening. Recent data reveal that it is not simply the decrease in capacity for DNA double-strand break repair, but also the altered response of some FA patients to the response to radiation with altered and intense production of inflammatory cytokines and other regulatory molecules that exacerbate the tissue injury [29–31]. Ionizing irradiation induces multiple changes in individual cells, tissues, and organs. Many of these alterations are not directly related to DNA double-strand break repair but involve physiologic changes in both the directly irradiated and unirradiated tissues. Inflammatory cytokines are produced and released from cells that do not die but do respond to radiation. These events include the swelling of endothelial cells (cells lining blood vessels) and the rapid infiltration of irradiated tissues through the circulation of inflammatory macrophages, neutrophils, and other cells that have been attracted by cytokines. Infiltrating cells also release cytokines, which exacerbate the injury site/irradiated site. Accordingly, physicians have approached treating cancer in FA patients with caution and also by adding anti-inflammatory drugs that dampen the cytokine release. Bone marrow transplantation in FA patients corrected the defect of anemia and suggested that it is the bone marrow, which mediates the FA patients' radiosensitivity [20]. However, new discoveries made by scientists funded by the Fanconi Anemia Research Fund (FARF) have revealed that there is a pleotropic effect of the FA genotype. The FA phenotype is broad and not all components are observed in every patient. These pleotropic effects of a mutated FA gene include changes in cell-to-cell communications [28] and defects in organ function at multiple levels. All of these changes cannot be simply explained by a defect in DNA double-strand break repair. As with many other genetic disorders, there are silent carriers of each FA gene such that the disease persists and continues to be diagnosed over multiple generations.

Not all FA patients show radiosensitivity, and, thus, clinical trials have been established to allow radiation oncologists to determine, who needs a specific decreased radiation fractionation or field size modification of their treatment plan, and who does not. Radiation protector and radiation mitigator drugs have been evaluated in FA patients and suggest that the sequelae of defective DNA double-strand break repair is followed by alterations in the oxidative stress response in cells such that the delivery of antioxidants can be used therapeutically to modify the sensitivity of these patients to ionizing irradiation [28–31].

Bloom's Syndrome is a radiosensitivity phenotype, which is associated with a defective helicase, another DNA repair enzyme [25]. The presentation of patients with Bloom's Syndrome is more difficult to diagnose, and there are fewer patients, but the same issues are present.

Nijmegen Break Syndrome is another defect associated with an altered DNA repair capacity that is caused by a mutation in a specific gene [17] and as with some FA patients is associated with physical and physiologic alterations including microcephaly (small brain and skull size) and predisposition to some cancers including lymphomas. Other disorders are attributable to increased chromosome breaks and altered DNA repair [7, 8] including Ataxia-Telangiectasia [26]. Disease states that display altered DNA repair [7, 8] all are rare, and other non-fatal genetic-mediated disorders that induce radiosensitivity will undoubtedly be reported in the future. The late effects of irradiation are more complex (Fig. 3.2) and involve multiple organ-to-organ communications. The acute effects of irradiation are seen in the sensitivity of Fanconi Anemia cell lines and tissue to radiation (Figs. 3.3, 3.4, and 3.5).

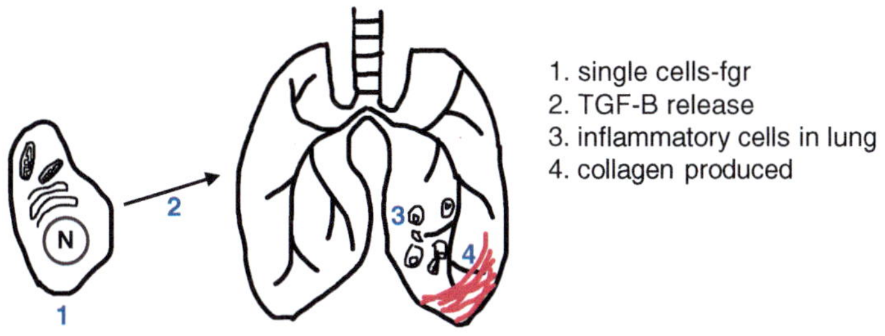

Fig. 3.2 Targets for decreasing radiation late effects. This figure demonstrates the targets of individual cells on the left, as well as, the organ-specific targets for secondary effects of irradiation. The figure demonstrates that single cells can release TGF-β, and other inflammatory cytokines that recruit inflammatory cells to the lung shown on the right [3]. The circulation [2] delivers cells and cytokines to the lungs. The final step in late effects is the deposition of collagen or other extracellular matrix proteins [4], casing fibrosis. All these steps are targets for radiation countermeasures, but also demonstrate the complexity of the late effects of irradiation

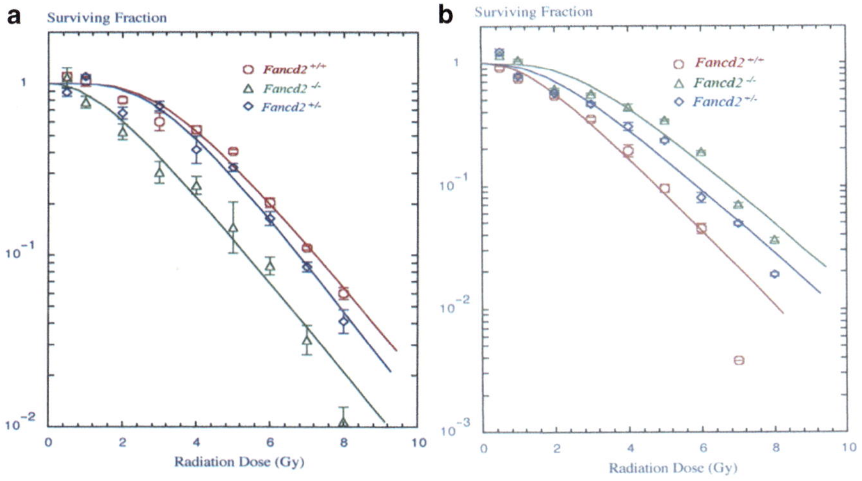

Fig. 3.3 Clonogenic radiation survival curves of *Fancd2−/−* (FVB/N) cell lines. Clonogenic radiation survival curves are shown for permanent bone marrow stromal (panel A) and interleukin 3 (IL-3)-dependent hematopoietic progenitor (panel B) cell lines derived from long-term bone marrow cultures established form whole bone marrow of 6- to 8-week-old [FVB/N (*Fancd2−/−*, *Fancd2+/−*, and *Fancd2+/+*)] mice. Cell lines were passaged in vitro for 2 months and clonal sublines established. Clonogenic radiation survival curves were performed using the single hit, multi-target model for bone marrow stromal cell lines (**panel a**) and IL-3-dependent hematopoietic progenitor cell lines (**panel b**). Results are shown in linear quadratic presentation as mean and standard error of the mean (SEM) of three separate experiments. D_0 and ñ were compared for statistically significant differences according to published methods [19]. From: Berhane H, Shinde A, Kalash R, et al. Amelioration of irradiation induced oral cavity mucositis and distant bone marrow suppression in *Fancd2−/−* (FVB/N) mice by intraoral JP4–039/F15. *Radiat Res.* 2014;182:35–49

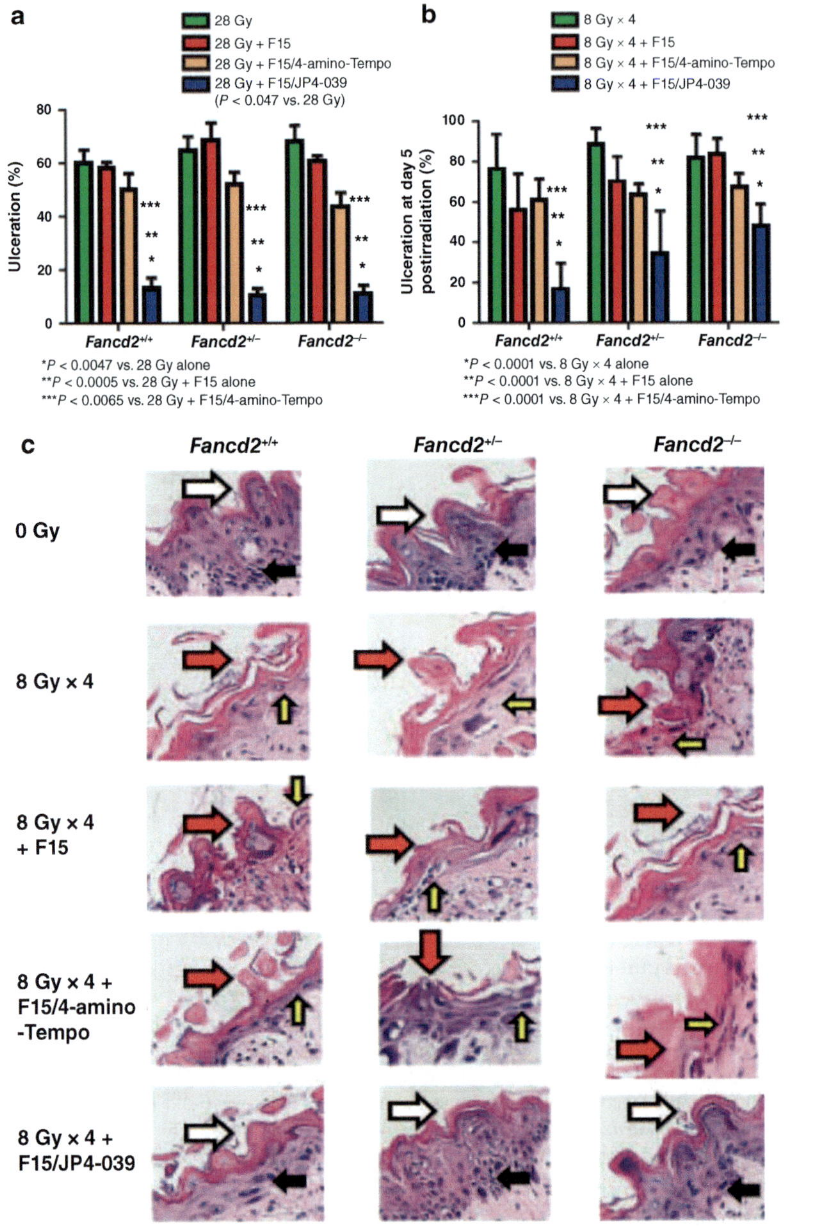

Fig. 3.4 F15/JP4–039 protects against mucositis induced by single fraction (28 Gy) and fractionated (8 Gy × 4) doses in *Fancd2−/−* mice. Nonirradiated tongue tissues were examined from *Fancd2+/+*, *Fancd2+/−*, and *Fancd2−/−* mice, as well as, tongue tissues irradiated with a single fraction (28 Gy, **panel a**) or fractionated dose (8 Gy × 4, **panel b**), with or without F15/JP4–039 pre-treatment (*$P < 0.0047$ compared with 28 Gy; *$P < 0.0001$ [20]). From: Shinde A, Berhane H, Rhieu BH, et al. Intraoral mitochondrial-targeted GS-nitroxide, JP4–039, radioprotects normal tissue in tumor-bearing radiosensitive *Fancd2−/−* (C57BL/6) mice. *Radiat Res.* 2016;185: 134–150

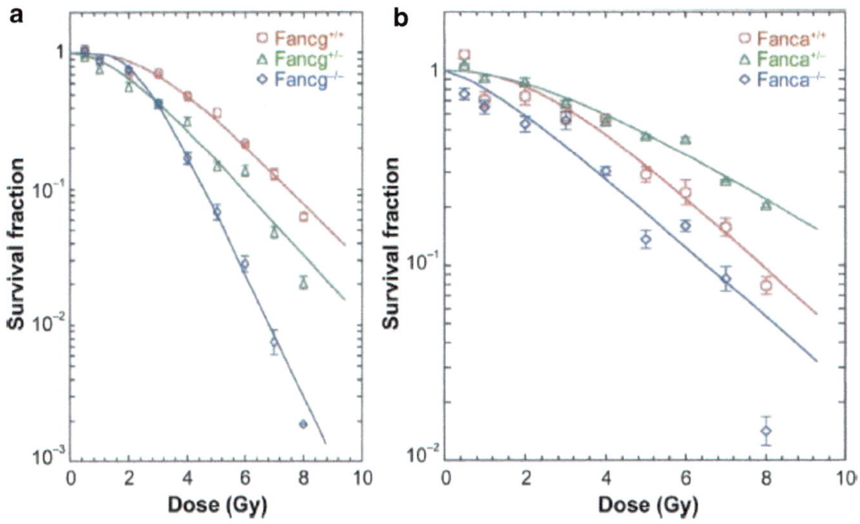

Fig. 3.5 Radiosensitivity of bone marrow stromal cell lines from Fancg−/− (**panel a**) and Fanca−/− (**panel b**) mice. Clonogenic radiation survival curves were performed, as described in Materials and Methods and shown in Table 3.1. From: Willis J, Epperly MW, Fisher R, et al. Amelioration of head and neck irradiation-induced mucositis and distant marrow suppression in Fanca−/− and Fancg−/− mice by intraoral administration of GS-nitroxide (JP4–039). *Radiat Res.* 2018;189: 560–578

Irradiation Hyper-Responders

Hyper-responder patients represent a category that is more complex. Radiation oncologists routinely document, during their weekly on-treatment visits, the presence of patients, who show radiation side effects earlier in a treatment course, and are, thus, labeled hyper-responders. The possible role of genetics in this category is much more difficult to elucidate since there is no association with one of the specific syndromes described above.

Current research with animal models may provide a clue to elucidating the mechanism of hyper-responders to therapeutic irradiation.

It is well known that inbred mouse and rat strains show different responses to total body irradiation. A series of experiments carried out with inbred mouse strains identified separate acute and late effects of irradiation [32]. Analysis of the genes involved in the late radiation fibrosis effect elucidated the chromosomal sites of genes that are associated with the radioresistance of C57BL/6 J mice compared to C3H/HeN mice. These two mouse strains have been widely used for decades in radiobiology experiments. The radioresistance of C57BL/6 J mice localizes to a segment of one chromosome by elegant experiments carried out by Travis et al. [33]. F1 hybrid mice (C57BL/6 J × C3H/HeN) F1, F2 hybrids, and backcrossed strains allowed her to find the focus on a specific chromosome, which predicted the radioresistance of C57BL/6 J mice. While the experiments did not lead to molecular cloning of the exact gene or genes on this site, the localization on this site of the gene for manganese superoxide dismutase (MnSOD) suggested that a difference in antioxidant functioning could explain the radioresistance of one mouse strain.

Oxidative stress is a known sequela of DNA double-strand breaks [34–44]. Cells that have an increased capacity to neutralize free radicals (created by the effective X-rays on water and oxygen) can decrease the number of DNA double-strand breaks, but also are involved in the production of oxidant molecules by dead and dying cells. Within irradiated tissues, there are cells that are repairing DNA single- and double-strand breaks and will display altered levels of biomarkers of oxidative stress [45–47]. These cells will release inflammatory cytokines that can induce DNA double-strand breaks in cells both close to irradiated tissue, but also at a distance arriving through the circulation. Thus, antioxidant therapies have been used to ameliorate ionizing radiation damaging effects. The first category of antioxidant responses in cells is the production of MnSOD [43]. This enzyme converts superoxide (a potent oxidative radical) to hydrogen peroxide, which is then acted upon by another enzyme catalase or glutathione peroxidase to form water [40]. Cells that are defective in MnSOD are radiosensitive [36]. Cells overexpressing MnSOD become normalized or radioresistant. To understand the action of an enzyme, which may confer radioresistance one must also understand the complexity of cellular responses to the absence of or the overproduction of a specific enzyme. The overexpression of one antioxidant enzyme may lead during gestation and animal development of the embryo, to the downregulation of other antioxidant molecules [38]. Thus, the condition of simply overexpressing MnSOD has been shown to in some cases not provide radioresistance.

During the gestation/embryogenesis of transgenic animals that overproduce increased levels of MnSOD, there may be downregulation of other antioxidant molecules such as catalase [40] or glutathione peroxidase [37] that are part of the natural response to oxidative stress. These enzymes function as a balanced system and in sequence. The overproduction of one component of the sequence may lead to compensatory decreased production in another so that the developing embryo can survive. This compensation is critically important, particularly, if increased levels of one component have deleterious effects on other developing systems.

Genetically Engineered Animals

The survival of a genetically engineered animal during embryonic development is complex; thus, an MnSOD overexpressing transgenic mouse may not be radioresistant due to the downregulation of other molecules [38]. The absence of MnSOD or another superoxide dismutase such as extracellular SOD or copper/zinc SOD (another metallo-enzyme) may lead to other possibilities of normalizing the overproduction of MnSOD [38] or the absence of MnSOD [39] (in the case of an engineered homologous recombinant negative-knockout mouse). What is apparent with transgenic and knockout animals is that the acute delivery of extra MnSOD to animals prior to

Table 3.1 Cell death pathways activated by ionizing irradiation

Pathways	Activator	Inhibitor	Reference
Apoptosis	Caspases	GS-Nitroxide	[51]
Necrosis	TNF-α	Necrostatin	[51]
Ferroptosis	15LOX/PEBP1	Bicalein Ferroloxin	[52]
Pyroptosis	Gastermin-0 Activator	Block Gastermin	[55]
Parthanatos	Mitochondrial PARP	Nito-targeted PARP inhibitor	[54]
Mitochondrial catastrophe	Caspase-2 activation	Caspase inhibitor	[56]

irradiation can be therapeutic and will overload them with a protective shield at just the correct time before exposure to irradiation [48, 49]. The animals that receive locally delivered MnSOD show a decreased toxicity of localized irradiation to that specific organ such as lung [36, 44], esophagus [43], intestine [46], bladder [49], or oral cavity [44]. Delivery of a radioprotective enzyme such as MnSOD or catalase acutely provides protection if delivered immediately before exposure to irradiation. Delivery of the protein MnSOD enzyme after irradiation is less effective than delivery of the transgene that produces RNA and protein inside the cells and suggests that it is functioning of MnSOD as a "shield," which should only be valuable if the shield is held up at the appropriate intracellular site, in the case of MnSOD; at the mitochondria, the cellular cytoplasmic organelle, which are the engines for the production of energy; and at the time of prior to irradiation. Thus, MnSOD delivered as a transgene is a radiation protector. In contrast, a radiation mitigator drug is that which is delivered after irradiation but before the development of major tissue injury and the associated symptoms of that injury. Radiation mitigators for humans represent a more complicated approach to understanding radioresistance or radiosensitivity because once irradiation has been delivered, DNA strand breaks and associated consumption of antioxidant stores begins to occur, the interruption of the process leading to cell, tissue, and organ death is more difficult to stop or to ameliorate. There are several pathways of radiation-induced cell death (Table 3.1) and small molecules have been developed to target and potentially neutralize each pathway [50–56]. New pathways are evolving [57] and may include some for for radioresistance as well as more complex biological processes [58].

Radiation Resistance

Radioresistance is much more difficult to define by genetic examples. Why are some animal and plant species resistant to irradiation? Unlike the clear mechanism of radiosensitivity by a defect in DNA double-strand break repair, radioresistance of an animal or plant is more difficult to explain. Background levels of irradiation have recently been studied [13] and increasing levels of exposure to 400 times background lead to little change in DNA double-strand breaks using current methods of calculation [13].

Attempts to associate animal or plant size with radioresistance have not led to a clear correlation. Insects show significant radioresistance (Phylum Arthropod); whereas other small animals including flatworms, roundworms, and segmented worms (phylum platyhelminthes, phylum rotundum, and phylum annilida, respectively) do not. Within each phylum, there are differences in the irradiation sensitivity of species. There has been relatively little research in these many areas since genetic analysis has been easier to approach by comparing human cells with those in very primitive single-celled organisms such as bacteria or yeast. The basis for the comparative study of single-celled organisms with humans, such a divergence of species, perhaps, can be explained by the conserved nature of many of the radiation repair genes and oxidative stress response genes [11]. Furthermore, the ability to rapidly clone and select bacteria and yeast led to the discovery of multiple gene categories that can be isolated in bacteria and yeast and also were found in human cells. Radioresistant bacteria and yeast have been the mainstay of the study of the molecular biology of DNA double-strand break repair [9]. As described in a previous chapter, the isolation of *Deinococcus radiodurans* [9] is a prime example of how the rapid proliferation and genetic selection in bacteria can be used to quickly isolate variance with the amplification of radiation repair genes. There are examples of radioresistance in other species. Studies with *Drosophila melanogaster* (Fruitfly) [11] and *Caenorhabditis elegans* [10] have also been valuable in the rapid selection of clonal variants with mutated radiation repair genes and the ease of selection and isolation of radiation resistance variants. Most recently, experiments with zebrafish [50] led to the isolation of ionizing radiation resistant variants and the demonstration that fish models can develop radiation fibrosis, a late effect of irradiation that can lead to genetic understanding of the mechanism of this late effect.

Most important to the understanding of radiation sensitivity and radioresistance in humans apart from the examples of genetic mechanisms is the observation of the effect of polypharmacy in humans. Most humans, who present to radiation oncologists for radiation therapy, are taking medication, and in some cases, have been on medications for decades. Patients with Diabetes Mellitus, Hypertension, and chronic auto-inflammatory diseases requiring steroidal or non-steroidal anti-inflammatory drugs may show different pattern of response to irradiation. Physicians have to carefully watch each patient separately and must be vigilant and aware of the presence of radiation side effects that can appear earlier than the typical time of presentation in most patients. Calling such a patient a hyper-responder would not apply to someone taking a chemotherapy drug (such as Mitomycin-C, Adriamycin, or Cis-Platinum), which is known to induce radiosensitivity. Other drugs taken for an unrelated clinical diagnosis can induce radiation sensitivity and cannot be related to a specific genetic disorder [23]. However, the knowledge that a patient has Fanconi Anemia or Bloom's Syndrome would alert the radiation oncologist to expect an earlier response and potentially change the treatment plan accordingly.

Radiosensitivity and radioresistance are very complicated phenomena, and the subject of multiple ongoing basic science and clinical/medical studies.

Complexity of Radiation Resistance

Even a specific genetic mutation that is associated with radiosensitivity may not show equivalent penetrance or clinical expression in different individuals. Genetic penetrance is described as the effect of a gene alteration on the phenotype of the individual. Some patients with Fanconi Anemia are diagnosed late in life, in the fourth or fifth decade of life, when they present with cancer that requires administration of a drug that kills cancer by DNA cross-linking. One such drug is Cis-Platinum. Several patients have been found to display a genetic pattern of alterations consistent with Fanconi Anemia after they have started treatment with Cis-Platinum for an unrelated disease [23]. Then, the patients are genotyped and found to display a pattern of Fanconi Anemia in their genotype. These patients may have lived for years with no anemia and no other phenotypic signs that are typical of the first pediatric patients diagnosed with FA as described above. Genetic penetrance is a phenomenon that complicates diagnosis of the mechanism of radiation sensitivity or radiation resistance.

As in many clinical disorders, physicians must be wary of individual patient responses to radiotherapy.

Further experiments with animal model systems should pave the way for elucidating many more aspects of radiosensitivity and radioresistance.

References

1. Robertson MP, Joyce GF. The origins of the RNA world. Cold Spring Harb Perspect Biol. 2012;4(5):a003608. https://doi.org/10.1101/cshperspect.a003608.
2. Steyskal GC. Trend curves of the rate of species description in zoology. Science. 1965;149(3686):880–2. https://doi.org/10.1126/science.149.3686.880.
3. Tessler M, Neumann JS, Kamm K, et al. Phylogenomics and the first higher taxonomy of Placozoa, an ancient and enigmatic animal phylum. Front Ecol Evol. 2022;10:1–18. https://doi.org/10.3389/fevo.2022.1016357.
4. Borovsky JE, Valdivia JA. The Earth's magnetosphere: a systems science overview and assessment. Surv Geophys. 2018;39(5):817–59. https://doi.org/10.1007/s10712-018-9487-x.
5. Gardner UG Jr, Wood SG, Chen EY, et al. Use of a therapeutic trial of graduated neoadjuvant radiotherapy for locally advanced esophageal cancer in a patient with Fanconi anemia. Adv Radiat Oncol. 2021;7(1):100810. https://doi.org/10.1016/j.adro.2021.100810.
6. Lewis LM, Tang AL, Wise-Draper TM, et al. Successful use of a therapeutic trial of graduated volume and dose escalation for postoperative head and neck radiotherapy in a Fanconi anemia patient. Head Neck. 2020;42(10):E16–22. https://doi.org/10.1002/hed.26395.
7. Burton GJ, Fowden AL. The placenta: a multifaceted, transient organ. Philos Trans R Soc Lond Ser B Biol Sci. 2015;370(1663):20140066. https://doi.org/10.1098/rstb.2014.0066.
8. Bennett CB, Lewis LK, Karthikeyan G, et al. Genes required for ionizing radiation resistance in yeast. Nat Genet. 2001;29(4):426–34. https://doi.org/10.1038/ng778.
9. Battista JR. Against all odds: the survival strategies of Deinococcus radiodurans. Ann Rev Microbiol. 1997;51:203–24. https://doi.org/10.1146/annurev.micro.51.1.203.
10. Ha NM, Tran SH, Shim Y-H, et al. Caenorhabditis elegans as a powerful tool in natural product bioactivity research. Appl Biol Chem. 2022;65:18. https://doi.org/10.1186/s13765-022-00685-y.

11. Tolwinski NS. Introduction: drosophila-a model system for developmental biology. J Dev Biol. 2017;5(3):9. https://doi.org/10.3390/jdb5030009.
12. Gogarten JP, Olendzenski L. Orthologs, paralogs, and genome comparisons. Curr Opin Genet Dev. 1999;9(6):630–6. https://doi.org/10.1016/s0959-437x(99)00029-5.
13. Olipitz W, Wiktor-Brown D, Shuga J, et al. Integrated molecular analysis indicates undetectable DNA damage in mice after continuous irradiation at −400-fold natural background radiation. Environ Health Perspect. 2012;120(8):1130–6. https://doi.org/10.1289/ehp.1104294.
14. Cannan WJ, Pederson DS. Mechanisms and consequences of double-strand DNA break formation in chromatin. J Cell Physiol. 2016;231(1):3–14. https://doi.org/10.1002/jcp.25048.
15. Kaina B. A genome-wide screening for DNA repair genes: much more players than hitherto known. Signal Transduct Target Ther. 2020;5(1):204. https://doi.org/10.1038/s41392-020-00314-4.
16. Hershberg R. Mutation-the engine of evolution: studying mutation and its role in the evolution of bacteria. Cold Spring Harb Perspect Biol. 2015;7(9):a018077. https://doi.org/10.1101/cshperspect.a018077.
17. Digweed M, Sperling K. Nijmegen breakage syndrome: clinical manifestation of defective response to DNA double-strand breaks. DNA Repair (Amst). 2004;3(8–9):1207–17. https://doi.org/10.1016/j.dnarep.2004.03.004.
18. Walden H, Deans AJ. The Fanconi anemia DNA repair pathway: structural and functional insights into a complex disorder. Annu Rev Biophys. 2014;43:257–78. https://doi.org/10.1146/annurev-biophys-051013-022737.
19. Alter BP, Giri N, McReynolds LJ, et al. Fanconi anaemia: a syndrome with distinct subgroups. Br J Haematol. 2022;197(4):467–74. https://doi.org/10.1111/bjh.18091.
20. Gluckman E, Auerbach AD, Horowitz MM, et al. Bone marrow transplantation for Fanconi anemia. Blood. 1995;86(7):2856–62.
21. Rodriguez A, Epperly M, Filiatrault J, et al. TGFβ pathway is required for viable gestation of Fanconi anemia embryos. PLoS Genet. 2022;18(11):e1010459. https://doi.org/10.1371/journal.pgen.1010459.
22. Rodriguez A, Zhang K, Farkkila A, et al. MYC promotes bone marrow stem cell dysfunction in Fanconi anemia. Cell Stem Cell. 2021;28(1):33–47. https://doi.org/10.1016/j.stem.2020.09.004.
23. Zatterale A, Calzone R, Renda S, et al. Identification and treatment of late onset Fanconi's anemia. Haematologica. 1995;80(6):535–8.
24. Rodriguez A, Yang C, Furutani E, et al. Inhibition of TGFβ1 and TGFβ3 promotes hematopoiesis in Fanconi anemia. Exp Hematol. 2021;93:70–84. https://doi.org/10.1016/j.exphem.2020.11.002.
25. Keller C, Keller KR, Shew SB, et al. Growth deficiency and malnutrition in bloom syndrome. J Pediatr. 1999;134(4):472–9. https://doi.org/10.1016/s0022-3476(99)70206-4.
26. Sirajwala AA, Khan S, Rathod V, et al. Ataxia-telangiectasia: a case report and a brief review. Cureus. 2023;15(5):e39346. https://doi.org/10.7759/cureus.39346.
27. Hasbaoui BE, Elyajouri A, Abilkassem R, et al. Nijmegen breakage syndrome: case report and review of literature. Pan Afr Med J. 2020;35:85. https://doi.org/10.11604/pamj.2020.35.85.14746.
28. Chihanga T, Vicente-Muoz S, Ruiz-Torres S, et al. Head and neck cancer susceptibility and metabolism in Fanconi anemia. Cancers (Basel). 2022;14(8):2040. https://doi.org/10.3390/cancers14082040.
29. Berhane H, Shinde A, Kalash R, et al. Amelioration of irradiation induced oral cavity mucositis and distant bone marrow suppression in Fancd2−/− (FVB/N) mice by intraoral JP4-039/F15. Radiat Res. 2014;182(1):35–49. https://doi.org/10.1667/RR13633.1.
30. Shinde A, Berhane H, Rhieu BH, et al. Intraoral mitochondrial-targeted GS-nitroxide, JP4-039, radioprotects normal tissue in tumor-bearing radiosensitive Fancd2−/− (C57BL/6) mice. Radiat Res. 2016;185(2):134–50. https://doi.org/10.1667/RR14035.1.

31. Willis J, Epperly MW, Fisher R, et al. Amelioration of head and neck irradiation-induced mucositis and distant marrow suppression in Fanca−/− and Fancg−/− mice by intraoral administration of GS-nitroxide (JP4-039). Radiat Res. 2018;189(6):560–78. https://doi.org/10.1667/RR14878.1.
32. Kalash R, Berhane H, Au J, et al. Differences in irradiated lung gene transcription between fibrosis-prone C57BL/6NHsd and fibrosis-resistant C3H/HeNHsd mice. In Vivo. 2014;28(2):147–71.
33. Haston CK, Travis EL. Murine susceptibility to radiation-induced pulmonary fibrosis is influenced by a genetic factor implicated in susceptibility to bleomycin-induced pulmonary fibrosis. Cancer Res. 1997;57(23):5286–91.
34. Kagan VE, Tyurina YY, Vlasova II, et al. Redox epiphospholipidome in programmed cell death signaling: catalytic mechanisms and regulation. Front Endocrinol (Lausanne). 2021;11:628079. https://doi.org/10.3389/fendo.2020.628079.
35. Rwigema J-CM, Beck B, Wang W, et al. Two strategies for the development of mitochondrial-targeted small molecule radiation damage mitigators. Int J Radiat Oncol Biol Phys. 2011;80(3):860–8. https://doi.org/10.1016/j.ijrobp.2011.01.059.
36. Epperly MW, Gretton JE, Bernarding M, et al. Mitochondrial localization of copper/zinc superoxide dismutase (Cu/ZnSOD) confers radioprotective functions in vitro and in vivo. Radiat Res. 2003;160:568–78.
37. Epperly MW, Melendez A, Zhang X, et al. Mitochondrial targeting of a catalase transgene product by plasmid liposomes increases radioresistance in vitro and in vivo. Radiat Res. 2009;171:588–95. https://doi.org/10.1667/RR1424.1.
38. Epperly MW, Travis EL, Whitsett JA, et al. Overexpression of manganese superoxide dismutase (MnSOD) in whole lung or alveolar type II (AT-II) cells of MnSOD transgenic mice does not provide intrinsic lung irradiation protection. Int J Cancer. 2001;96(1):11–21. https://doi.org/10.1002/1097-0215(20010220)96:1<11::aid-ijc2>3.0.co:2-r.
39. Epperly MW, Epstein CJ, Travis EL, et al. Decreased pulmonary radiation resistance of manganese superoxide dismutase (MnSOD)-deficient mice is corrected by human manganese superoxide dismutase-plasmid/liposome (SOD2-PL) intratracheal gene therapy. Radiat Res. 2000;154(4):365–74. https://doi.org/10.1667/0033-7587(2000)154[0365:dprrom]2.0.co:2.
40. Nandi A, Yan L-J, Jana CK, et al. Role of catalase in oxidative stress- and age-associated degenerative diseases. Oxidative Med Cell Longev. 2019;2019:9613090. https://doi.org/10.1155/2019/9613090.
41. Epperly MW, Travis EL, Sikora C, et al. Magnesium superoxide dismutase (MnSOD) plasmid/liposome pulmonary radioprotective gene therapy: modulation of irradiation-indued mRNA for IL-1, TNF-α, and TGF-β correlates with delay of organizing alveolitis/fibrosis. Biol Blood Marrow Transplant. 1999;5(4):204–14. https://doi.org/10.1053/bbmt.1999.v5.pm10465100.
42. Epperly MW, Defilippi S, Sikora C, et al. Intratracheal injection of manganese superoxide dismutase (MnSOD) plasmid/liposomes protects normal lung but not orthotopic tumors from irradiation. Gene Ther. 2000;7(12):1011–8. https://doi.org/10.1038/sj.gt.3301207.
43. Stickle RL, Epperly MW, Klein E, et al. Prevention of irradiation-induced esophagitis by plasmid/liposome delivery of the human manganese superoxide dismutase (MnSOD) transgene. Radiat Oncol Investig. 1999;7(4):204–17. https://doi.org/10.1002/(SICI)1520-6823(1999)7:4<204::AID-RO12>3.0.CO:2-S.
44. Guo HL, Seixas-Silva JA, Epperly MW, et al. Prevention of irradiation-induced oral cavity mucositis by plasmid/liposome delivery of human manganese superoxide dismutase (MnSOD) transgene. Radiat Res. 2003;159(3):361–70. https://doi.org/10.1667/0033-7587(2003)159[0361:porioc]2.0.co:2.
45. Carpenter M, Epperly MW, Agarwal A, et al. Inhalation delivery of manganese superoxide dismutase-plasmid/liposomes (MnSOD-PL) protects the murine lung from irradiation damage. Gene Ther. 2005;12(8):685–93. https://doi.org/10.1038/sj.gt.3302468.

46. Guo HL, Wolfe D, Epperly MW, et al. Gene transfer of human manganese superoxide dismutase protects small intestinal villi from radiation injury. J Gastrointest Surg. 2003;7(2):229–35. https://doi.org/10.1016/s1091-255x(02)00186-5.
47. Greenberger JS, Epperly MW. Radioprotective antioxidant gene therapy: potential mechanisms of action. Gene Therapy Mol Biol. 2004;8:31–44.
48. Epperly MW, Bray JA, Kraeger S, et al. Prevention of late effects of irradiation lung damage by manganese superoxide dismutase gene therapy. Gene Ther. 1998;5(2):196–208. https://doi.org/10.1038/sj.gt.3300580.
49. Kanai AJ, Zeidel ML, Lavelle JP, et al. Manganese superoxide dismutase gene therapy protects against irradiation-induced cystitis. Am J Physiol Renal Physiol. 2002;283(6):F1304–12. https://doi.org/10.1152/ajprenal.00228.2002.
50. Epperly MW, Bahary N, Quader M, et al. The zebrafish—Danio rerio—is a useful model for measuring the effects of ionizing irradiation. In Vivo. 2012;26(6):889–97.
51. Steinman J, Epperly M, Hou W, et al. Improved total-body irradiation survival by delivery of two radiation mitigators that target distinct cell death pathways. Radiat Res. 2018;189(1):68–83. https://doi.org/10.1667/RR14787.1.
52. Thermozier S, Hou W, Zhang X, et al. Anti-ferroptosis drug enhances total body irradiation mitigation by drugs that block apoptosis and necroptosis. Radiat Res. 2020;193(5):435–50. https://doi.org/10.1667/RR15486.1.
53. Simeonov A, Marugan J, Mallampalli RK, et al. Discovering selective antiferroptotic inhibitors of the 15LOX/PEBP1 complexes non-interfering with biosynthesis of lipid mediators. Proc Natl Acad Sci USA. 2023;120(25):e2218896120. https://doi.org/10.1073/pnas.2218896120.
54. Krainz T, Du L, Lewis T, et al. Synthesis and evaluation of a mitochondria-targeting poly(ADP-ribose) polymerase-1 inhibitor. ACS Chem Biol. 2018;13(10):2868–79. https://doi.org/10.1021/acschembio.8b00423.
55. Man SM, Karki R, Kanneganti T-D. Molecular mechanisms and functions of pyroptosis, inflammatory caspases and inflammasomes in infectious diseases. Immunol Rev. 2017;277(1):61–75. https://doi.org/10.1111/imr.12534.
56. Castedo M, Perfettini J-L, Roumier T, et al. Cell death by mitotic catastrophe: a molecular definition. Oncogene. 2004;23(16):2825–37. https://doi.org/10.1038/sj.onc.1207528.
57. Grandchamp A, Berk K, Dohmen E, et al. New genomics signals underlying the emergence of human proto-genes. Genes (Basel). 2022;13(2):284. https://doi.org/10.3390/genes13020284.
58. Stankowski S, Zagrodzka ZB, Garlovsky MD, et al. The genetic basis of a recent transition to live-bearing in marine snails. Science. 2024;383(6678):114–9. https://doi.org/10.1126/science.adi2982.

Chapter 4
Approaches to Understanding Radiobiologic Consequences of Space Travel: Shuttle Missions, International Space Station, and NASA Approach to Research TRISH Programs

The issue of space radiation is prominent as a focus for research at multiple levels. For the present geopolitical situation, planned space travel and planning for space missions are critical to the national interest. The issue is important because of the military consequences of a potential organized or terrorist threat to the satellite programs in the United States, which are necessary for communications and management of both domestic and military event coordination. The issue is also critical to all scientists, who explore new avenues of discovering alternative fuel supplies by mining operations on the moon and distant sites and for learning how to plan for human life in extra-terrestrial environments. In the past decades, the focus on lunar landings has included the potential for use of the moon as a strategic base for launching space missions of longer duration, but also for mining operations. There is increasing interest in the moon as a source of minerals and potential fuel supplies for dwindling resources on planet Earth has been a priority. The planning for a human Mars mission has been discussed at many levels [1–5]. At present, the consensus is that the next NASA-funded mission will be for a lunar landing and associated missions with multiple sorties from a habitat to explore other regions on the moon. The next space missions that are conducted under the auspices of NASA), another national or international consortia of nations, or even the private sector collaborations will require planning for the effects of space radiation.

There are over 100 individuals, who have experienced long exposure to space radiation [6–11]. These are the astronauts, who have spent time on the International Space Station (the longest duration being over 1 year), and others, who have carried out space shuttle missions and, of course, the Apollo astronauts, who carried out the first moon landings. These individuals have been exposed to irradiation sources outside the magnetosphere on the Earth, and their medical follow-up is providing valuable information on the consequences of radiation exposure. Cataract formation has been a common medical observation, and the concern for potential earlier neurocognitive deficits and induction of cancer has been a focus of the physicians, who continue surveillance programs on astronauts [12–18]. While there have been no

J. Greenberger, *Radiation Oncology and Radiation Biology*,
https://doi.org/10.1007/978-3-031-66300-0_4

reports of unexpected medical effects of space radiation exposure to date, there remains concern of a magnitude enough to motivate some scientists to predict that "humans can never live in space" [19].

Countermeasures for Space Radiation

What are the major issues regarding space radiation and the development of countermeasures? Humans have demonstrated resilience to adapt to harsh environments on Earth. These examples include adaptation to low oxygen concentrations from mountain living and living at high altitudes, such as Leadville, CO, or a high altitude at other locations on Earth including the Himalayas, and Tibet [15, 20–23]. Adaptation to life in low oxygen concentration is associated with an increase in hemoglobin production by red cells from the bone marrow to improve the oxygenation kinetics of hemoglobin. However, there are examples of the failed ability of humans to adapt to harsh environments. Individuals living in areas that have been contaminated by biological waste, chemical spills, or biological agents, as in the case of infectious agent pandemics during the recent COVID-19 pandemic have shown difficulty in adaptation [24]. Of particular concern is the issue of continuous low-dose rate radiation exposure [25–29].

History reveals the challenges for humans. Records of the plagues caused by *Yersinia pestis* including that in Drobrovnek, the introduction of a novel pathogen into an environment can result in a disastrous loss of life including an estimated reduction of one-third of the European population in the thirteenth century. Contagious agents have contributed to genocide in the case of the spread of smallpox, Typhus, and other agents throughout the indigenous people (Native Americans) in populations of the United States in the years following 1870. While the analogy to infectious agents may seem inappropriate as a comparison for space irradiation, the adaptation of humans to a foreign environment does not always occur spontaneously and efficiently as in the high-altitude adaptation of humans to low oxygen concentrations.

Adaptation of humans to space irradiation will present several novel problems. For those astronauts, who lived on the International Space Station for periods as long as a year, their successful adaptation to weightlessness, isolation, and space radiation is encouraging. However, this one-year radiation exposure must be contrasted to the several billion years of the evolution of life on planet Earth, which led to the evolution of mammals and *Homo sapiens*. This evolution was dictated in part by the concept of "survival of the fit" and natural selection. Natural selection was associated with the selection of genes for survival but some of these gene functions have led to deleterious but nonlethal consequences. One recent example is the published information on genes associated with the extinct Homo Neanderthal population. Genes that were associated with the adaptation of Neanderthals to low temperature and harsh environmental conditions that were passed down through the intra-breeding of Neanderthals with *Homo Sapiens* have been shown to be associated with psychiatric and other medical disorders.

During the billions of years of evolution on Earth, some species have become extinct and usually demonstrated a history of inability to survive in an environment in which other environmental changes produced new predators, or there was climate change or significant change in the food supply. Not all adaptations to a changing environment have been successful and the reasons may not be easily attributable to one factor.

The presence of natural selection has led to the creation of new species or other evolutionary changes, which may take hundreds of thousands of generations. The example of natural selection of a radioresistant bacteria *Deinococcus radiodurans* is one example, but thousands of generations of bacteria were required to select the radioresistant variant. With single-cell bacteria and a doubling time of 4 h, the selection could be achieved within weeks to months. Because of the doubling time of this bacterial strain, which is hours, the "evolution" was fast. In contrast, multicellular mollusks (snail) ware demonstrated to transition from egg laying to live generation by a process calculated to take over 200,000 generations. Thus, in the animal kingdom adaptation is an evolutionary process as documented by not only the fossil record but also laboratory experiments. In contrast, the adaptation of humans to life at high altitudes or in a toxic environment may not easily occur in a single generation.

Challenges for Astronauts

Astronauts, who will be on the space vessel for the first mission to Mars will experience at least 836 days outside the Earth's magnetosphere according to the estimate in the publication on the Mars Curiosity Mission [8–10, 30–33]. While this duration may only be twice that of the longest space mission to date on the International Space Station, the Mars Mission will undoubtedly produce data that will be of value for future missions that go even further and will be of longer duration. The development of radiation countermeasures will focus on expectations from prolonged exposure to space ionizing irradiation [25]. Two concepts should be of continual focus: (1) duration of exposure [6, 7, 18] and (2) quality of irradiation [34–44]. There have been experiments on exposure to continuous low-dose rate irradiation [25]. In experimental systems in which animals were exposed to continuous low-dose rate irradiation, these experiments used gamma irradiation emitting isotopes or X-rays [25]. The duration of these experiments was long enough to provide useful information but was limited to gamma radiation (X-rays). Using higher daily dose exposure for periods over 2 years, the work at Argonne Laboratories in the 1980s giving 3–5 Roentgens in air (3–5 rad per day) to out-bred beagle dogs provided more alarming and serious information since two thirds of the animals died within 2 years of bone marrow failure or leukemia. These experiments were carried out with a gamma irradiation emitter source from a centrally located Cobalt 60 radiation isotope.

Continuous low dose rates and sporadic exposure to proton irradiation and heavy charged particles as in the case of galactic cosmic irradiation (GCR) have not been studied in experimental animals for reasons of both cost and practicality. Therefore, the first data that will be obtained from prolonged exposure (over 1 year) to space radiation will be derived from the coming human space missions. What are the radiobiological concerns? The best data on the radiobiological effects of different forms of ionizing irradiation have come from clinical radiotherapy [34–46].

Even the robust data from clinical use of different radiation sources cannot simulate the data expected from long-term exposure to sporadic GCR. Given that the magnetosphere channels charged particles to the poles, one would expect that there might be data from those species that lived in these polar environments. Are there data on the radiobiology of penguins, leopard seals, and other species that have existed in the polar regions of the Earth? Is there information suggesting that species, that live in these regions, where charged particles have been funneled by the magnetosphere for millennia, have expression of genes that have been selected for radioresistance to GCR)? Such data would be useful information.

Even the best radiobiology experimental data would be of limited use since conditions of natural selection and evolution would not apply to the astronauts spending over 1 year in space, on the Martian surface, or in more distant locations. What is known about GCR is that the admixture of charged particles ranges from carbon, iron, silicone, and other elements. The best data are coming from the mixed beam experiments at Brookhaven National Laboratories in which acute exposure of cells or experimental animals is yielding some useful information on the response to this form of irradiation. However, the plans for a Mars Mission to follow the Lunar Sorties Mission must deal with the challenge that we must provide an environment for astronauts that is as safe as possible.

The research effort for a Mars mission must include protection and mitigation of radiation damage from the quality of radiation that has not been experienced by humans on Earth: solar protons, galactic cosmic irradiation, and the neutrons generated by (GCR) hitting the elements in the spacecraft. One useful approach has been that of materials scientists. The discovery of graphene, and other materials that are both light and attenuate ionizing irradiation, will undoubtedly help in the design of a spacecraft. Furthermore, the focus on shielding materials will be prominent with respect to minimizing the creation of neutrons by interaction with galactic cosmic irradiation charged particles. Shielding will be a very important part of the approach to protecting the astronauts [47–51].

It has been 55 years since Neil Armstrong set foot on the moon and proclaimed, "One Small Step for Man, One Giant Leap for Mankind." What has happened to the United States space program since then? Looking back even further, the decision to make the space program independent of the United States Military led to the creation of the National Aeronautic and Space Administration (NASA), by then President Dwight D. Eisenhower which has received varying levels of funding from Congress yearly since its inception and led us to the planned Mars Mission [7–9]. The decision to keep the space program independent of the military was based upon fears, generated during the "Cold War" competition between the United States and the Soviet

Union (and its other, then perceived enemies) that might have led to the militarization of the space program. Political factors continue to remain intertwined with science. This intermingling of politics with science in the United States is still evident with the varying levels of funding for the National Institutes of Health (NIH), the Center for Disease Control (CDC), and other federal agencies, as well as, NASA. There remains a reality that the space program and funding for NASA must continue for a variety of reasons, including the importance of the Space Program to National Military Defense.

There is a growing consensus among members of the scientific community that mining operations on the moon and eventually other planets in our solar system can provide a source of valuable materials and even sources of energy for Earth [2]. The recent plans to place a robotic "peregrine" moon lander on the lunar surface by a collaboration between NASA and Pittsburgh-based company Astrobiotic [2] was in part based on the need to collect information on the components of lubricants for mining machines. The potential of the moon to provide not only minerals but fuel sources is real. Energy remains a major concern for National priorities since fossil fuels will eventually run out, and the alternative sources nuclear, solar, geothermal, wind, water power, and others cannot meet current needs. This reality regarding the relevance of the moon to solve future energy needs is independent of military issues related to the importance of the moon for the U.S. space program. There is a concern about global climate change on Earth and the continuing dependence of most nations upon fossil fuels. Some prominent scientists have even issued alarm warnings that the human population must seek colonization of other moons or planets within the next 100 years since the Earth will eventually become uninhabitable [19]. Finally, there is the continuing push by scientists (supported by science fiction cinema in the entertainment industry) to stress the importance of space travel and exploration of other planets in our own solar system, then travel to potentially habitable planets and moons outside our solar system. Recent evidence from the Juno Satellite Mission points to Eurora, a moon of Jupiter, which has been reported to have evidence of water [3]. Science fiction can lead the way to both positive and negative eventual realities. However, it is the creativity of humans that will be the factor that drives the space program forward. The space program for a planned Mars Mission now faces three prominent obstacles to overcome: (1) fuel to reach and return from Mars; (2) the materials with which to construct the space vehicle; and (3) countermeasures to ensure the safety of the astronauts on what is projected to be a 860 day mission [7–10]. A major component of the third issue will be radiation protection.

History reveals that military conflict (war) can lead to great advances in technology [47]. The discovery of the airplane and heavier than air flight by the Wright brothers [6] followed by the application of "heavier than air" flight to routine mail delivery [47] was a relatively slow first step that led to innovations and improvements in airplane design. Airplane wing design and engine efficiency were accelerated by World War I and led to the rapid development of airplanes that could carry greater weights including bombs to deliver lethal force. Airplanes led to efficient troop deployment and then eventually commercial passenger transport and delivery of goods. Within 100 years of discovery, airplanes changed again from primitive gasoline-fueled single-engine biplanes to the creation of jet-powered airplanes with afterburners to increase speed [49], and, ultimately, rocket-powered engines to deliver weapons at hypersonic speeds [49]. At a recent Radiation Research Society Meeting in Hawaii, a previous United States astronaut described the strategy of his current company to develop an engine, which could reliably propel a spacecraft for 1000 h without failure [34, 49]. He discussed the current decision not to consider the use of a nuclear-powered engine due to the fear of contamination of the atmosphere with radioactive materials should the engine fail. He also discussed the relative inefficiency of current solar-powered or battery-powered engines. Thus, the current plans by NASA for a Mars Mission considered the use of solid fuel powered engines, in part due to the fear of an accident regarding nuclear-powered spacecraft. The situation is clearly different from the current acceptance of nuclear power for submarines and ships. The difference may be the concern for unplanned nuclear isotope contamination of the atmosphere in the event of a spacecraft accident during liftoff or return to Earth. What about the concern for radioisotope exposure to astronauts (galactic cosmic irradiation) during space travel? This issue is of major importance for NASA and for radiobiology.

There was a recent article in the journal *Scientific American* entitled "Why We'll Never Live in Space" [19]. It is the purpose of the present chapter to discuss the possible reasons for the conclusions made in that publication to be incorrect [19].

Humans have been naturally curious and inventive since the first recorded history. However, to begin to understand the challenges of human space travel, one must first recognize the incompleteness of our available data on the potentially greatest threat: radiation.

The current plans by NASA and other governmental agencies to plan first for a staged preparation for the Mars Mission. The first stage will be a longer duration mission to the moon. The mission to Mars must focus on the challenge of adapting to space radiation. So, the next Lunar Mission will address the issue of radiation exposure of longer duration. Building a habitat on the moon will require radiation shielding, but first understanding the components of radiation including X-rays, solar protons, galactic cosmic irradiation, and neutrons that are created by GCR hitting the materials in the habitat (Fig. 4.1). Research on this challenge has provided information as to the complexity of dealing with radiation exposure.

The available evidence from past NASA) orbital missions including the Gemini and Apollo Missions has stressed the importance of correct quantitation of irradiation exposure to astronauts [7–10]. Accurate quantitation requires dosimeters that can record not only the time and intensity of exposure, but information on the quality of the irradiation gamma ray, X-ray, proton, high linear energy transfer particles-radioisotopes from galactic cosmic irradiation (GCR) (supernovaes), and neutrons (Fig. 4.1).

Once, humans are outside the magnetosphere, the protective Van Allen Belt [24], and, therefore, are outside the magnetosphere-mediated protection from charged particles (the solar proton events and galactic cosmic irradiation), there now is a critical need to understand the radiobiology of charged particles and neutrons. It is important to first understand the types and magnitude of irradiation that are detectable outside the magnetosphere. Data on radiation exposure that were obtained from the space

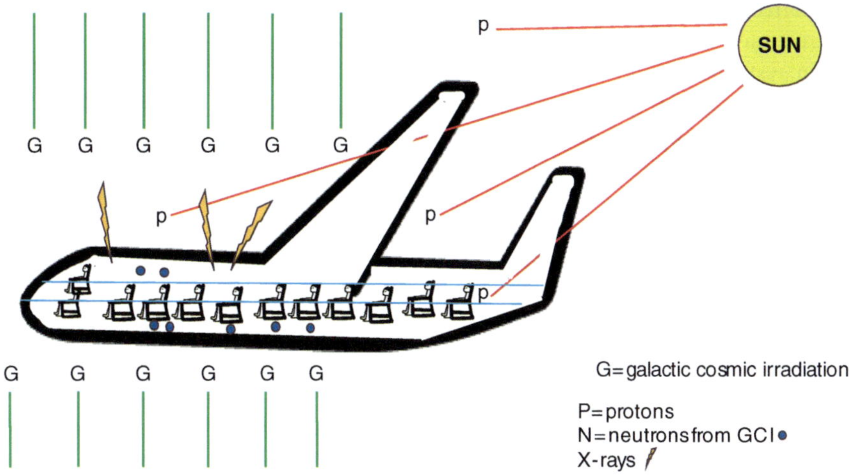

Fig. 4.1 Astronauts in a spacecraft will be subjected to multiple forms of irradiation. The figure demonstrates astronauts sitting inside a spacecraft, who will be subjected to solar proton events (P) coming from sunspots on the sun, galactic cosmic irradiation (G), GCI which represent high LET particles or ionized atoms, such as Iron[59], Carbon[14], and neutrons, which arise from the GCR hitting the elements of the spacecraft (blue dots), and finally X-rays (wavy golden lines), which are coming from both the galactic cosmic radiation events and also preceding the arrival of protons from the sunspots

shuttle and International Space Station Missions have revealed that solar proton events are seasonal and directional. Their presence can be predicted by the telescopic observation of sunspots on the surface of the sun, and the gamma ray bursts that are detectable on Earth and which precede the emission of protons [8–10]. Thus, astronauts can be alerted from Earth that a proton fluence is coming. In contrast, GCR is constant and from all directions [8]. There then follows the need for shielding. The space vehicle must then be prepared to sustain the oncoming GCR and proton fluence. But, how does one prepare a spacecraft for proton shielding?

Blocking protons is not a trivial event. Protons can be shielded by the same materials that are used to shield the body from X-rays; however, these shielding materials must be constructed of heavy materials, and weight alone makes shielding a challenge for the space vehicle. The shielding of an entire vehicle may be cost ineffective [27]. Furthermore, the fuel required to deliver the shielding material from the Earth's surface to the site of assembly of a space vehicle at a space station would cost levels that may not be sustained by current budgets allocated to the space program. One strategy has been the rotation of the astronauts on a serial basis, to enter a relatively protective structure for one person at a time; perhaps, during a 6–8 h sleep interval. The rotation of individuals in sequence to a protected substructure in the space vehicle is one option that has been used by NASA to limit the number of hours per day of exposure, but the effect of the relative shielding area may prove to be inadequate for prolonged exposures (months to years) and may still be ineffective. Another fact is that proton irradiation has a significantly increased relative biologic effect (RBE) as do neutrons [20–23] on most human organs and organ systems compared to X-rays (Figs. 4.2, 4.3, and 4.4). Thus, protection from the biological consequences of solar proton events remains a major challenge for planning a safe future moon mission. Furthermore, the construction of a safe lunar habitat will be critical. The moon does not have a protective magnetosphere, so protons, as well as, other charged particles will hit the lunar surface unattenuated.

The issue of galactic cosmic irradiation (GCR) is even more complex and potentially a more critical biologic factor that should not be under estimated [8]. Unlike solar proton events, which are directional and seasonal and varying in magnitude (depending on the size of solar storms—sunspots); the galactic cosmic irradiation is constant, even though the series of events is sporadic and unpredictable. GCR is a result of supernovae (the death of stars) from outside our solar system, and is the result of events that may have occurred light years ago and distances far away from the spacecraft and its human occupants. Current measuring devices include the Hubble and Webb telescopes [50] have allowed astronomers and astrophysicists to determine the numbers of GCR sources and where supernovae have occurred in stars and solar systems that are hundreds of light years away from Earth. While the fact may sound encouraging as to events that occurred yesterday as opposed to 100 light years ago, the charged particles, which arose from any supernovae no matter where and when originated are here now and cause damage. One published estimate suggests that there are thousands of supernovae every day [9]. The Webb Telescope, which replaced the Hubble Telescope as the most sensitive source of data in the

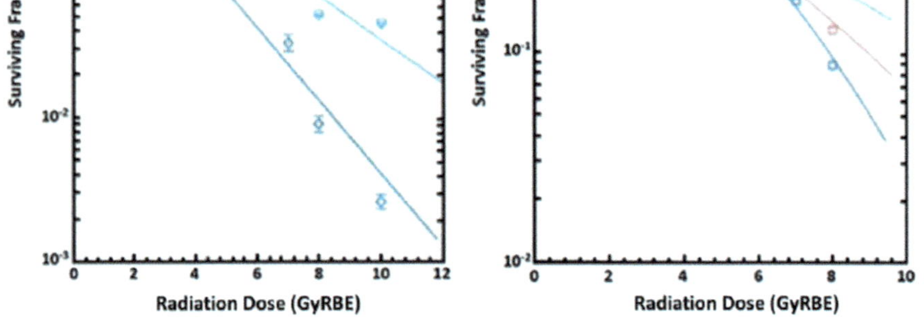

Fig. 4.2 Clonogenic survival curves for Fanca−/− and Fanca+/+ BMSCs treated with either proton therapy (**a**) or photon therapy (**b**) in the presence or absence of JP4–039 (27). From: Quinn TJ, Ding X, Li X, et al. Amelioration of mucositis in proton therapy of Fanconi Anemia Fanca−/− mice by JP4–039. In Vivo. 2019;33: 1757–1766

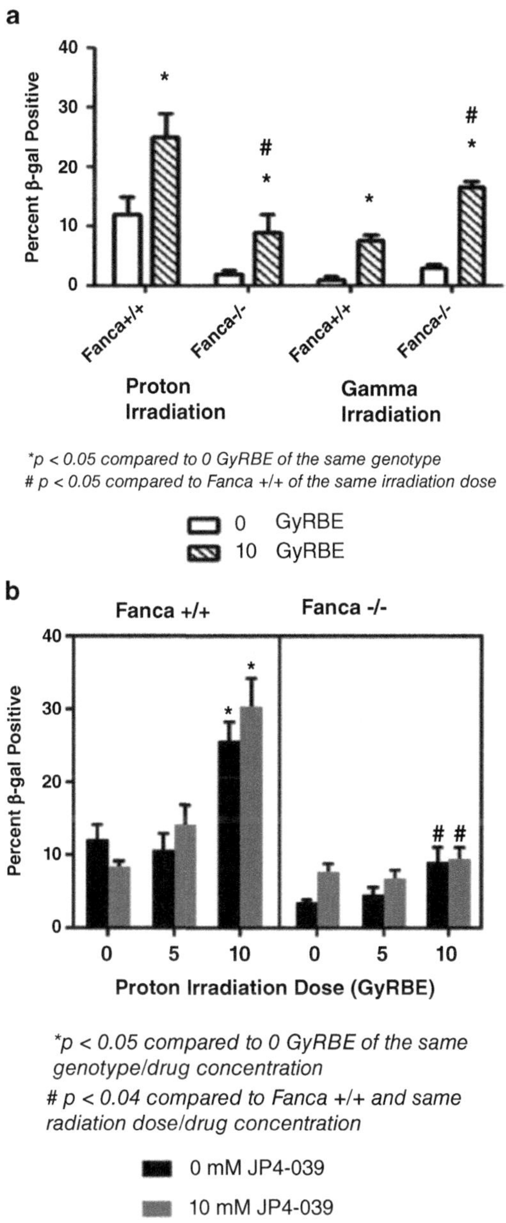

Fig. 4.3 B-Galactosidase assay for Fanca+/+ or Fanca−/− BMSCs following (**a**) proton or photon radiation therapy. Effect of (**b**) JP4039 on proton-induced senescence in both FA models [27]

universe, has expanded our understanding of the number of stars and, thus, the potential number of supernovae [50]. The physical expansion of the universe is now quantifiable more precisely than that of 10 years ago. The distance between stars is increasing over time and indicates that the universe is expanding [50]. This means

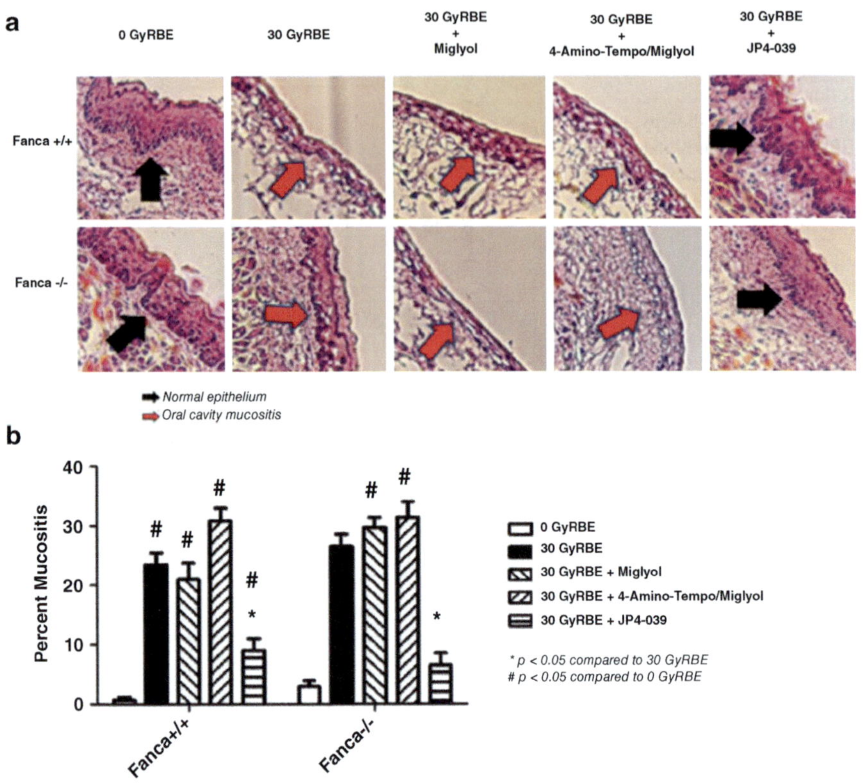

Fig. 4.4 Fanca+/+ and Fanca−/− mice were irradiated with 30 GyRBE to the oral cavity, in the presence or absence of vehicle, non-targeted 4-AT or JP4–039, and the percent of mucositis was assessed (**a**, **b**) [27]

that there is an outward movement away from the Earth of all solar systems. This fact might suggest that there will be a limit to the number of GCR sources generating events because the stars will be further away. However, other data collected with the Webb Telescope indicate that there are more stars and more solar systems than predicted by the Hubble Telescope [50]. These data indicate that there will likely not be a decrease in the frequency or magnitude of supernovae that are detected over the next 100 years. Therefore, advances in the design and building of a spacecraft must consider shielding against GCR for transporting of humans to and from Mars. Then, NASA will be able to plan for a successful Mars Mission, correct? However, we must face the unavoidable conclusion that the effects of GCR-charged particles including the generation of neutrons in the space vehicle from GCR hitting the materials in the vehicle may prove to be more deleterious and even prohibitive. We have much to learn about neutrons (Tables 4.1 and 4.2). Of great concern is the effect of radiation on the immune function during long exposure times [12, 13], and teratogenesis and reproductive health [15–18].

Table 4.1 Components of galactic cosmic irradiation during transit to and on the surface of Mars

Radiation type	Estimated dose (milliren)	Source	Estimate of RBE
1. Ɣ-rays	See total	Sun	1.0
2. Protons	See total	Sun and GCR	1.1
3. GCR: Carbon Silicon Iron Others	1.69–1.80 m/Sv/day	Supernovae from all directions	Not corrected for dose rate
4. Neutrons	Not known	GCR particles hitting the spacecraft materials	Not given
5. Total	0.66 ± 0.12 Sievert	Total	253 day cruise to Mars × 2

Table 4.2 Components of galactic cosmic radiation on Martian surface

Radiation type	Estimated dose (millirem)	Estimate of RBE
1. X-rays	Variable	1.0
2. Protons	Variable	1.1
3. GCR	0.64 ± 0.12 MSV/day	Dose rate 180–225 uGy/day[a]
4. Neutrons	20% of the dose	
5. Total	300 days observation.	Dose rate 190–202 uGy/day [40]

[a] 300 days @ 200 uG/day = 6 × 10^4 uGy = 60 mGy/but not dose rate—or RBE adjusted

To approach the consequences of space irradiation, one must first understand the methods that are available to address the problem. The article in *Scientific American* entitled "Why We'll Never Live in Space" [19] listed some of the factors that are prominent in the minds of NASA scientists. These factors include prolonged human isolation for a Mars Mission during the anticipated 18–24 months away from Earth; the psychological effects of prolonged weightlessness; the biological changes in human organ systems that will occur (including changes in bone formation and destruction (turnover) leading to degradation of the skeleton, neurologic consequences of weightlessness, and cardiovascular changes) [10]. The author of the article [10] suggested that one major factor; namely, "the consequences of irradiation was yet to be addressed" [19].

Given that radiation detectors have provided useful data on solar proton events, galactic cosmic irradiation, and the creation of neutrons by charged particles hitting a spacecraft, we may now begin to approach the radiobiology of each of these forms of irradiation and gain some insight into the magnitude of the problem. The physical units of measurement are listed in Table 4.3.

Table 4.3 Glossary of terms (SI science international units)

Gray = 1 joule/kg—Energy absorbed = 100 rad
Rad = cGy = 100 ergs per gram absorbed = 0.01 joule/kg = (0.01 Gy)
Roentgen = radiation in air—Ionization chamber reading of electric static unit per cc = 2.50 × 10^4 Coul-mb pe kg of air
Rem = Eose equivalent in absorbed dose in rads with a quality factor of (1 rem = 0.015v)
Sievert = product of absorbed dose in grays and quality factor (1 SV = 100 rem)
Curie = 3.7 × 10^{10} disintegrations/second
Bacquerel = 1 disintegration (radioisotope) per second
RBE = relative biological effect: Varies to/each organ and organ system. Varies by dose rate and energy of machine relative to X-ray photons. GCR can vary by ion: Helium, iron, neon, silicon, carbon. Neutron can vary form 1.0–3.5 for effect on ovary. Electron (Beta particle) 1.1–3.5 for ovary

Consequences of Proton Irradiation from Solar Proton Events

The radiobiologic effect of protons has been studied intensively in the past decades. This is primarily because of the use of therapeutic proton irradiation to treat cancer [27]. The number of clinical proton delivery programs in cancer centers throughout the world from the first in the 1970s to the present has increased dramatically. Proton irradiation is now available to nearly all citizens in the United States, Europe, and many other countries. Proton irradiation has been very successful in targeting tumor volumes deep in the body, and the precision of dose delivery has been shown to exceed that of all available X-ray delivery systems using linear accelerators. However, the radiobiology of protons has provided some potentially alarming data with respect to their relative biological effect (RBE) [27]. The RBE is defined as the relative biological consequences that are detectable with one physical unit of irradiation compared to X-rays. The RBE studies with protons were initially carried out in basic science laboratories and looked at several sources of irradiation that were then being considered for therapeutic use in Radiation Oncology Departments. RBE studies were carried out with protons and also with other potentially therapeutic radiation beams delivering protons [26, 37, 38], neutrons [28], pi-mesons [29], helium nuclei (alpha particles) [45, 46], and carbon ions [42, 43] all delivered by novel accelerator treatment devices. RBE experiments were usually conducted with cells in culture (in vitro) using clonogenic radiation survival curves with cancer permanent murine or human cell lines that were irradiated in tissue cultures [27]. These RBE studies were also carried out by giving total body irradiation (TBI) to experimental animals, usually to genetically inbred strains of mice [27]. While there is controversy over the actual number for the RBE of protons the number is not universally agreed upon. The data do uniformly agree that protons have a greater RBE compared to X-rays. The physical unit of measure for delivery of irradiation is calculated by a physical unit as the amount of energy delivered to a cell or tissue. The metric allows one to compare each form of irradiation with X-rays by physical principles of ergs per milligram or Joules per gram of tissue. The RBE is a different issue. The data have always shown that there is an increase in RBE for protons compared to X-rays for the same physical unit. The measurement of protons in each of several units, RADS, Gray, and Roentgen equivalent man (REM) as it relates to RBE, has been to date focused for application to clinical radiotherapy.

When one attempts now to apply these metrics of proton levels from clinical radiotherapy to solar proton events (SPE) that apply to space irradiation, the situation becomes more complex. Radiobiology experiments that were carried out to prepare for clinical use of protons in radiotherapy were controllable with respect to dose, dose rate, and energy of the protons. Protons are created for clinical use by cyclotrons [27]. The dose delivered by protons in vitro or in vivo to animals was and is reliably quantitated. The time of exposure, volume of tissue treated, and dose delivered can be measured accurately and can be delivered in a single exposure or timed planned fractionated exposures [27]. The problem in translating clinical data with proton radiotherapy to space radiation proton exposure is that there is no research system available for sporadic delivery of protons of different energies and at different intervals. What is available? There are systems that could be designed for the study of this delivery of continuous low-level proton exposure but these are not yet available [25]. Continuous low-dose exposure has been done with the 60x background irradiation levels of gamma rays [25]. However, continuous low-dose exposure differs from sporadic exposure, and varying times between each exposure are separated by varying periods of no detectable exposure. No such data has been published to date. Why is this important? Because of the radiation damage repair mechanism in cells, tissues, and organs.

Challenges to Simulate Space Radiation

The repair of continuous low-level irradiation is never complete and does leave residual effects [25]. Cells in culture, as well as, experimental animals are known to adapt to proton irradiation and gamma irradiation/X-rays. However, the X-ray/γ-ray adaptation is a product of the evolutionary biology of all organisms leading up to humans over billions of years, as was described in Chap. 1. During evolution on Earth, solar protons were diverted to the poles by the magnetosphere. So, developing organisms did so without protons in their environment. Therefore, there is an expectation that the consequences of sporadic exposure of asronauts to protons, even if predictable by measuring gamma irradiation bursts during solar proton events (SPEs), will be the same as those for X-rays. This expectation may prove to be wrong based upon the absence of availability of data. At the present time, there is limited data on the specific effect of sporadic proton irradiation with respect to the parameters that would likely affect astronauts including neurocognitive changes, bone marrow suppression, intestinal stem cell damage, liver damage, lung damage, carcinogenesis and cardiac damage. However, we do have data for the current follow-up of the estimated 150 humans, who have experienced space radiation in the space program, which includes exposure to soar protons. The NASA-funded research in radiobiology has considered all of the components of space irradiation to be paramount in the design of both the spacecraft and the development of countermeasures for the Mars Mission.

The published information on the effects of protons, and the energy ranges that would be expected for protons coming from SPEs lead to the unavoidable consequence that the radiobiology of protons will be a major issue for both the upcoming moon habitat "Lunar Sorties" missions and the Mars Mission.

Radiobiologic Effects of Galactic Cosmic Irradiation (GCI)

Sensitive detection systems in unmanned space probes and, most recently, the Curiosity Rover [8–10] experiments of robot level on the Martian surface have provided valuable information on the magnitude of GCI. These data have revealed not only the detection of 1000 supernovae per day but also the kinds of particles that will come from each GCI event. The charged particles that are detected include a spectrum of ions from silicon, carbon, iron, and others (Table 4.1). To approach the radiobiology of GCI, the Brookhaven National Laboratory has developed a GCI Irradiation System that will deliver a spectrum of different charged particles [14]. Initial studies were done with Iron 59 particles and radiobiology indicated a significant increase in the RBE for these charged particles [14]. Experiments with cells in culture and with TBI delivery to animals confirmed these differences. However, due to the expense of setting up an experiment for the delivery of charged particles and the difficulty of keeping the delivery system functioning was a challenge. It is not possible to deliver fractionated irradiation that would be comparable to the sporadic detection of GCI that would be experienced by astronauts during a prolonged space mission. Therefore, the available data must be used for predictions of the magnitude of the problem. The concept of a "mixed-beam" of the different atoms in the charged particles that comprise GCI presents another unavoidable issue [14].

Astronauts will experience bursts of gamma radiation from sunspots that precede the solar proton events, then proton irradiation, and also will be exposed to sporadic GCI that contains isotopes of many elements from each supernova, and neutrons generated from the GCI atoms hitting the materials in the space craft. Some experiments have been carried out with mixed beams of simulated GCI and are very difficult to interpret [14]. The concept of mixed beam irradiation is not new. It is now used clinically in patients, who may receive electron beam (beta particle) irradiation simultaneously with each fraction of x-irradiation [27]. These controlled studies provided some useful information that may help the design of mixed beam experiments for application in space radiation. However, electrons have a relatively low RBE due to the small particle size of electrons [40]. The energy level of clinical electrons, as with X-ray photons, can be precisely controlled, as can the depth dose characteristics and volume of tissue treated. The level of control in clinical radiotherapy as with clinical protons is great [27]. Extrapolation of these data to the mixed beam of sporatic space radiation is not possible. There are varying energies of X-rays, protons, and charged particles of many isotopes, and these levels may change over time.

One exception to the absence of clinical data on GCR is the use of carbon ion radiotherapy [42, 43]. In Germany and Japan, linear accelerators have delivered carbon-ion high LET radiation and there is an estimate of RBE. The current evidence indicates that GCR will be a significant and prominent factor in the radiation of space travel. As will be discussed in the next chapter, the development of countermeasures for radiation exposure must take into account the components of GCR.

Neutron Irradiation

Neutrons have a prominent radiobiological effect on cells in culture and in animals. Clinical use of neutrons was limited to relatively few treatment centers, one in Seattle, Washington [28]. As with clinical proton delivery systems, the RBE was a factor that was prominent. Neutron irradiation has a greater RBE than protons due to the increased size of the neutron particle.

The detection systems for neutrons are more complicated [44]. Clinical radiation physicists first detected neutron irradiation coming from the collimator of linear accelerators. Neutron irradiation was detected when X-rays above the energy level of 12 MeV hit the clinical linear accelerator collimators, which are usually constructed of depleted uranium, and the magnitude of neutrons was found to be increased with greater photon (X-ray) energy [44]. Currently, the commissioning of new linear accelerators is accompanied by a single quantitation of neutron levels during X-ray delivery. The systems for the detection of neutrons are complex, expensive, and difficult to administer [44]. Continual measurement of neutrons in clinical radiotherapy centers is not required at the present time. The magnitude of neutron production and their monitoring is also not currently required. Many radiation oncology physicists and radiation oncologists recognize neutron measurements as a potential requrement for the future, particularly, with regard to the concern for the contribution of neutrons to carcinogenesis by x-irradiation [8, 45–52]. If neutron irradiation is deemed to be "insignificant," or at least at a level that does not require continuous monitoring today, then one does not have to consider that radiotherapy using X-ray energies above 12 MeV is, in fact, a form of "mixed beam" irradiation. For patients receiving TBI with photons, if the energy is above 12 MeV, it may not require that clinical physicists quantitate the contribution of neutrons to the total body irradiation fraction delivered. TBI is still used, although in fewer clinical protocols than in the past, to prepare patients for bone marrow transplantation by clearing out the hosts' bone marrow space to receive the donor bone marrow transplanted stem cels. TBI is also used in combination with chemotherapy to destroy cancer cells in the body. Quantitation of x-irradiation currently does not take into account the contribution of neutrons to the dose delivered.

Why are neutrons relevant to space radiation? Neutrons occur when high LET particles, charged particles from supernovae (galactic cosmic irradiation) hit metallic objects [10] (Fig. 4.1). The composition of a spacecraft for the Mars Mission and for missions beyond Mars will undoubtedly contain metals, carbon fibers, or other materials that will generate neutrons when hit with GCE. The physics of the creation of neutrons by GCI is a very interesting area of study now and new literature is forthcoming. By the time of the Mars Missions, there will be data available to help design not only a spacecraft that minimizes neutron creation by GCR, but also medical countermeasures that can protect astronauts not only from X-rays and protons but also from GCR and neutrons.

References

1. Patel ZS, Brunstetter TJ, Tarver WJ, et al. Red risks for a journey to the red planet: the highest priority human health risks for a mission to Mars. NPJ Microgravity. 2020;6(1):33. https://doi.org/10.1038/s41526-020-00124-6.
2. Macktoobian M, Gillet D, Kneib J-P. Astrobotics: swarm robotics for astrophysical studies. IEEE Robot Automat Mag. 2021;28(3):92–101.
3. Menou K. Climate stability of habitable earth-like planets. Earth Planet Sci Lett. 2015;429:20–4.
4. Hall DT, Strobel DF, Feldman PD, et al. Detection of an oxygen atmosphere on Jupiter's moon Europa. Nature. 1995;373(6516):677–81. https://doi.org/10.1038/373677a0.
5. Bish DL, Blake DF, Vaniman DT, et al. X-ray diffraction results from Mars science laboratory: mineralogy of rocknest at gale crater. Science. 2013;341(6153):1238932. https://doi.org/10.1126/science.1238932.
6. Liu H, Yao Z, Fu Y, Feng J. Review of research into bioregenerative life support system(s) which can support humans living in space. Life Sci Space Res (Amst). 2021;31:113–20. https://doi.org/10.1016/j.lssr.2021.09.003.
7. Jones JA, Montesinos C, Karouia F, et al. Space radiation protection countermeasures in microgravity and planetary exploration. (Abstract) 16th Annual World Cancer Congress, Budapest, Hungary, June 12–14, 2024.
8. Cucinotta FA, Durante M. Cancer risk from exposure to galactic cosmic rays: implications for space exploration by human beings. Lancet Oncol. 2006;7(5):431–5. https://doi.org/10.1016/S1470-2045(06)70695-7.
9. Durante M, Cucinotta FA. Heavy ion carcinogenesis and human space exploration. Nat Rev Cancer. 2008;8(6):465–72. https://doi.org/10.1038/nrc2391.
10. Durante M, Cucinotta FA. Physical basis of radiation protection in space travel. Rev Mod Phys. 2011;83(4):1245–50.
11. Wilson JW, Thibeault SA, Cucinotta FA, et al. Issues in protection from galactic cosmic rays. Radiat Environ Biophys. 1995;34(4):217–22. https://doi.org/10.1007/BF01209745.
12. Cassatt DR, Winters TA, PrabhuDas M. Immune dysfunction from radiation exposure. Radiat Res. 2023;200(4):389–95. https://doi.org/10.1667/RADE-22-00197.1.
13. Hollingsworth BA, Aldrich JT, Case CM, et al. Immune dysfunction from radiation exposure. Radiat Res. 2023;200(4):396–416. https://doi.org/10.1667/rade-22-00004.1.
14. Brown K, Ahrens L, Chiang IH, et al. The NASA space radiation laboratory at Brookhaven national laboratory: preparation and delivery of ion beams for space radiation research. Nucl Instrum Methods Phys Res, Sect A. 2010;618(1–3):97–107.
15. Montesinos CA, Khalid R, Cristea O, et al. Space radiation protection countermeasures in microgravity and planetary exploration—a review for special issue on space life science in life. Life (Basel). 2021;11(8):829. https://doi.org/10.3390/life11080829.
16. Zeitlin C, Hassler DM, Cucinotta FA, et al. Measurements of energetic particle radiation in transit to Mars on the Mars science laboratory. Science. 2013;340(6136):1080–4. https://doi.org/10.1126/science.1235989.

17. Ehresmann B, Hassler DM, Zeitlin C, et al. Charged particle spectra measured during the transit to Mars with the Mars science laboratory radiation assessment detector (MSL/RAD). Life Sci Space Res (Amst). 2016;10:29–37. https://doi.org/10.1016/j.lssr.2016.07.001.
18. Hassler DM, Zeitlin C, Wimmer-Schweingruber RF, et al. Mars' surface radiation environment measured with the mars science laboratory's curiosity rover. Science. 2014;343(6169):1244797. https://doi.org/10.1126/science.1244797.
19. Scoles S. Why we'll never live in space. Scientific American. 2023:22.
20. Acharya MM, Baulch JE, Klein PM, et al. New concerns for neurocognitive function during deep space exposures to chronic low dose-rate, neutron radiation. eNeuro. 2019;6(4):ENEURO.0094-19. https://doi.org/10.1523/ENEURO.0094-19-2019.
21. Wang B, Yasuda H. Relative biological effectiveness of high LET particles on the reproductive system and fetal development. Life (Basel). 2020;10(11):298. https://doi.org/10.3390/life10110298.
22. Maglieri R, Licea A, Evans M, et al. Measuring neutron spectra in radiotherapy using the nested neutron spectrometer. Med Phys. 2015;42(11):6162–9. https://doi.org/10.1118/1.4931963.
23. Exposito MR, Sanchez-Nieto B, Terron JA, et al. Neutron contamination in radiotherapy: estimation of second cancers based on measurements in 1377 patients. Radiother Oncol. 2013;107(2):234–41. https://doi.org/10.1016/j.radonc.2013.03.011.
24. Bannova O, Bell L. Radiation shielding design strategies for lunar minimal functionality habitability element. Acta Astronaut. 2010;67(9–10):1103–9.
25. Olipitz W, Wiktor-Brown D, Shuga J, et al. Integrated molecular analysis indicates undetectable DNA damage in mice after continuous irradiation at –400-fold natural background radiation. Environ Health Perspec. 2012;120(8):1130–6. https://doi.org/10.1289/ehp.1104294.
26. Paganetti H, Niemierko A, Ancukiewicz M, et al. Relative biological effectiveness (RBE) values for proton beam therapy. Int J Radiat Oncol Biol Phys. 2002;53(2):407–21. https://doi.org/10.1016/s0360-3016(02)02754-2.
27. Quinn TJ, Ding X, Li X, et al. Amelioration of mucositis in proton therapy of Fanconi anemia Fanca–/– mice by JP4-039. In Vivo. 2019;33(6):1757–66. https://doi.org/10.21873/invivo.11666.
28. Baiocco G, Barbieri S, Babini G, et al. The origin of neutron biological effectiveness as a function of energy. Sci Rep. 2016;6:34033. https://doi.org/10.1038/srep34033.
29. Yuhas JM, Li AP, Kligerman MM. Present status of the proposed use of negative pi mesons in radiotherapy. In: Lett JT, editor. Advances in radiation biology, vol. 8. Academic Press; 2013. p. 52–83.
30. Baker DN. Wave-particle interaction effects in the Van Allen belts. Earth Planets Space. 2021;73(1):189. https://doi.org/10.1186/s40623-021-01508-y.
31. Dikpati M, McIntosh SW, Wing S. Simulating properties of "seasonal" variability in solar activity and space weather impacts. Front Astron Space Sci. 2021;8:688604.
32. Prantzos N, Boissier S. On the relative frequencies of core-collapse supernovae sub-types: the role of progenitor metallicity. Astron Astrophys. 2003;406:259–90.
33. Ver Steeg G, Menicucci NC. Entangling power of an expanding universe. Phys Rev. 2009;D79:044027.
34. Arunan S, Satish R. Mars orbiter Mission spacecraft and its challenges. Curr Sci. 2015;109(6):1061–9.
35. Kamada T, Tsujii H, Blakely EA, et al. Carbon ion radiotherapy in Japan: an assessment of 20 years of clinical experience. Lancet Oncol. 2015;16(2):e93–e100. https://doi.org/10.1016/S1470-2045(14)70412-7.
36. Schulz-Ertner D, Nikoghosyan A, Thhilmann C, et al. Results of carbon ion radiotherapy in 152 patients. Int J Radiat Oncol Biol Phys. 2004;58(2):631–40. https://doi.org/10.1016/j.ijrobp.2003.09.041.
37. Kim J-W. Magnetic fields and beam optics studies of a 250 MeV superconducting proton radiotherapy cyclotron. Nucl Instrum Methods Phys Res, Sect A. 2007;582(2):366–73.

38. Raju MR. Proton radiobiology, radiosurgery, and radiotherapy. Int J Radiat Biol. 1995;67(3):237–59. https://doi.org/10.1080/09553009514550301.
39. Wahl AC. Production of Fe^{59} by the Co^{59} (n,p) reaction in the Brookhaven reactor. J Chem Phys. 1953;21:182.
40. Bellamy M, Eckerman K. Relative biological effectiveness of low-energy electrons and photons. In: Letter Report Office of Radiation and Indoor Air U.S. Environmental Protection Agency (EPA). Oak Ridge National Laboratory; 2013.
41. Svendsen K, Guenot D, Svensson JB, et al. A focused very high energy electron beam for fractionated stereotactic radiotherapy. Sci Rep. 2021;11(1):5844. https://doi.org/10.1038/s41598-021-85451-8.
42. Malouff TD, Krishnan S, Seneviratne DS, et al. Carbon ion therapy: a modern review of an emerging technology. Front Oncol. 2020;10:82. https://doi.org/10.3389/fonc.2020.00082.
43. Lazar AA, Schulte R, Faddegon B, et al. Clinical trials involving carbon ion radiation therapy and the path forward. Cancer. 2018;124(23):4467–76. https://doi.org/10.1002/cncr.31662.
44. Gomez F, Sanchez-Doblado F, Iglesias A, et al. Active on-line detector for in-room radiotherapy neutron measurements. Radiat Meas. 2010;45(10):1532–5.
45. Bloomer WD, McLaughlin WH, Wolf A, et al. Astatine-211-Tellurium radiocolloid cures experimental malignant ascites. Science. 1981;212(4492):340–1. https://doi.org/10.1126/science.7209534.
46. Bloomer WD, Lipsztein R, Dalton JF. Antibody-mediated radiotherapy. Cancer. 1985;55(9 Suppl):2229–33. https://doi.org/10.1002/1097-0142(19850501)55:9+<2229::aid-cncr2820551427>3.0.co:2-x.
47. Hansen JR. Aviation history in the wider view. Technol Cult. 1989;30(3):643–56.
48. King MK. Boron ignition and combustion in air-augmented rocket afterburners. Combust Sci Technol. 1972;5(1):155–64.
49. Reshotko E. Transition issues at hypersonic speed. 44th AIAA Aerospace Sciences Meeting and Exhibit, 9-12 January, 2006, Reno, Nevada. 2006.
50. Kalirai J. Scientific discovery with the James Webb space telescope. Contemp Phys. 2018;59(3):251–90.
51. Sivananthan A, Shields D, Fisher R, et al. Continuous 1 year oral administration of the radiation mitigator, MMS350, after total body irradiation restores bone marrow stromal cell proliferative capacity and reduces age-related senescence in Fanconi anemia (Fanca−/−) mice. Radiat Res. 2019;191(2):139–53. https://doi.org/10.1667/RR15199.1.
52. Leatherbarrow EL, Harper JV, Cucinotta FA, et al. Induction and quantification of y-H2AX foci following low and high LET-irradiation. Int J Radiat Biol. 2006;82(2):111–8. https://doi.org/10.1080/09553000600599783.

Chapter 5
Strategies for Radioprotection of Astronauts

Currently available information indicates that there will be at least four sources of continuous, but sporadic irradiation exposure to astronauts, either in a space vehicle or on the surface of the moon or Mars. These four sources are as follows: (1) X-rays (gamma rays) [1], (2) solar proton events (proton irradiation) [2, 3], (3) high linear energy transfer particles (galactic cosmic irradiation (GCR)) [4, 5], and (4) neutrons both from space and generated in the space vehicle or on the Lunar or Martian surface by GCR hitting the components of the vehicle or habitat [6]. The relative levels of each form of radiation that will be sustained on a daily, weekly, or monthly basis are likely to fluctuate based on many factors. There are seasonal variations in the appearance of sunspots (solar proton events), and these are directional—depending upon where the solar storm arises on the surface of the sun relative to the location of the moon or the Martian orbit. The data are based upon our current ability to detect X-ray bursts from the sun, which precede the solar proton emission [2, 3]. Other available evidence comes from multiple sources, most prominently, the data collected by long-duration robotic space vehicle mission(s) to the Martian surface [7–10]. These data provide valuable information because of the duration of the time of collection. With an expected 6-month (180 days) travel time from Earth to Mars, multiple months on the Martian surface (510 days), and an equal 6 months or more for return to Earth, astronauts will experience chronic accumulation of at least 860 days irradiation damage [7]. The space vehicle shielding capabilities, at the present time, while attenuating some of the irradiation cannot eliminate it [7].

The radiobiology of space travel will rely heavily upon three sets of data that are published: 1) the first is from the decades of experience with clinical radiation therapy. These data report both acute and late effects of clinical radiotherapy that are observed in cancer patient survivors. The second source of data is the available information from the long-term survivors of the Hiroshima and Nagasaki bombing events in 1945 and their progeny [11, 12]. Finally, there is information from survivors of nuclear reactors and other military irradiation accidents [9–31]. While much of these data are from survivors of much higher doses of irradiation that were

J. Greenberger, *Radiation Oncology and Radiation Biology*,
https://doi.org/10.1007/978-3-031-66300-0_5

delivered in a short time, it is relevant to the types of irradiation that will be experienced, and over a long duration by astronauts. There are some data from the follow-up of the nearly 100 astronauts, who experienced the space shuttle and space station missions [9, 10], as well as, Apollo astronauts [9].

The, perhaps, most relevant information to the human radiation biology of space travel is that obtained from irradiated nonhuman primates. Data from the Wake Forest Non-Human Primate Center has provided information on the effects of irradiation on many organ systems that were thought previously to be unaffected or minimally affected by ionizing irradiation including the pancreas (with the development of diabetes) [13, 14], the brain (with neurocognitive defects) [13], and the heart with new data showing radiation-induced fibrosis [14]. Therefore, an approach to radiation protection for astronauts must take into account the accumulating evidence that nearly all organs and organ systems in humans will be at risk for both acute and late radiation effects. Furthermore, since the irradiation will be continuous, the concept of radiation protective countermeasures (delivered before exposure) vs. radiation mitigators (delivered after exposure) will not be clear cut as it is in the case of clinical radiotherapy [15, 16]. First responders are those people coming to the site of a nuclear accident or war fighters entering a contaminated zone in the military scenario will need countermeasurers [15].

NASA (National Aeronautics and Space Administration) and other research agencies have focused on the known acute dangers of ionizing radiation exposure: namely, the Hematopoietic Acute Radiation Syndrome (H-ARS) and the Gastrointestinal Acute Radiation Syndrome (GI-ARS). The Hematopoietic Syndrome is caused by damage to the bone marrow and is well established. Several radiobiology textbooks cite the LD50/30 (lethal dose for 50% of individuals including humans that are exposed to total body irradiation (TBI)) and die within 30 days. For human adults, this dose for X-rays is estimated to be around 3–4.5 Gy and is not corrected for dose rate (cGy/minute). Higher dose rates delivering each dose are more lethal. These data come from single fraction X-ray (gamma ray) exposure experiments that were extrapolated from multiple experiments including those with rodent and nonhuman primate models [13]. These data cannot be reliably translated to an approach for radiation protection/mitigation of astronauts because the dose was a single fraction and was delivered at a relatively high dose rate (100–200 cGy/min). Thus, the published literature on the human LD50/30 is not necessarily indicative of the expected conditions of radiation exposure of astronauts.

Radiation damage is continually repaired in cells, organs, and organ systems. It is well known that experimental animals can adapt to continuous low-dose radiation exposure [17–19]. The adaptation to irradiation is not the same in all animals. Even with genetically in-bred mouse strains, there are strain-specific differences [20]. Furthermore, with out-bred animals, such as beagle dogs in the Argonne Laboratory, publications from the 1980s, there were markedly different responses of subsets of animals to continuous ɣ-ray irradiation [21].

During the 1980s, the period of the "Cold-War," much research was carried out in animal model systems that were designed to mimic continuous relatively low-dose exposure of humans that would be experienced during years of living in a region of fallout from thermonuclear weapons detonation [21]. The survivors of a single exposure to radiation from a fission bomb or thermonuclear (fusion) bomb would be living in a radiation-contaminated environment from a fallout. Such individuals would have been far enough away from the hypocenter of the detonation to survive the acute explosion. The studies in out-bred beagle dogs that were carried out at Argonne National Laboratories were pioneered by Thomas Fritz and Thomas Seed [21]. The datas was collected with animals receiving 3–5 Roentgens in the air (roughly 3–5 RAD total body dose per day) were in a room, where the cages of animals were in a circle surrounding a central Cobalt 60 source [21]. The Cobalt 60 source was above ground for 20 h per day and was lowered onto the floor for 4 h daily to allow cleaning of the room and feeding animals. The cages were rotated to allow a homogeneous TBI to be delivered. The experiment was over a two-year duration [21].

These experiments at Argonne National Laboratories were to simulate the conditions on Earth after a thermonuclear bomb explosion and soil contamination by fallout. The dogs displayed three different patterns of response to the radiation environment. These out-bred beagle dogs in these experiments were at the time the closest available animal model for the nonuniform (out-bred) human civilian population genetics. The experimental model, although, not designed to mimic space irradiation could today be interpreted to reflect multiple genetic background differences in the crew of a spacecraft.

In the study with beagle dogs [21], one-third of animals developed bone marrow suppression and died over time months/years of aplastic anemia (lack of red blood cells and white blood cells). Another third of animals went on to develop malignancy, the most prominent was acute erythroleukemia [21], which is in the category of acute leukemias and was different from the chronic myeloid leukemia originally reported to have presented in the survivors of the Hiroshima and Nagasaki bombings [12]. The final third of animals, which may be most relevant to the present discussion of radiation protection for astronauts, developed what was termed "radio-accommodation" [21]. These animals revealed the capacity to adapt to continuous low-dose (3–5 Roentgen in air) radiation exposure [21].

The adaptation to ionizing irradiation exposure first came from original studies by Elkind [22] and Puck [23]. These studies reported the importance of fractionation (time interval separating multiple radiation exposures) in the response of cells to radiation. A dose of radiation that was followed by a period of no exposure revealed the capacity of cells in tissue culture to repair irradiation damage, such that the second dose of irradiation, when delivered to the same cells in culture, was not directly additive [22, 23]. These studies suggested that the cells repaired radiation damage. Some cell line phenotypes, such as lymphocytes have less ability to repair, while others (malignant melanoma tumor cells) have a great capacity to repair [22, 23]. Studies reported over the decades following these original experiments showed that there was measurable repair of radiation damage.

More recently, the experiments with *Deinococcus radiodurans* [24] which were built upon the original cell culture observations revealed that bacteria could adapt to very high doses of irradiation by the processes of both radiation repair and natural selection of genetically modified radioresistant variants [25]. The *Deinococcus radiodurans* bacteria that survived over weeks of high-dose exposure, in the end had a chromosome essentially filled with naturally selected radiation repair genes and antioxidant genes [26]. The adaptation of bacteria with a doubling time of hours was much faster than the doubling time of the bone marrow stem cells in the Argonne Laboratory out-bred beagle dogs, and the dogs had no rapid proliferation of successive animal generations to select variants as did the bacteria [21]. Instead, dogs revealed what one generation experienced. The doubling time of marrow stem cells takes much longer in mammals like dogs and is very complex. Given the prominence of research on the hematopoietic syndrome and gastrointestinal syndrome (in which bone marrow stem cells and intestinal stem cells respectively are studied), there are fewer mechanisms by which mammalian tissue stem cells in a single generation can adapt to ionizing irradiation. To evolve a change in phenotype one estimate for the primitive Mollusk (snail) was that 200,000 generations would be required [27]. A single-cell *Deinococcus radiodurans* could generate 200,000 generations in a much shorter time than the multicellular Mollusk. Clearly, radiation protection/mitigation for astronauts could not be achieved by the process of natural selection.

Most of the experimental evidence on radiation protectors/mitigators comes from mouse models and shows that under the conditions of radiation exposure the most primitive stem cells resist damage by maintaining a state of quiescence (non-dividing state) [28].

In the experiments reporting the effect of irradiation on synchronized cells in the different phases of the cell cycle, the cells in the mitosis phase and the gap phase immediately following mitosis (G2) were found to be the most radiosensitive [29]. This study with synchronized cell lines is consistent with the knowledge that during mitosis chromatin is most susceptible to DNA double-strand break damage from irradiation [29]. Furthermore, the activation of radiation repair enzymes would be not be expected to be higher in mitosis. Adding to this knowledge of DNA repair, there is information about antioxidant stores, which are the "first defense" against irradiation damage [30–35]. One would expect that during specific phases of the cell cycle, both DNA repair enzymes and antioxidant stores would be most capable of resisting the molecular biologic effects that follow exposure to ionizing irradiation, while the other cell cycle phases would not be as capable. Overall, these studies were carried out in a controlled environment where the irradiation source was turned on or off and the dose was precisely monitored.

In the case of sporadic irradiation exposure and with varying and unpredictable mixtures of X-rays/protons/GCR and neutrons from the spacecraft, the situation would be expected to be more complex. Using all of the available data, radiation biologists have focused on developing radiation protectors and mitigator agents. (Mitigators are those given after irradiation exposure but before the presence of symptoms of irradiation damage.) The Radiation Countermeasures Program of NIAID/NIH focuses on two major effects of ionizing radiation damage; namely, consumption of antioxidant stores [33] and DNA double-strand breaks [32]. So, a radiation countermeasure would be focused on: (1) keeping antioxidant levels high and/or (2) repairing DNA double-strand breaks. There are other avenues of radiation countermeasure development; namely: (3) reducing the inflammatory response

Table 5.1 Categories of radiation countermeasures to protect and/or mitigate the deleterious effects of space radiation

Category of countermeasure	Examples of protector/mitigator
Reduce DNA double Strand breaks	Caffeine
Replenish antioxidant stores	Diet Vitamin C, vitamin E MnSOD-PL Catalase-PL GS-Nitroxide TTP-Nitroxide
Reduce inflammation	Corticosteroids Non-steroidal anti-inflammatory drugs IL-22 IFN-β
Stimulate stem cell repopulation in situ	G-CSF GM-CSF

to irradiation and (4) reducing cell trafficking that communicates damage and increases cell death [36–38] (Table 5.1).

The discovery and development of radiation protectors/mitigators for space irradiation must address both protection and mitigation since protection against the first radiation exposure would be followed by mitigation of that first exposure but also must focus on protection from the next radiation exposure. Therefore, the discovery, development, and administration of radiation countermeasures for application to space irradiation must focus on both protection and mitigation capacity [39–41].

Antioxidants as Radiation Countermeasures

The first events in ionizing irradiation exposure are those associated with either direct DNA double-strand break damage or indirect damage through the production of free radicals in the cells that are derived from the ionization of major components in cells, oxygen, and water [42–53]. The discovery of antioxidants as radiation countermeasures raises a concern that those radiation sources, which produce direct DNA double-strand breaks (not going through free radical steps), might not be effectively countered by antioxidants [30–33]. However, recent evidence indicates that proton irradiation is also mitigated by an antioxidant drug (JP4-039—a GS-nitroxide) [34]. Other drugs with antioxidant capacity have also been shown to both protect and mitigate the lethality of protons and high LET particles [35]. How can this be the case? The answer may involve the production by dying cells of factors that consume antioxidants in other nonirradiated or surviving cells [36].

Consumption of antioxidant stores in cells, tissues, and organs leads to cell death and tissue lethality [33]. Therefore, increasing the capacity of molecular targets to withstand irradiation by having higher levels of antioxidants present was the first strategy for the development of radiation countermeasures [16, 38, 39]. Increasing the antioxidant capacity by dietary changes or delivery of antioxidant nutrients (vitamin E, vitamin C, and foods with high antioxidant capacity [40] (Table 5.1) was the first strategy. NASA-funded research demonstrated the capacity of this approach to protect against ionizing irradiation damage in model systems [40, 41]. Information on the effectiveness of antioxidants as a countermeasure has extended to experimental models of each of the multiple forms of expected space irradiation exposure: protons, galactic cosmic irradiation mediated by LET particles (GCR), and neutrons (from the GCR hitting the metallic and other components of the spacecraft). In each of these systems, an antioxidant approach to protection/mitigation showed some promise [37–41].

The capacity of organisms and animal models to increase their antioxidant stores revealed cautionary notes. The phenomenon of homeostasis has been established in multiple biological systems [42, 43]. A perturbation of antioxidant stores including the increase in levels would be expected to result in an adjustment by each organism and animal model to downregulate other systems to counteract the increased presence of antioxidants. This phenomenon has been demonstrated with transgenic animals, that were designed to overproduce a major antioxidant, manganese superoxide dismutase (MnSOD) [44] or Catalase [45]. These animals adapted to the overproduction of one antioxidant by potentially downregulating other oxidative stress defense mechanisms [44]. Furthermore, continuous overproduction or increased production of antioxidants had other deleterious effects, particularly, in the setting of developmental biology. Some transgenic mice suffered lethality or significant neurological damage by the overproduction of an antioxidant (Cu/ZnSOD) during gestation [46]. This phenomenon will be described in the section on Genetic Engineering. Scientists must be cognizant of the significant effects of overexpression of an antioxidant on the developing embryo.

Overproduction of a particular antioxidant may be deleterious during an embryonic developmental stage. Approaches to test this hypothesis have been to use a cre-flox system [47] to turn on the production of an antioxidant at high levels after successful gestation and after birth [48]. The ability to regulate the delivery of antioxidants is one goal of current research [46] With respect to solar proton events and exposure of spacecraft and astronauts to protons, the ability to predict an increase in proton exposure by the detection on Earth of the preceding gamma ray burst could lead to a system in which astronauts would be advised by Earth observers to administer an antioxidant stimulant supply at the time of a gamma ray burst, telling them that the proton fluence is coming. Rapid elevation of antioxidant stores at that time (rather than continually) could lead to radiation protection at the appropriate time without causing an adaptive change of the balance of homeostasis of the antioxidant stores that could persist after the solar proton event had passed.

A potential experimental model system would be one in which a continuous delivery of a radiation countermeasure at baseline levels [48] could be administered and then when an solar proton event (SPE) was expected, an additional bolus of another radioprotective agent could be delivered [47]. Such an experiment is logical and can be carried out in mouse models.

Radiation Countermeasures That Target DNA Repair and Minimize DNA Damage

A second logical target for the discovery and development of radiation countermeasures against space irradiation would focus on DNA double-strand break damage and its repair. Much evidence indicates that cells from animals with genetic causes of defective DNA repair are more radiosensitive, as are their tissues, organs, and organ systems (Table 5.1). Animal models of Fanconi Anemia (FA), Nijmegan Break Syndrome, Bloom's Syndrome, and Ataxia Telangiectasia are radiosensitive (see Chap. 3). Model systems in which overexpression of DNA repair enzymes or other mediators of double-strand break repair have been more difficult to study. In the case of the absence of a DNA repair enzyme leading to incomplete repair of DNA, the system may lead to the expression of an alternate pathway to provide such repair. However, this phenomenon is less efficient than the other cases of overexpression of a repair enzyme. Systems in which overexpression of a DNA repair enzyme had shown compensatory downregulation of other protective systems result in a normalization or homeostasis [42, 43]. The reason for this disparity in the response to a genetic modification in one direction is not obvious. One can hypothesize that during embryonic development, as well as, during post-partum growth, there is a need for a response to environmental DNA-damaging agents including irradiation. It may be necessary for tissues and organ systems to eliminate DNA damage to cells as part of an organized strategy to return to baseline homeostasis. Blocking the organisms need for elimination of defective or injured cells can be deleterious.

Animal models of enzyme deficiency [49] lead the animals to be vulnerable to the absense of the ability to eliminate cell populations during development. There followed a significant developmental defect [48]. In one case, hyperplasia of the developing brain and nervous system was seen in Caspase-1 knockout mice. Further research demonstrated that developing tissues during gestation must be able to eliminate defective cells by Caspase-mediated apoptosis [49]. Blocking this process of apoptotic cell death from irradiation could also lead to abnormalities in growth and development in fetal animals [47]. Further studies must be carried out to test this hypothesis.

The development of mouse embryos that are irradiated in utero is associated with damage to the central nervous system if the irradiation is delivered at that time during gestation when the brain and blood vessels are developing [50]. Targeting a developing mouse embryo with an antioxidant drug (JP4-039), which was delivered to the mother and can cross the placenta and enter the developing brain, resulted in the amelioration of damage to both the brain and the blood vessels [50]. However, in one study, the irradiated surviving animals did have neurocognitive defects suggesting that radiation protection might induce other unexpected events and, thus, be expected to be incomplete [50].

For radiation countermeasures that target DNA double-strand breaks and induce repair, it is also important to recognize the ability of cells, tissues, organs, and organ systems to adapt even during gestation. The DNA repair defect that is found in Fanconi Anemia mice (as described in a previous Chap. 3) leads to the hematopoietic system defects. FA animals (Fancd2−/−) that were genetically engineered to have an absent critical component of the DNA repair scaffold (namely, Fancd2) were shown to display bone marrow failure that was mediated by hypersensitivity of their bone marrow stem cells to the suppressive cytokine; namely, TGF-β [51]. It was hypothesized that creating a situation in which Fancd2−/− mice were also defective in TGF-β signaling might restore normal hematopoiesis [52]. These animals might not have the anemia that is displayed in Fancd2−/− mice. When double-knockout mice were created that were missing both Fancd2 and SMAD3 (a critical component of TGF-β signaling), these animals showed the opposite effect; namely, death during fetal gestation [52]. Analysis of the mechanism of this unexpected result was enlightening. The Fancd2−/− mice are defective in the DNA repair mechanism known as homologous recombination [52]. They survived by their capacity to rely during gestation on the alternative mechanism to repair DNA double-strand breaks; namely, nonhomologous end-joining (NHEJ) [52]. An unexpected effect of adding the SMAD3−/− genotype to the Fancd2−/− genotype was that there was a suppression of the NHEJ repair mechanism, leaving the developing embryos with no way to repair DNA double-strand breaks [52]. Most embryos died in utero. Given that there are over 1000 DNA double-strand breaks detected during every cell division, cells must have some way to repair this form of damage. The importance of this experimental result with double-knockout (DKO) Fancd2−/− SMAD3−/− mice [52] is relevant to space radiation and the use of countermeasures. Approaches must take into account the consequences of delivering a countermeasure, which, while appearing as a simple and direct approach, may lead to unexpected consequences caused by the ability of the body to downregulate compensatory and, thus, critical processes for survival.

Radiation Countermeasures Focused on Cytokines and the Inflammatory Response

There is much evidence that both acute ionizing irradiation damage and chronic damage are accompanied by an inflammatory response [53]. The response is radiation dose and radiation quality dependent. Administration of cytokines that can suppress the effects of those that are induced by irradiation has been a highly effective strategy for developing new radiation countermeasures (Table 5.1). For example, the increase in production of irradiated cells and tissues of IL-1, TNF-α, TGF-β, and others [48–53] can be countered by the administration of cytokines that reverse the suppressive effects of these inflammatory cytokines on the bone marrow. The use of stimulatory agents that counteract these cytokines such as G-CSF does work (Table 5.1).

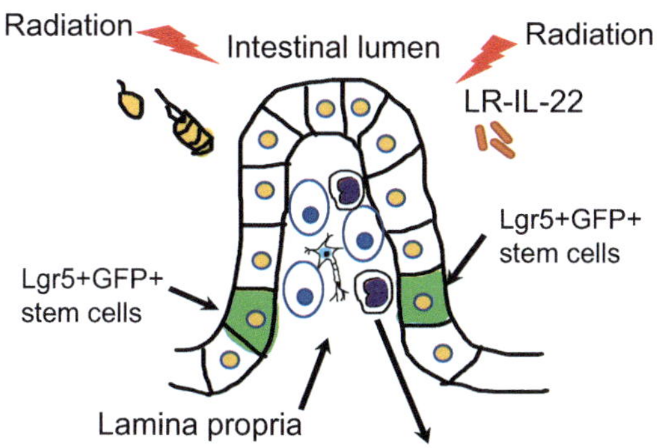

Fig. 5.1 Novel genetically engineered Lactobacillus reuteri delivering IL-22 to the radiation exposed intestine is a mitigator. The intestinal villi are shown in the figure and the intestinal stem cells, which in the mouse model are Lgr5 + gfp + (green). These cells are hit by irradiation and are damaged. Delivering the protective and mitigative cytokine IL-22 by Lactobacillus reuteri (genetically engineered, refs. 56–58) stimulates protection of the green intestinal stem cells and also regeneration of the intestinal cripts

Strategies to Discover and Develop New Radiation Countermeasures Against Space Irradiation

Given that it will be very challenging to detect changes in the background levels of space irradiation and the relative components from X-ray, proton, GCI mediated high energy particles, and neutrons, given the problem that the administration of countermeasures could lead to adaptation of humans to agents delivered, the issue of safety must be first and prominent in this area of research. Agents to maintain and replenish antioxidant stores appear to be a logical focus of research. Similarly, agents that minimize DNA double-strand break damage or stimulate repair also appears as a sound approach. While each of these biological approaches continues, there are also other places, where radiation countermeasures can be developed. The most novel and potentially existing approach is to use genetically engineered bacteria to deliver by swallowing radiation countermeasures to the intestine [50–54] (Fig. 5.1). This GI-ARS countermeasure appears to deliver mitigation to the bone marrow, which makes it a possible multi-system radiation mitigator [54–58].

Preventing Biologic Effects of Space Radiation by Shielding

The materials used to construct a space vehicle (such as graphene) have been tested for their ability to limit the transit of each form of irradiation [59]. New materials that are of lightweight, but also can resist each form of irradiation are being developed and represent an ideal strategy for protecting and mitigating space-radiation damage [59] which appears to be one such system. It appears that radiation countermeasures must include both physical modification of the spacecraft, particularly, to limit neutron production but also radiobiological agents that can correct or reduce the damage to cells, tissues, organs, and organ systems [60, 61].

References

1. Guo J, Zeitlin C, Wimmer-Schweingruber RF, et al. Radiation environment for future human exploration on the surface of Mars: the current understanding based on MSL/RAD dose measurements. Astron Astrophys Rev. 2021;29:article #8.
2. Wang L, Zhang Z, Shen X, et al. Effects of solar proton events associated with X-ray flares on near-Earth electron and proton fluxes based on ZH-1 satellite observations. Frontiers. Earth Sci. 2022;10:article 895561.
3. Gopalswamy N, Makela P, Yashiro S, et al. Source of energetic protons in the 2014 September 1 sustained gamma-ray emission event. Sol Phys. 2020;295(2):18. https://doi.org/10.1007/s11207-020-1590-8.
4. Norbury JW, Schimmerling W, Slaba TC, et al. Galactic cosmic ray simulation at the NASA space radiation laboratory. Life Sci Space Res (Amst). 2016;8:38–51. https://doi.org/10.1016/j.lssr.2016.02.001.
5. Barthel J, Sarigul-Klijn N. Radiation production and absorption in human spacecraft shielding systems under high charge and energy galactic cosmic rays: material medium, shielding depth, and byproduct aspects. Acta Astronaut. 2018;144:254–62.
6. Litvak ML, Mitrofanov IG, Sanin AB, et al. Observations of neutron radiation environment during odyssey cruise to Mars. Life Sci Space Res (Amst). 2021;29:53–62. https://doi.org/10.1016/j.lssr.2021.03.003.
7. Heldmann JL, Marinova MM, Lim DSS, et al. Mission architecture using the SpaceX starship vehicle to enable a sustained human presence on Mars. New Space. 2022;10(3):259–73. https://doi.org/10.1089/space.2020.0058.
8. Bromet EJ. Emotional consequences of nuclear power plant disasters. Health Phys. 2014;106(2):206–10. https://doi.org/10.1097/HP.0000000000000012.
9. Voorhies AA, Ott CM, Mehta S, et al. Study of the impact of long-duration space missions at the international space station on the astronaut microbiome. Sci Rep. 2019;9(1):9911. https://doi.org/10.1038/s41598-019-46303-8.
10. Delp MD, Charvat JM, Limoli CL, et al. Apollo lunar astronauts show higher cardiovascular disease mortality: possible deep space radiation effects on the vascular endothelium. Sci Rep. 2016;6:29901. https://doi.org/10.1038/srep29901.
11. Douple EB, Mabuchi K, Cullings HM, et al. Long-term radiation-related health effects in a unique human population: lessons learned from the atomic bomb survivors of Hiroshima and Nagasaki. Disaster Med Public Health Prep Suppl. 2011;1(01):S122–33. https://doi.org/10.1001/dmp.2011.21.
12. Moloney WC, Kastenbaum MA. Leukemogenic effects of ionizing radiation on atomic bomb survivors in Hiroshima city. Science. 1955;121(3139):308–9. https://doi.org/10.1126/science.121.3139.308.
13. Olson JD, Schaaf GW, Elgohari BA, et al. Radiation-induced pulmonary fibrosis in non-human primates (NHPs) is preceded by cellular senescence and upregulation of tyrosine kinase Fgr, which is detectable by bronchial alveolar (BAL) gavage. Radiat Res. 2024. (in press).
14. Cohen EP, Hankey KG, Bennett AW, et al. Acute and chronic kidney injury in a non-human primate model of partial-body irradiation with bone marrow sparing. Radiat Res. 2017;188(6):661–71. https://doi.org/10.1667/RR24857.1.
15. Raviraj J, Bokkasam VK, Kumar VS, et al. Radiosensitizers, radioprotectors, and radiation mitigators. Indian J Dent Res. 2014;25(1):83–90. https://doi.org/10.4103/0970-9290.131142.

16. Greenberger JS. Radioprotection. In Vivo. 2009;23(2):323–36.
17. Farhood B, Goradel NH, Mortezaee K, et al. Intercellular communications—redox interactions in radiation toxicity; potential targets for radiation mitigation. J Cell Commun Signal. 2019;13(1):3–16. https://doi.org/10.1007/s12079-018-0473-3.
18. Smith LE, Nagar S, Kim GJ, et al. Radiation-induced genomic instability: radiation quality and dose response. Health Phys. 2003;85(1):23–9. https://doi.org/10.1097/00004032-200307000-00006.
19. Limoli CL, Corcoran JJ, Milligan JR, et al. Critical target and dose-rate responses for the induction of chromosomal instability by ionizing radiation. Radiat Res. 1999;151(6):677–85.
20. Jackson IL, Vujaskovic Z, Down JD. Revisiting strain-related differences in radiation sensitivity of the mouse lung: recognizing and avoiding the confounding effects of pleural effusions. Radiat Res. 2010;173(1):10–20. https://doi.org/10.1667/RR1911.1.
21. Seed TM, Kaspar LV. Changing patterns of radiosensitivity of hematopoietic progenitors from chronically irradiated dogs prone either to aplastic anemia or to myeloproliferative disease. Leuk Res. 1990;14(4):299–307. https://doi.org/10.1016/0145-2126(90)90156-4.
22. Elkind MM, Sutton-Gilbert H, Moses WB, et al. Radiation response of mammalian cells grown in culture: V. temperature dependence of the repair of X-ray damage in surviving cells (aerobic and hypoxic). Radiat Res. 1965;25:359–76.
23. Puck TT, Marcus PI. Action of X-rays on mammalian cells. J Exp Med. 1956;103(5):653–66. https://doi.org/10.1084/jem.103.5.653.
24. Krisko A, Radman M. Biology of extreme radiation resistance: the way of Deinococcus radiodurans. Cold Spring Harb Perspect Biol. 2013;5(7):a012765. https://doi.org/10.1101/cshperspect.a012765.
25. Liu F, Li N, Zhang Y. The radioresistant and survival mechanisms of Deinococcus radiodurans. Radiat Med Protect. 2023;4(2):70–9.
26. Daly MJ. A new perspective on radiation resistance based on Deinococcus radiodurans. Nat Rev Microbiol. 2009;7(3):237–45. https://doi.org/10.1038/nrmicro2073.
27. Stankowski S, Zagrodzka ZB, Butler RK, et al. The genetic basis of a recent transition to live-bearing in marine snails. Science. 2024;383(6678):114–9. https://doi.org/10.1126/science.adi2982.
28. Ploemacher RE, van der Sluijs JP, Voerman JS, et al. An in vitro limiting-dilution assay of long-term repopulating hematopoietic stem cells in the mouse. Blood. 1989;74(8):2755–63.
29. Bernhard EJ, Maity A, Muschel RJ, et al. Effects of ionizing radiation on cell cycle progression. Radiat Environ Biophys. 1995;34(2):79–83. https://doi.org/10.1007/BF01275210.
30. Stockwell BR, Friedmann Angelli JP, et al. Ferroptosis: a regulated cell death nexus linking metabolism, redox biology, and disease. Cell. 2017;171(2):273–85. https://doi.org/10.1016/j.cell.2017.09.021.
31. DiCarlo AL, Hatchett RJ, Kaminski JM, et al. Medical countermeasures for radiation combined injury: radiation with burn, blast, trauma, and/or sepsis. Report of an NIAID workshop, march 26-27, 2007. Radiat Res. 2008;169(6):712–21. https://doi.org/10.1667/RR1295.1.
32. Jackson S. Sensing and repairing DNA double-strand breaks. Carcinogenesis. 2002;23(5):687–96. https://doi.org/10.1093/carcin/23.5.687.
33. Vertuani S, Angusti A, Manfredini S. The antioxidants and pro-antioxidants network: an overview. Curr Pharm Des. 2004;10(14):1677–94. https://doi.org/10.2174/1381612043384655.
34. Fink MP, Macias CA, Xiao J, et al. Hemigramicidin-TEMPO conjugates: novel mitochondria-targeted antioxidants. Crit Care Med. 2007;35(9 Suppl):S461–7. https://doi.org/10.1016/j.bcp.2007.05.019.
35. Quinn TJ, Ding X, Li X, et al. Amelioration of mucositis in proton therapy of Fanconi anemia fanca−/− mice by JP4-039. In Vivo. 2019;33(6):1757–66. https://doi.org/10.21873/invivo.11666.
36. Korystov YN. Contributions of the direct and indirect effects of ionizing radiation to reproductive cell death. Radiat Res. 1992;129(2):228–34.

37. Greenberger JS, Epperly MW. Radioprotective antioxidant gene therapy: potential mechanisms of action. Gene Ther Mol Biol. 2004;8:31–44.
38. Greenberger JS, Epperly MW. Pleiotrophic stem cell and tissue effects of ionizing irradiation protection by MnSOD-plasmid liposome gene therapy. In: Columbus F, editor. Progress in gene therapy. Nova Science Publications; 2005. p. 110–8.
39. Greenberger JS, Epperly MW. Antioxidant therapeutic approaches toward amelioration of the pulmonary pathophysiological damaging effects of ionizing irradiation. Curr Respir Med Rev. 2007;3:29–37.
40. Epperly MW, Wang H, Jones J. Antioxidant-chemoprevention diet ameliorates late effects of total body irradiation and supplements radioprotection by MnSOD-plasmid liposome administration. Radiat Res. 2011;175(6):759–65. https://doi.org/10.1667/RR2398.1.
41. Epperly MW, Epperly LD, Zhang X, et al. Overexpression of MnSOD transgene product protects cryopreserved bone marrow hematopoietic progenitor cells from ionizing irradiation. Radiat Res. 2007;168(5):560–6. https://doi.org/10.1667/RR1071R.1.
42. Puelles VG, Huber TB. Kidneys control inter-organ homeostasis. Nat Rev Nephrol. 2022;18(4):207–8. https://doi.org/10.1038/s41581-022-00549-0.
43. Selye H. Homeostasis and heterostasis. Perspect Biol Med. 1973;16(3):441–5. https://doi.org/10.1353/pbm.1973.0056.
44. Chen Z, Siu B, Ho Y-S, et al. Overexpression of MnSOD protects against myocardial ischemia/reperfusion injury in transgenic mice. J Mol Cell Cardiol. 1998;30(11):2281–9. https://doi.org/10.1006/jmcc.1998.0789.
45. Chen X, Liang H, Van Remmen H, et al. Catalase transgenic mice: characterization and sensitivity to oxidative stress. Arch Biochem Biophys. 2004;422(2):197–210. https://doi.org/10.1016/j.abb.2003.12.023.
46. Dal Canto MC, Gurney ME. Neuropathological changes in two lines of mice carrying a transgene for mutant human Cu,Zn SOD, and in mice overexpressing wild type human SOD: a model of familial amyotrophic lateral sclerosis (FALS). Brain Res. 1995;676(1):25–40. https://doi.org/10.1016/0006-8993(95)00063-v.
47. Hoess RH, Abremski K. The Cre-lox recombination system. In: Eckstein F, Lilley DMJ, editors. Nucleic acids and molecular biology 4. Berlin, Heidelberg: Springer-Verlag; 1990. p. 99–109.
48. Rhieu BH, Shinde A, Epperly MW, et al. Organ-specific responses of total body irradiated doxycycline-inducible manganese superoxide dismutase Tet/Tet mice. In Vivo. 2014;28(6):1033–43.
49. Le H-V, Minn AJ, Massague J. Cyclin-dependent kinase inhibitors uncouple cell cycle progression from mitochondrial apoptotic functions in DNA-damaged cancer cells. J Biol Chem. 2005;280(36):32018–25. https://doi.org/10.1074/jbc.M504689200.
50. Wu YL, Christodoulou AG, Beumer JH, et al. Amelioration of fetal irradiation injury form mid-gestation total body radiation with maternal administration of the mitochondrial-targeted GS-nitroxide JP4-039. Radiat Res. 2024.
51. Rodriguez A, Yang C, Furutani E, et al. Inhibition of TGFβ1 and TGFβ3 promotes hematopoiesis in Fanconi anemia. Exp Hematol. 2021;93:70–84. https://doi.org/10.1016/j.exphem.2020.11.002.
52. Rodriguez A, Epperly M, Filiatrault J, et al. TGFβ pathway is required for viable gestation of Fanconi anemia embryos. PLoS Genet. 2022;18(11):e1010459. https://doi.org/10.1371/journal.pgen.1010459.
53. Stromsnes K, Correas AG, Lehmann J, et al. Anti-inflammatory properties of diet: role in healthy aging. Biomedicines. 2021;9(8):922. https://doi.org/10.3390/biomedicines9080922.
54. Zhang X, Fisher R, Hou W, et al. Second generation probiotics producing IL-22 increase survival of mice after total body irradiation. In Vivo. 2020;34(1):39–50. https://doi.org/10.21873/invivo.11743.

55. Liu H-Y, Giraud A, Seignez C, et al. Distinct B cell subsets in Peyer's patches convey probiotic effects by *Limosilactobacillus reuteri*. Microbiome. 2021;9(1):198. https://doi.org/10.1186/s40168-021-01128-4.
56. Espinal A, Epperly MW, Mukherjee A, et al. Intestinal radiation protection and mitigation by second-generation probiotic *Lactobacillus reuteri* engineered to deliver Interleukin-22. Int J Mol Sci. 2022;23(10):5616. https://doi.org/10.3390/ijms23105616.
57. Hamade DF, Espinal A, Yu J, et al. Lactobacillus reuteri releasing IL-22 (LR-IL-22) facilitates intestinal radioprotection for whole-abdomen irradiation (WAI) of ovarian cancer. Radiat Res. 2022;198(1):89–105. https://doi.org/10.1667/RADE-21-00224.1.
58. Hamade DF, Epperly MW, Fisher R, et al. Release of interferon-β (IFN-β) from probiotic Limosolactobacillus reuteri-IFN-β (LR-IFN-β) mitigates gastrointestinal acute radiation syndrome (GI-ARS) following whole-abdominal irradiation. Cancers (Basel). 2023;15(6):1670. https://doi.org/10.3390/cancers15061670.
59. Mbayachi VB, Ndayiragije E, Sammani T, et al. Graphene synthesis, characterization and its applications: a review. Results Chem. 2021;3:100163.
60. Kagan VE, Wipf P, Stoyanovsky D, et al. Mitochondrial targeting of electron scavenging antioxidants: regulation of selective oxidation vs. random chain reactions. Adv Drug Deliv Rev. 2009;61(14):1375–85. https://doi.org/10.1016/j.addr.2009.06.008.
61. Shinde A, Epperly MW, Cao S, et al. Effects of the radiation mitigator bifunctional sulfoxide MMS350 on hematopoiesis and long-term bone marrow cultures. In Vivo. 2014;28(4):457–65.

Chapter 6
Prolonged Effects of Physiological Change, Psycho-Social Stress, Zero Gravity, Alterations in the Intestinal Microbiome, and Metabolism on the Response to Space Irradiation

It is no surprise that the majority of research and media publications on space travel focus on topics of concern for the health and welfare of astronauts separate from the concern about irradiation exposure [1–4]. The relative lack of attention to space irradiation is in part attributable to the fact that the majority of data published to date focuses on the more obvious concerns for astronauts, who will be spending significant time outside the Earth's atmosphere. These other nonradiation concerns include weightlessness [5–7]; social isolation; diet-induced changes [8–10]; possible trauma [11]; fractures [12]; infections [13, 14]; cancer [15, 16]; and aging [17–20]. Physiologic changes in the body called "adaptation," lack of exercise, and changes in metabolism that are attributable to the altered diet will include changes in the microbiome [8–10]. Also, there is concern about the effects of drugs used in first aid following injuries [11, 12] and infections [13, 14]. While ionizing irradiation is now clearly recognized as a major concern for planning lunar habitat missions and the Mars Mission, the other factors, in addition, have brought to light a new concern; namely, their interaction with ionizing irradiation [1–3]. Unlike the results of combined injury in the case of acute radiation exposure from a terrorist event, the combined injury of radiation during space travel will be relative to continuous low-dose effects.

The discovery and development of radiation countermeasures by the NIAID-funded Radiation Countermeasures Program, terms this phenomenon "combined injury" (Table 6.1). The latest countermeasures are orally injected genetically engineered bacteria [21–23], which may alter the microbiome [8–10]. Experiments carried out at the Armed Forces Radiological Institute (AFRRI) over the past decades revealed the profound effects of combined injury with ionizing irradiation. Prominent have been the physiologic changes that will occur during space travel [24–28]. There has been recognition of multiple independent physiologic factors on increasing the magnitude of damage by adding radiation to bone wound healing [12], recovery from infection [13, 14], soft tissue wound healing [11], blunt force trauma [11], concussion, and aging [17–20]. There is general agreement among

J. Greenberger, *Radiation Oncology and Radiation Biology*,
https://doi.org/10.1007/978-3-031-66300-0_6

Table 6.1 Potential "Combined Injury" effects that may exacerbate space radiation

Category	Example
Zero-gravity	Weightlessness
Social isolation	PTSD, Shell shock
Infection	Viral illness
Thermal burn	Electrical burn
Concussion	Trauma
Bone loss	Osteoporosis
Muscle-loss	Lack of exercise
Aging	Cell senescence accumulates
Polypharmacy	Pain medicine Antibiotic Phenergan for adaptation

radiation oncologists that comorbid medical conditions exacerbate ionizing irradiation effects with respect to both acute and late radiation-induced cell damage and cell death pathways [14, 15]. Cancer risk for astronauts is a major concern [16] and has been ever since radiation was linked to cancer in humans [17]. There is clearly a uniform concern about accelerated aging during space travel [18–20].

There is also emerging evidence that the female gender provides a relative radioresistance; although, the mechanism is not currently understood [19, 20, 25–27]. Estrogen has significant positive effects on several aspects of the physical stamina of muscles, the amelioration of bone degradation, estrogen positivity effects utilization of endocrine hormones, as well as, cardiac and pulmonary health [25, 26]. Estrogen also has distinct effects on altering the intestinal microbiome, and, potentially, stimulating the overabundance of specific bacterial taxa that contribute to a more balanced metabolic control of nutrition [27–33].

There are several categories of concern about combined injury involving radiation and also the impact of prior genetic and medical conditions on radiation tolerance, as it relates to the health of astronauts and their capacity to resist the deleterious effects of radiation exposure. Microgravity may affect the treatments delivered for infections [29–34]. Gene regulation is altered by microgravity [35, 36]. Astronauts themselves report the need for exercise equipment during prolonged missions since physical health is critical to all other challenges [37].

Effect of Weightlessness on Ionizing Irradiation-Induced Damage

Animal experiments carried out in the space shuttle and the International Space Station confirmed prior studies with cells in culture including mammalian cells, bacteria, and yeast with respect to changes in basic principles of cell function under conditions of weightlessness [5–7]. Zero gravity alters chemical reactions. Zero gravity alters chemical reactions, as it relates to Materials Science and Metallurgy. In a recent publication concerning Materials Science, the chemistry of the assembly of materials has been shown to be different in the absence of gravity [28]. The evolution of life on Earth began with biochemical processes that led to the creation of nucleic acids, the building blocks of DNA and RNA. In more complex multicellular animals, as well as, in Eukaryotes, that contain the organelles including cytoplasmic mitochondria; the transport of newly synthesized proteins from the nucleus to mitochondria evolved as chemical reactions and physiologic functions all in the oxygenated environment of gravity on Earth. The biology of bacteria, fungi, and other human symbiotes and pathogens is different in microgravity [29–36].

When basic chemical processes were studied under the condition of weightlessness, the results were different. In the case of the construction of graphene (a synthetic biomaterial that is being considered for the construction of space vehicles due to its resilience to extremes of temperature and also it radiation resistance, there was improved molecular assembly under the conditions of weightlessness) [28]. There is current concern that these materials science experiments will also impact and alter the basic cellular biochemical reactions and may also, ultimately, the functioning of cells [29–37]. Human tissues and organs, as well as, symbiotic and pathogenic microbes may function differently under conditions of prolonged weightlessness.

The longest space missions to date, in which astronauts have lived in the International Space Station for periods of months, have demonstrated profound physiologic changes in the human body that are attributable to weightlessness. A basic principle is that the human body, like that of experimental animals, functions differently in the absence of gravity. One of the first observations with astronauts in the International Space Station was the phenomenon of bone loss in zero-gravity environment. Space mission astronauts requested the availability of an exercise bike or exercise equipment to allow muscle contraction on bones and joints to reduce bone loss [37]. It has been established that hospitalized patients on prolonged bed rest display significant bone loss, as well as, pressure-produced ulceration of skin, underlying subcutaneous fat, and musculature. The phenomenon of cachexia from cancer is known to be exacerbated by prolonged bed rest [37–41]. Exercise is known to stimulate wound healing and recovery from trauma.

How does weightlessness affect the ionizing irradiation responses? Ionizing irradiation induces a rapid consumption of antioxidant stores in cells due to the production of radical oxygen species (ROS) (ionization of water and oxygen). The biochemical events associated with response to oxidative stress include activation of the cellular antioxidant system [42]. Glutathione is a small molecule, whose presence throughout the microanatomy of cells is responsible for the neutralization of free radicals. Induction of antioxidant enzymes including superoxide dismutase, catalase, and glutathione peroxidase also occurs rapidly after irradiation exposure and is a continual course of antioxidant responses to all forms of inflammation including that induced by ionizing irradiation [43–45].

Biochemical reactions that control the production of glutathione and other components of the antioxidant defense system are altered in the absence of gravity [42,

43]. The magnitude of changes is known to increase over time. Physiologic changes that have been reported to occur after prolonged weightlessness can be in part managed by providing dietary supplements that can increase levels of antioxidants and facilitate resistance to irradiation. Whether the zero-gravity atmosphere alters the process is a subject of current research. Diet changes and providing exercise equipment and other methods by which to keep muscles active can prevent loss of bone, health of joints, and both the axial and peripheral skeleton strength to allow normal activities such as those on the Earth's surface [40–43].

A challenge for NASA and other scientists working on the TRISH Program (Translational Research Institute for Space Health Program) in designing experimental systems to stimulate the effects of prolonged weightlessness and life outside the magnetosphere has been the difficulty in stimulating a zero-gravity atmosphere on Earth [43]. One method that was studied was that of the "suspended limb" model. In these experiments, one hind limb of a rodent was maintained suspended in the air above the animal and kept in a state where the action of muscles on joints and bones could be eliminated. This system, while known to be imperfect, has been used widely due to the convenience of the establishment of the model. Experiments with weightlessness in animals can be simulated by placing them in a centrifuge environment to counteract the effects of gravity. These experiments have also revealed profound differences in cellular, tissue, organs, and organ system functioning [43]. The available published data on the effects of weightlessness on radiobiology are limited. Basic radiation survival curves and radiation chemistry experiments cannot efficiently be carried out on the space station in a zero-gravity atmosphere. Complicating this focus of research is the need for providing either artificial gravity or simulation of the effects of gravity on the skeleton and other organ systems for the astronauts' health and the maintenance of a good environment in which to carry out the weightlessness experiments. The available evidence indicates that the radiobiology of X-rays is altered by weightlessness, though, the magnitude and the conditions are yet to be defined [43]. Less data are available on protons, GCI, or neutrons in part due to the expense of producing these radiation sources.

Psychosocial Effects of Stress on the Response to Space Irradiation

The pathophysiology of stress has been a subject of intense investigation primarily in the accumulating information with military veterans returning from combat and those, who have survived terrifying conditions of war. The phenomenon was termed "shell-shock" experienced by World War I veterans, "battle fatigue" experienced by World War II veterans, and "Post-Traumatic Stress Disorder" (PTSD) in veterans of the Vietnam War and missions in Iraq and Afghanistan. The data from all generations have confirmed the profound physiologic changes that follow these stress experiences. The stress experienced by those in social isolation has also been studied. Prisoners in solitary confinement, miners trapped in collapsed mine environments, and those living in social isolation have provided data on the physiologic changes, including steroid hormone levels that accompany social isolation. Do these conditions affect the ionizing irradiation response? It is known that steroid hormone elevation reduces the production of inflammatory cytokines in radiotherapy patients, who receive steroids to reduce edema of the irradiated brain, spinal cord, or lung [46]. There is a rebound effect of irradiation when the steroids are withdrawn or tapered, and the symptoms and edema can return sometimes in a more severe pattern [47].

There is some available information from experiments with rodents that are maintained in single animal metabolic cages, compared to those maintained in communities. Those in isolation have different levels of plasma hormones, detectable differences in endocrine function, metabolism, and serum/plasma levels of other cytokines as well. To extrapolate these changes to the response to ionizing irradiation, there are many complicating factors. As described in earlier chapters, space irradiation is a combination of a mixed beam effect (protons, high LET particles including ionized atoms from galactic cosmic irradiation, X-rays, and neutrons). Furthermore, the levels of exposure to space irradiation are changing in quality and changes are sporadic. While there is a chronic low level of cumulative exposure, the fact that this occurs at unpredictable times and the intervals between significant levels of exposure are unpredictable. Therefore, to study the physiologic changes that result from an experimental model cannot be assumed to be the same in the setting of chronic and sporadic mixed beam irradiation.

Effect of Polypharmacy on Space Irradiation

The effects of administration of small molecule therapeutics including stimulants and suppression of any biochemical processes may be exacerbated by ionizing irradiation [44–45]. A common factor with conditions that may merit the administration of a drug during a space mission: (infection, pain, and trauma) is that of drug effects on inflammatory cytokine release. The stress of prolonged social isolation and limited socialization for astronauts may also contribute to altered or elevated levels of inflammatory cytokines and hormones [46, 48]. One study has been focused on the pituitary peptide hormone, oxytocin, a peptide that is released following the action of a "releasing factor" that is made in the hypothalamus. Oxytocin has been shown to be elevated during maternal–child interactions [49], and other positive social eye-contact interactions [49]. Oxytocin levels increase following eye contact with other individuals in social groups, and have recently been shown to be reduced in people with social-developmental disorders including autism [49]. This hormone has been used to treat autistic children to stimulate interaction with other people. Oxytocin levels increase in both humans and dogs during the eye contact of positive interactions [49]. Oxytocin levels in astronauts and in experimental animal studies have been shown to be altered by the conditions of space travel [50]. How oxytocin levels affect the irradiation response has been studied in some experiments. Oxytocin, as well as, other peptide hormones, and hormone-releasing factors have been studied with respect to the basic radiation survival curves, as well as, measures of irradiation-induced cell death [50].

Irradiation Induction of Cell Death or Senescence and Late Effects

Radiation-induced cell death overlaps with cell death induced by a variety of factors that are present in "combined injury."

At least six forms of cell death have been described: apoptosis, necroptosis, ferroptosis, parthanatos, pyroptosis, and intra-mitotic death [44, 45]. Each of these forms of cell death is induced by ionizing irradiation and is also induced by other factors, which may contribute to the environment of astronauts during a prolonged space mission. Each of these forms of cell death can also lead to the condition of cellular senescence in which cells neither die nor recover the ability to proliferate, but rather sit in tissues and elaborate proteins known, and the senescence-associated secretory phenotype (SASP) [51–53]. The production of some SASP proteins can induce inflammation. Senescence has been investigated with respect to other forms of stress, but not all have been studied with respect to combination with ionizing irradiation. The irradiation-induced stimulation of these cell death pathways in specific organs by factors other than irradiation can occur during a prolonged space mission and may influence not only the bone marrow and intestinal repair capacities from irradiation exposure but also have effects on other organ systems.

Not all people can be astronauts. The ability to adapt to the psychosocial changes of a prolonged space mission, as well as, weightlessness has been studied in astronauts, who are selected for space missions by their psychosocial, as well as, physiologic screening to estimate their capacity to endure a stressful environment. Managing the challenges of controlling the environment in an unpredictable situation presents a need to adapt to stress. Simply having individuals, who are skilled in managing stress levels and who are conditioned for prolonged space missions does guarantee their successful coping with events that are associated with psychosocial stress. The effects of space radiation must be studied relative to changes in hormone levels, the changes in cytokine levels, and the effect of mixed beam irradiation in both the acute and chronic paradigms.

Effects of Infection on the Response to Space Radiation

There is ample evidence that the balance, as well as, the types of bacterial, viral, fungal, and other agents causing infections change after the irradiation exposure responses [34, 54]. Published data report the profound effects of infection and/or anti-bacterial agents on radiation responses of cells in culture and also in animals [55–57]. Astronauts will be taking with them complex microbiome. Meta-analysis of the intestinal microbiome has now been elevated to the level of hoarding the distribution of taxa of bacteria, as well as, viruses and fungi in the intestine [34, 54]. Changes in the relative distribution of taxa, termed alpha and beta diversity [54], have been shown to affect intestinal metabolism and communication of inflammatory events in the intestine (infection, as well as, response to ionizing irradiation) to other organs and organ systems.

Studies were carried out on germ-free mice, as well as, mice maintained on constant treatment with antimicrobials with respect to irradiation response. These data have shown that both the infectious agents, and the administration of antimicrobial agents alters radiosensitivity [55, 56]. In the confined space of a space vehicle or space station, better conditions of maintenance of appropriate levels of oxygen and carbon dioxide in the ambient air, there will be a potential for transmission of infectious agents. There is no logical or practical way to "sterilize" astronauts for a prolonged space mission. Therefore, individuals will carry with them not only their own intestinal microbiome (which varies between individuals and is associated with prior dietary history, as well as, levels of production of digestive hormones and other historical factors) but also their own aerodigestive tract microbiome [54]. One of the challenges for NASA has been to establish what medical equipment, drugs, and other countermeasures can be reasonably stored and provided on a space vehicle. Discussions about which antibiotics, what anti-inflammatory agents, and what drugs should be included in the "medical kit" on a space vehicle are ongoing.

Effect of Diet on Response to Space Radiation

Control of the diet of astronauts, in the zero-gravity environment, has been a subject of intense investigation over the decades since the first manned space vehicle experiments. Liquid food materials have been defined. Studies of the changes in the human microbiome between individuals that would occur during weeks/months of confinement in a space vehicle have been studied [8, 57]. The microbiome does change and specific diets could alter it [8, 21–23, 34, 54]. However, studies in humans, particularly, those with chronic infections such as that in *Clostridium difficile* (*C. diff*) have revealed individual responses to a specific pathogen [54]. Experiments with the radiation survival of animals given radiation countermeasures that target each of the cell death pathways have been carried out and can alter the microbiome is the lung and potentially alter the intestine [34, 54] resulting in a change in the intestinal microbiome.

There has been a recent interest in "elite survivors" of total body irradiation [34] looking at the effect of the change in the microbiome on those animals that survive a dose of irradiation, which is expected to kill 50% of animals. The specific bacterial taxa that have been associated with survival have been reported [54]. There is a consensus that infection will alter ionizing irradiation response in both experimental animals and in humans. How these infections will translate to alterations in the functioning of critical organs is not known.

Combinations of Multiple Components of Combined Injury

Each of several categories of potential factors that react with ionizing irradiation has been discussed individually. Publications of experiments with each of the above factors combined with irradiation have been helpful but have limited predictive value. Combinations of the effects of multiple factors with radiation require a more complex analysis. The presence of simultaneous ionizing irradiation, zero gravity, social isolation, and infection may occur in varying patterns. The phenomenon of wound healing and trauma must be addressed when combined with the other factors listed above. More intensive research must follow with respect to animal model systems, but also with the analysis of the evidence from prolonged space missions. Administration of radiation countermeasures against chronic mixed beam exposure must be determined to be safe in the polypharmacy of treatment of the various confounding components of combined injury. For example, an infection sustained by an astronaut during a space mission may require administration of an antibiotic drug. The response to a drug may alter the irradiation response [54, 55]. Several antibiotics have been shown to have separate actions as radiation protectors or mitigators [55]. Future studies will undoubtedly address the complexity of managing the effects of space irradiation in the complex environment of space travel.

References

1. Ehresmann B, Hassler DM, Zeitlin C, et al. Charged particle spectra measured during the transit to Mars with the Mars science laboratory radiation assessment detector (MSL/RAD). Life Sci Space Res (Amst). 2016;10:29–37. https://doi.org/10.1016/j.lssr.2016.07.001.
2. Zeitlin C, Hassler DM, Cucinotta FA, et al. Measurements of energetic particle radiation in transit to Mars on the Mars science laboratory. Science. 2013;340(6136):1080–4. https://doi.org/10.1126/science.1235989.
3. Hassler DM, Zeitlin C, Wimmer-Schweingruber RF, et al. Mars' surface radiation environment measured with the Mars science laboratory's curiosity rover. Science. 2014;343(6169):1244797. https://doi.org/10.1126/science.1244797.
4. Tachibana K, Tachibana S, Inoue N. From outer space to earth-the social significance of isolated and confined environment research in human space exploration. Acta Astronaut. 2017;140:273–83.

5. Vico L, Lafage-Proust MH, Alexandre C. Effects of gravitational changes on the bone system in vitro and in vivo. Bone. 1998;22(5 Suppl):95S–100S. https://doi.org/10.1016/s8756-3282(98)00017-9.
6. Nixon JV, Murray RG, Bryant C, et al. Early cardiovascular adaptation to simulated zero gravity. J Appl Physiol Respir Environ Exerc Physiol. 1979;46(3):541–8. https://doi.org/10.1152/jappl.1979.46.3.541.
7. Baldwin KM, Herrick RE, Hyina-Kakueva E, et al. Effects of zero gravity on myofibril content and isomyosin distribution in rodent skeletal muscle. FASEB J. 1990;4(1):79–83. https://doi.org/10.1096/fasebj.4.1.2136840.
8. Epperly MW, Wang H, Jones J, et al. Antioxidant-chemopreventive diet ameliorates late effects of total body irradiation and supplements radioprotection by MnSOD-plasmid liposome administration. Radiat Res. 2011;175(6):759–65. https://doi.org/10.1667/RR2398.1.
9. Voorhies AA, Lorenzi HA. The challenge of maintaining a healthy microbiome during long-duration space missions. Front Astron Space Sci. 2016;3:23.
10. Siddiqui R, Akbar N, Khan NA. Gut microbiome and human health under the space environment. J Appl Microbiol. 2021;130(1):14–24. https://doi.org/10.1111/jam.14789.
11. Alexander DJ. Trauma and surgical capabilities for space exploration. In: Gilman LM, Widder S, Blaivas M, Karakitsos D, editors. Trauma team dynamics. Cham: Springer International Publishing; 2016. p. 253–66.
12. Gokhale AS, Epperly M, Glowacki J, et al. Small molecule GS-nitroxide and MnSOD gene therapy ameliorate ionizing irradiation-induced delay in bone wound healing in a novel murine model. In Vivo. 2010;24(4):377–85.
13. Taylor PW, Sommer AP. Towards rational treatment of bacterial infections during extended space travel. Int J Antimicrob Agents. 2005;26(3):183–7. https://doi.org/10.1016/j.ijantimicag.2005.06.002.
14. Dar HH, Epperly MW, Tyurin VA, et al. *P. aeruginosa* augments irradiation injury via 15-lipoxygenase-catalyzed generation of 15-HpETE-PE and induction of theft-ferroptosis. JCI Insight. 2022;7(4):e156013. https://doi.org/10.1172/jci.insight.156013.
15. Samhan-Arias AK, Ji J, Demidova OM, et al. Oxidized phospholipids as biomarkers of tissue and cell damage with a focus on cardiolipin. Biochim Biophys Acta. 2012;1818(10):2413–23. https://doi.org/10.1016/j.bbamem.2012.03.014.
16. Brenner DJ, Doll R, Goodhead DT, et al. Cancer risks attributable to low doses of ionizing radiation: assessing what we really know. Proc Natl Acad Sci USA. 2003;100(24):13761–6. https://doi.org/10.10703/pnas.2235592100.
17. Pierce DA, Shimizu Y, Preston DL, et al. Studies of the mortality of atomic bomb survivors. Report 12, Part 1. Radiat Res. 1996;146(1):1–27.
18. Wang E. Age-dependent atrophy and microgravity travel: what do they have in common? FASEB J. 1999;13(Suppl):S167–74. https://doi.org/10.1096/fasebj.13.9001.s167.
19. Epperly MW, Smith T, Wang H, et al. Modulation of total body irradiation induced life shortening by systemic intravenous MnSOD-plasmid liposome gene therapy. Radiat Res. 2008;170(4):437–43. https://doi.org/10.1667/rr1286.1.
20. Zhou S, Greenberger JS, Epperly MW, et al. Age-related intrinsic changes in human bone marrow-derived mesenchymal stem cells and their differentiation to osteoblasts. Aging Cell. 2008;7(3):335–43. https://doi.org/10.1111/j.1474-9726.2008.00377.x.
21. Hamade DF, Epperly MW, Fisher R, et al. Release of interferon-β (IFN-β) from probiotic Limosilactobacillus reuteri-IFN-β (LR-IFN-β) mitigates gastrointestinal acute radiation syndrome (GI-ARS) following whole abdominal irradiation. Cancers (Basel). 2023;15(6):1670. https://doi.org/10.3390/cancers15061670.
22. Espinal A, Epperly MW, Mukherjee A, et al. Intestinal radiation protection and mitigation by second-generation probiotic Lactobacillus-reuteri engineered to deliver Interleukin-22. Int J Mol Sci. 2022;23(10):5616. https://doi.org/10.3390/ijms23105616.

23. Hamade DF, Espinal A, Yu J, et al. Lactobacillus reuteri releasing IL-22 (LR-IL-22) facilitates intestinal radioprotection for whole-abdomen irradiation (WAI) of ovarian cancer. Radiat Res. 2022;198(1):89–105. https://doi.org/10.1667/RADE-21-00224.1.
24. Patterson AM, Vemula S, Plett PA, et al. Age and sex divergence in hematopoietic radiosensitivity in aged mouse models of the hematopoietic acute radiation syndrome. Radiat Res. 2022;198(3):221–42. https://doi.org/10.1667/RADE-22-00071.1.
25. Gilligan DM, Quyyumi AA, Cannon RO 3rd. Effects of physiological levels of estrogen on coronary vasomotor function in postmenopausal women. Circulation. 1994;89(6):2545–51. https://doi.org/10.1161/01.cir.89.6.2545.
26. Ruggiero RJ, Likis FE. Estrogen: physiology, pharmacology, and formulations for replacement therapy. J Midwifery Womens Health. 2002;47(3):130–8. https://doi.org/10.1016/S1526-9523(02)00233-7.
27. Baker JM, Al-Nakkash L, Herbst-Kralovetz MM. Estrogen-gut microbiome axis: physiological and clinical implications. Maturitas. 2017;103:45–53. https://doi.org/10.1016/j.maturitas.2017.06.025.
28. Chen C, Feng S, Peng H, et al. Thermocapillary convection flow and heat transfer characteristics of graphene nanoplatelet based nanofluid under microgravity. Microgravity Sci Technol. 2021;33:article #40.
29. Tirumalai MR, Karouia F, Tran Q, et al. Evaluation of acquired antibiotic resistance in *Escherichia coli* exposed to long-term low-shear modeled microgravity and background antibiotic exposure. MBio. 2019;10(1):e02637. https://doi.org/10.1128/mBio.02637-18.
30. Tirumalai MR, Karouia F, Tran Q, et al. The adaptation of *Escherichia coli* cells grown in simulated microgravity for an extended period is both phenotypic and genomic. NPJ Microgravity. 2017;3:15. https://doi.org/10.1038/s41526-017-0020-1.
31. Hammond TG, Stodieck L, Birdsall HH, et al. Effects of microgravity on the virulence of Listeria monocytogenes, Enterococcus faecalis, Candida albicans, and Methyicillin-resistant Staphylococcus aureus. Astrobiology. 2013;13(11):1081–90. https://doi.org/10.1089/ast.2013.0986.
32. Rosenzweig JA, Ahmed S, Eunson J Jr, et al. Low-shear force associated with modeled microgravity and spaceflight does not similarly impact the virulence of notable bacterial pathogens. Appl Microbiol Biotechnol. 2014;98(21):8797–807. https://doi.org/10.1007/s00253-014-6025-8.
33. Knox BP, Blachowicz A, Palmer JM, et al. Characterization of *Aspergillus fumigatus* isolates form air and surfaces of the international Space Station. mSphere. 2021;1(5):e00227–16. https://doi.org/10.1128/mSphere.00227-16.
34. Guo H, Chou W-C, Ting JPY, et al. Multi-omics analyses of radiation survivors identify radioprotective microbes and metabolites. Science. 2020;370(6516):eaay9097. https://doi.org/10.1126/science.aay9097.
35. Bijlani S, Stephens E, Singh NK, et al. Advances in space microbiology. iScience. 2021;24(5):102395. https://doi.org/10.1016/j.isci.2021.102395.
36. Corydon TJ, Schulz H, Richter P, et al. Current knowledge about the impact of microgravity on gene regulation. Cells. 2023;12(7):1043. https://doi.org/10.3390/cells12071043.
37. Glover EI, Phillips SM. Resistance exercise and appropriate nutrition to counteract muscle wasting and promote muscle hypertrophy. Curr Opin Nutr Metab Care. 2010;13(6):630–4. https://doi.org/10.1097/MCO.0b013e32833f1ae5.
38. Deuster PA, Morrison SD, Ahrens RA. Endurance exercise modifies cachexia of tumor growth in rats. Med Sci Sports Exerc. 1985;17(3):385–92.
39. Evans WJ, Morley JE, Argiles J, et al. Cachexia: a new definition. Clin Nutr. 2008;27(6):793–9. https://doi.org/10.1016/j.clnu.2008.06.013.
40. Galvao DA, Newton RU. Review of exercise intervention studies in cancer patients. J Clin Oncol. 2005;23(4):899–909. https://doi.org/10.1200/JCO.2005.06.085.

41. Dimeo F, Stieglitz RD, Novelli-Fischer U, et al. Correlation between physical performance and fatigue in cancer patients. Ann Oncol. 1997;8(12):1251–5. https://doi.org/10.1023/a:1008234310474.
42. Stein TP. Space flight and oxidative stress. Nutrition. 2002;18(10):867–71. https://doi.org/10.1016/s0899-9007(02)00938-3.
43. Herranz R, Anken R, Boonstra J, et al. Ground-based facilities for simulation of microgravity: organism-specific recommendations for their use, and recommended terminology. Astrobiology. 2013;13(1):1–17. https://doi.org/10.1089/ast.2012.0876.
44. Steinman J, Epperly M, Hou W, et al. Improved total-body irradiation survival by delivery of two radiation mitigators that target distinct cell death pathways. Radiat Res. 2018;189(1):68–83. https://doi.org/10.1667/RR14787.1.
45. Thermozier S, Hou W, Zhang X, et al. Anti-ferroptosis drug enhances total body irradiation mitigation by drugs that block apoptosis and necroptosis. Radiat Res. 2020;193(5):435–50. https://doi.org/10.1667/RR15486.1.
46. Galhardo L, Oliveira RF. The effects of social isolation on steroid hormone levels are modulated by previous social status and context in a cichlid fish. Horm Behav. 2014;65(1):1–5. https://doi.org/10.1016/j.yhbeh.2013.10.010.
47. Azria D, Magne N, Zouhair A, et al. Radiation recall: a well recognized but neglected phenomenon. Cancer Treat Rev. 2005;31(7):555–70. https://doi.org/10.1016/j.ctrv.2005.07.008.
48. Rasmusson AM, Marx CE, Pineles SL, et al. Neuroactive steroids and PTSD treatment. Neurosci Lett. 2017;649:156–63. https://doi.org/10.1016/j.neulet.2017.01.054.
49. Lee H-J, Macbeth AH, Pagani JH, et al. Oxytocin: the great facilitator of life. Prog Neurobiol. 2009;88(2):127–51. https://doi.org/10.1016/j.pneurobio.2009.04.001.
50. Desai RI, Limoli CL, Stark CEL, et al. Impact of spaceflight stressors on behavior and cognition: a molecular, neurochemical, and neurobiological perspective. Neurosci Biobehav Rev. 2022;138:104676. https://doi.org/10.1016/j.neubiorev.2022.104676.
51. Mukherjee S, Epperly MW, Fisher R, et al. Inhibition of tyrosine kinase Fgr prevents radiation-induced pulmonary fibrosis (RIPF). Cell Death Discov. 2023;9(1):252. https://doi.org/10.1038/s41420-023-01538-3.
52. Mukherjee A, Epperly M, Shields D, et al. Ionizing irradiation induced Fgr in senescent cells mediates fibrosis. Cell Death Discov. 2021;7(1):349. https://doi.org/10.1038/s41420-021-00741-4.
53. Mukherjee A, Epperly MW, Fisher R, et al. Silica-induced lung fibrosis is associated with senescence, Fgr, and recruitment of bone marrow monocyte/macrophages. In Vivo. 2021;35(6):3053. https://doi.org/10.21873/invivo.12601.
54. Li K, Epperly M, Greenberger J, et al. Longitudinal fecal microbiome study of total body irradiated mice treated with radiation mitigators identify bacterial associations with survival. Front Cell Infect Microbiol. 2021;11:715396. https://doi.org/10.3389/fcimb.2021.715396.
55. Epperly MW, Franicola D, Shields D, et al. Screening for in vitro radiation protection and mitigation capacity of antimicrobial agents including those used in supportive care regimens for bone marrow transplant recipients. In Vivo. 2010;24(1):9–19.
56. Greenberger JS, Clump D, Kagan V, et al. Strategies for discovery of small molecule radiation protectors and radiation mitigators. Front Oncol. 2012;1:59. https://doi.org/10.3389/fonc.2011.00059.
57. Montesinos CA, Khalid R, Cristea O, et al. Space radiation protection countermeasures in microgravity and planetary exploration. Life (Basel). 2021;11(8):829. https://doi.org/10.3390/life11080829.

Chapter 7
Lunar Exploration and Lessons Learned

The planning for the next Lunar Mission by NASA will take into account many challenges. After the first successful moon landing in 1969 by the Apollo Mission and follow-up missions, there have been lessons learned from these brief, but historic moon landings. The lessons have emphasized many important factors regarding the next lunar mission, but also for space travel in general. The environment inside the spacecraft and moon lander suggests that a future moon habitat, from which the planned lunar sorties missions will initiate, must be designed to accommodate the basic needs of astronauts, most importantly, oxygen, environmental temperature control, water, and food and medical supplies that are necessary for living. Designing appropriate solutions to these challenges has been possible due to the successful preparations for the past missions. NASA is planning for a lunar habitat from which astronauts, even for as few as four individuals, will reside between sortie missions. If these people are going to be on the lunar surface for days/weeks, there are several major issues to address one of which is the radiation exposure that will be sustained [1–17].

Shielding from Lunar Radiation Exposure

Shielding from ionizing irradiation is achieved by two general categories of approaches: shielding of radiation and radiation countermeasures. This chapter will address the importance of the upcoming lunar sorties mission. Shielding of the astronauts in the moon lander and in the habitat from each of the four sources of ionizing irradiation will be one issue to address. There will undoubtedly be significant solar proton events preceded by gamma ray increases in exposure [1–3]. Galactic cosmic irradiation (GCR) is known to be constant with respect to the known measuring devices; however, varying compositions of the ionized particles and energy levels may vary [4–8]. Finally, neutron generation in the moon lander

J. Greenberger, *Radiation Oncology and Radiation Biology*,
https://doi.org/10.1007/978-3-031-66300-0_7

and in the spacecraft by GCR hitting the components of the structures will be another source of radiation [10–13]. All forms of irradiation can be addressed with shielding. However, the requirements for shielding differ based on the source of the irradiation. Gamma rays, protons, and GCR can be shielded by materials usually of high molecular weight and physical weight [14–17]. This issue of shielding, in itself, is a major challenge since getting materials from the Earth to the moon requires fuel, significant expense to transport, and, above all, the feasibility of getting enough material for a shelter device to provide some shielding. Neutron shielding is much more difficult. Obvious sources include water and graphite, which are used in the control rods in thermonuclear energy plants. Graphite is much lighter, and there is encouraging information from new Material Sciences approaches to developing graphene and other relatively lightweight materials that can be assembled in a zero-gravity environment and shown to provide much better radiation shielding [14–17].

A second major approach to managing the radiation sources that would be encountered on the lunar surface is that of radiation countermeasures [18–24]. NASA has funded many projects seeking to develop pharmacologic methods to minimize radiation damage in real time and on a continuous basis. Current radiation countermeasures [18, 19] and the development of new ones will be described in later chapters of this book. However, two general strategies for this approach include one being the continuous administration of a dietary or pharmacologic agent that will increase antioxidant stores and the capacity for cells to resist radiation damage. The second is to provide astronauts with information about the ongoing increase in solar proton events [2], such that they could migrate quickly from a lunar sortie mission into a relatively shielded environment to decrease exposure to solar protons (Fig. 7.1).

Lunar Mission to Precede Mars Mission

Why is the lunar sortie mission so important? NASA and the general scientific community are becoming more concerned about the duration of radiation exposure, which will increase as the length of a space radiation mission is increased. The Mars Mission to place humans on the Martian surface has been calculated to be one that would last for 860 days or longer [25–32]. This length of time out of the Earth's atmosphere and away from the protective magnetosphere will expose astronauts to continuous GCR, solar proton events, and neutrons generated in the spacecraft. The materials, which have been designed to transport and protect astronauts during space travel and on Lunar or Martian surface, must be durable and effective [14]. For the Lunar Mission, it will be very important to gain information on days/weeks of exposure to these forms of irradiation before a longer duration mission can be planned. Space exploration has been established as a top priority for the United States and originated with the elegant speeches made by John F. Kennedy in the 1960s. One of the major reasons for the Apollo mission to land astronauts on the

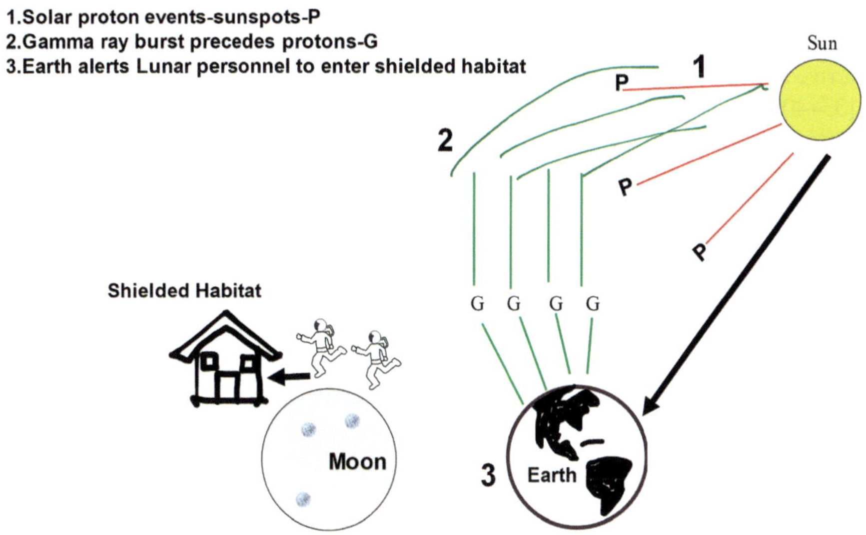

Fig. 7.1 Lunar sorties mission managing radiation exposure from solar protons. Astronauts on the lunar surface will be alerted from Earth (3) that there is a solar proton event impending. The sun has storms on the solar surface (sunspots). These release a gamma-ray burst shown as curved G lines (letter G) followed by proton events (P). The Earth alerts astronauts on the lunar surface to seek shelter in the habitat, which is shielded (4). Information system will decrease astronaut exposure to solar protons

lunar surface was to initiate space exploration. The moon provides a potential source of minerals and energy, which will continue to be a major concern for the next 100 years. As the conversion from fossil fuel energy sources to alternate energy sources continues on Earth, there will be an increased need to discover and develop other sources of energy. Mining operations on the lunar surface are a priority. To be able to fulfill the requirements of a multiday-week lunar operation, astronauts must be supplied with food and new sources of water [33–40]. The issue of water will be critical not only for the lunar mission but also for the Mars Mission and following missions.

Astronauts Require Water and Oxygen and Temperature Control

Water can be synthesized by biochemical reactions, but the reagents for such synthesis and the scale of reagents for the chemistry required to deliver enough water per individual may be substantial. One of the reasons that robotic satellite probes of the solar system have been so important is to discover places, where water may be an intrinsic part of the constituents of each potential site of a future space mission. Recent data have suggested that the one moon of Jupiter, Europa, may contain water

[1, 41, 42]. Studies of the Martian environment have provided conflicting evidence as to the past or present source of water [43]. Current evidence suggests that water arrived on Earth, delivered by meteorites at some point prior to the origin of life [33–40]. These same meteorites may have hit the lunar surface at some point in its history, and the search for subterranean deposits of water is continuing. In the event that there is no detectable source of water on the moon, facilities must be developed to generate water for any future long-duration lunar expeditions. If we are focused on developing mining operations on the lunar surface and construction of complex habitats in the future, then the engineering required for a water production plant must be considered. These next steps cannot be planned until it is clear from lunar exploration whether there is a source of water on the moon. Given the need for lunar exploration to prepare for mining operations, but also to understand the challenges for longer-duration space missions, NASA and associate scientific groups are planning for the logistics of the lunar sortie events.

Logistics of Lunar Sorties Mission and Space Radiation

Will lunar sorties be carried out by astronauts moving on foot or in a lunar exploration vehicle? Getting this vehicle (Moon-Buggy) will itself produce a challenge. The exploration from the lunar habitat out on the sorties will be limited by multiple factors. If the missions will be by foot, then the distance from the habitat must be calculated to allow individuals to quickly return in the event that solar proton events are detected by the gamma-ray preceding burst on Earth [2]. The energy of protons in the SPE will be a significant factor. Low-energy protons with reduced penetration capacity would penetrate the spacesuit and potentially produce skin burns on the astronauts, while high-energy protons could go deep into tissues and be part of the generation of the H-ARS (Hematopoietic-Acute Radiation Syndrome), which has been considered to be once possible to astronauts [21, 44–46]. If communication from the Earth to the astronauts indicates that an SPE is in progress (Fig. 7.1), the order of events will be first getting back into the habitat, which would have greater shielding than the spacesuits. The distance traveled on foot would be much less than that in a vehicle, and the speed of the vehicle returning to the habitat would be considered. These factors will go into mission planning to determine where the habitat will be placed. Ground-penetrating surveillance missions on the moon have suggested places, where mining operations or water exploration would be most productive. Placing the habitat near such a geographic region would be important so that sorties could be made safe for the astronauts. Predictions of solar proton events would also be important if the medical countermeasures for astronauts would be a consideration [18, 19, 44]. Predicting changes in GCR levels would be more difficult, but recent data suggest that the level is constant [47–49].

Knowing that an SPE is coming, astronauts could take a second medical countermeasure, which would be designed to mitigate the effects of acute proton radiation exposure [18, 19]. Given that the relative biological effect of protons is higher than that of gamma rays (X-rays), the maintenance of surveillance and communication about SPs will be key for astronauts. The lessons learned from past lunar missions, while brief, are important.

Issues of Gravity and Oxygen and Water Relative to Radiation

The gravity on the lunar surface, although one-sixth of that gravity on the Earth, will still provide astronauts with some ability that is absent from the weightless, zero-gravity environment of the spacecraft [50–54]. How this fact impacts human physiology will be important to determine from the lunar sortie mission. The sorties will produce some exercise, which will decrease bone degeneration and provide some stabilization for cardiovascular health [44]. How this will impact the transition from reduced gravity to zero-gravity back on the spacecraft is not known. The medical monitoring techniques for astronauts have been developed, and these will be utilized including real-time observations of levels of blood oxygenation, pulse, blood pressure, respiratory rate, body temperature, and other measures of physiologic function. Radiation exposure levels must be measured [15, 45, 46, 48, 55]. The longer the mission, the more data will be collected. Another reason for the importance of the lunar sortie mission is the relative closeness of the moon to Earth. In the event that a need for a planned shortening of the mission arises (medical emergency for the astronauts or some other event), the transport time back to the planet will be manageable relative to the durations for a space mission of longer duration and with a target further from Earth. Lessons learned from real time monitoring of the astronauts on the lunar sorties mission will be critical to plan for future missions to more distant targets.

What Is Known About Radiation Exposure Levels from Space Radiation

The wealth of data coming in yearly from unmanned space probes have provided valuable information, as well as to NASA, to the general scientific literature [25–43]. The scientists and engineers who pioneered the Voyager satellite programs provided valuable details concerning our solar system as far out as planet Neptune and the best available true data about Pluto, which may not be a true planet [52]. The decision by NASA to continue the Voyager program and continue to collect data as the satellite leaves our solar system is an important decision [51]. As data from these programs continue to come in, NASA has also focused on plans for Lunar exploration as a stepping stone to the Mars Mission [25]. It appears that there will be a staged Lunar program with a more distant goal being the human exploration of Mars [53]. Perhaps, there will be a "stop" at a lunar assembly facility for preparation of the Mars spacecraft, or will the assembly be carried out at a space station orbiting the Earth? There are now fewer discussions about going directly from Earth to Mars, with no intermediate stop, in part because of the expense, but also because of the need to obtain answers about many precautionary factors, including how to deal with space radiation. The Lunar Sortie Mission is a logical next step [17].

As the discussions about Lunar exploration continue, there are many topics about which there is great interest (Table 7.1). Among these topics is the need to deal with continuous exposure of astronauts to space irradiation. The travel to and from Mars and that sustained by humans spending prolonged time on the Martian surface will lead to many challenges, many of which can be answered by Lunar exploration including both historical and planned missions. Ultimately, data on how decisions will be made regarding a staging process for the Mars Mission will certainly be valuable. The Lunar Missions must provide data on the search for water [33–40] and the methods by which to deal with continuous low-dose radiation [23, 24]. The Lunar Missions to follow will also answer several key questions about not only the Mars Mission, but also whether the moon is a valuable source of minerals and new ways to generate energy. Some data are already available on radiation biology relative to each of the options currently being discussed to ensure the health and safety of astronauts. Basic radiobiology experiments established that cells do repair

Table 7.1 Challenges to insure a safe and informative lunar mission

Issue	Direction for the solution	Yet unresolved
Fuel and energy	Solid fuel for the mission	Battery power and solar energy
Transportation for the sorties	Lunar dune buggy	One or two vehicles
Oxygen	Renewable source: Oxygen chemistry	Spacesuits Transport vehicles Habitat
Water	Renewable source or all carried from earth	Water—Chemistry
Communication with earth	Warning of solar flares and proton flumace	Spacesuit and vehicle shielding
Supplies for the mission	Duration of mission, medical supplies, pharmacy, emergency management	Triage procedures Early abortion and early return
Radiation shielding	Materials for spacecraft moon lander, vehicle, habitat	How to shield against radiation?
Radiation countermeasures	What will be taken: LR-IFN-B? Potassium iodide, Prussian blue, chelator drugs, antioxidants	What to take and when
Diet and microbiome	What to measure for diet effects?	Where to sample and how to interpret results?
Monitor radiation levels	Badge dosimeter, Ionization chambers Curiosity rover dosimeters	What data frequency and response to increase over expected

radiation damage if given time to repair [56, 57]. But the unknown factors that lead to late effects are the real challenge [26–28], as is the danger of a combined injury effect [44].

Life Outside the Earth

NASA has released several RFAs (requests for applications) [54] offerings over the years concerning how to deal with the radiation exposure of astronauts, who will be tasked with each of a series of missions ranging from life in a lunar habitat to sorties to different areas on the lunar surface. How this plan evolves and when it will be realized are still subjects of debate. The discussions about the radiobiology of the "Lunar-Sorties" Mission have revealed several challenges for ensuring the safety of the astronauts (Fig. 7.1, Table 7.1) [45, 46].

In one series of discussions, NASA scientists suggested that there would be a plan to have a group of astronauts on the lunar surface perhaps for some period of time, and that they would periodically leave a protected environment (lunar habitat), which provides shelter between "sorties" (walking or vehicle driven missions from the habitat out into different directions) (Fig. 7.1). The site on the lunar surface where the habitat will be constructed is still being discussed. Why discuss such a strategy? In one series of discussions, there was a question about the radiation levels that would be expected and doses sustained by astronauts on the lunar surface. There is no protective magnetosphere on the moon [58]. There would be no expectation that there will be protection from galactic cosmic irradiation (GCR) (charged heavy ion molecules from distant supernovae-death of stars) hitting the lunar surface. There is no protective particle deflection by a Van-Allen Belt [58] or other components of the magnetosphere to funnel charged particles to the North or South poles, as there is on Earth. In addition, there is no expectation that any rotation of the moon on its axis would contribute to any form of periodic radiation protection from the solar release of protons (SPE-Solar Proton Events), which are directional, but also charged particles that will hit the astronaut on the lunar surface. The lack of rotation of the moon is obvious from the earliest human observations of the lunar surface and the description of the stable observation of large craters. The names given to surface features include the "Sea of Tranquility," where Neil Armstrong landed in 1969 and communicated "This is Tranquility Base, the Eagle has Landed." Improved orbiting of Earth's telescopes [41, 42] has mapped the structure of many of the objects on the moon and these have been largely unchanged for observers over hundreds of years. The absence of significant mountain ranges on the moon eliminates the option of using the geology to shield the habitat from SPEs.

Earth telescopes have greatly improved the details of these pockmarks on the lunar surface and become more real as geographic locations, but even the Hubble [41] and Webb [42] orbiting telescopes have provided details. Observations of the "bright side of the moon" are detailed. What also was clear is that details about the "dark side" of the moon have not allowed discussions about putting the "habitat" in a safe location. The dark side of the moon may be invisible to Earth observers, but it is bombed by GCR and protons and gamma rays, the same as the light side. A lunar habitat will face the sun and will sustain repeated solar proton events (SPEs) from repeat irradiation events. While the same side of the moon always faces the Earth, and we have named it the "dark side of the moon," that dark side, in fact, does face the sun during part of the lunar day. Therefore, the idea of building a habitat on what we call the dark side will, in fact, not shield the astronauts from protons during the times that we perceived the existence of a dark side. How are there ways to predict increased SPEs? They are seasonal [2] and deliver a gamma-ray burst that precedes the protons and is detectable on Earth, in time to warn the members of the Lunar Sortie to shelter (Fig. 7.1), but how can they reach a shelter fast enough, and what will be the materials comprising the shelter?

Communication with Earth

One of the strategies toward building some type of safe shelter structure on the moon was to allow astronauts on sorties to return to it based upon the prediction of SPEs from real-time observations of solar proton events (sunspots) on Earth (Fig. 7.1). The observers on Earth would communicate to the lunar astronauts that a gamma-ray burst had been detected, and that a solar proton event or increase in proton irradiation would follow. Theoretically, this strategy would allow astronauts a warning to return to that structure and seek protection from solar proton irradiation. The paucity of data on total body irradiation exposure from protons, particularly, at varying energies, varying dose rates, and at varying separated intervals between fractionation exposures makes it difficult to define the radiobiology and medical sequalae. There are some data on the effects of total body protons [3]. However, the dosimetry of human exposure to solar proton events has been difficult to quantify. The available data from Mars unmanned-Rover experiments [55] and the evidence from the limited time humans have spent on the lunar surface, going back to 1969, have provided some information. What medical countermeasures and physical protective strategies will be provided to the lunar sorties astronauts based on the radiobiology of the effects of estimated exposure to the lunar surface environment [18, 19]? How can we plan for a habitat and for the Lunar-Sortie missions?

Transportation: The Moon "Dune Buggy"

Physicists and radiation biologists must design a model lunar habitat; wherein, human exposure to solar protons and galactic cosmic irradiation can be mitigated, which will be the construction materials [4]. To build a structure one must deliver the building materials. Is there a light alternative to lead, depleted uranium, and other common Earth shielding materials [5]. The baseline background gamma ray

(X-ray) exposure must first be factored into mathematical modeling and calculating exposure from SPEs and GCI. AI (artificial intelligence) algorithms, perhaps, can be used to design models that would be potentially helpful to first determine the dose. The seasonal variation in sunspots and SPEs can be modeled, but there is no known seasonal variation in GCRs [47]. Would there be a reduction in radiation exposure from GCRs if a habitat were to be constructed on the surface of one region of the moon? Is there a mountain or deep crater? Another question is whether the core of the moon contains any significant levels of radium or other radioactive isotopes, as does the planet Earth that would emit gamma rays that must be factored into the calculations of cumulative exposure levels. Does the Rover data provide answers [6]? If there are planned missions to establish mineral mining operations on the moon, this question about how to quantify cumulative radiation exposure levels must be answered [45, 46].

The structure of a lunar surface habitat is a subject for both Engineering and Materials Scientists. What materials could this structure be fashioned out of? There is new information about the assembly of graphene-based structures in a zero-gravity environment [8, 9] that have intrinsic resistance to extremes of temperature.

Transport and Assembly of Radiation Shielding Materials

Do the best lightweight and practical materials for the lunar habitat have the capacity for radiation shielding? Perhaps, the materials for the habitat, which must be designed to be lightweight, can also be radiation resistant (against GCR solar protons and X-rays of varying energies and penetration capacity). The Materials Science experiments may be designed and construction could be carried out at a space station, and then materials transported to the lunar surface. There are data showing that materials construction in zero gravity conditions yields more resilient products. (The materials being researched include: silicon carbide and gallium nitride.) [8]. Construction of the lunar habitat would be limited by the same factors that have gone into solving problems for the International Space Station. What would be the materials used in the construction? What materials are available that would be of the appropriate lightweight for transport from the Earth's surface to the assembly site (whether it be a space station or a lunar surface habitat)? Most importantly, what materials will be both practical and cost effective? If one carries out these calculations, one must also consider that chosen materials should attenuate space radiation exposure. Thus, the list of candidate materials may be limited.

Calculating the radiation biological effects on human exposure on a lunar mission, whether it be prolonged residence inside a habitat, or accompanied by lunar sorties—will require knowledge of the planned times outside the habitat. The materials used to construct the habitat must take into account the generation of neutrons from GCR hitting the materials and released within the habitat. The habitat will be constantly hit by galactic cosmic irradiation. When charged particles hit the elements of the structure, neutrons will be generated [9, 10].

There is some information available on which materials generate more neutrons when struck by the ions that comprise GCR [9] charged particles components of GCR include silicon, carbon, iron, and others. The radiobiology of total body neutrons is limited, but some measurements have been derived [10]. The dose rate varies from the exposed low dose rate of GCR hitting the habitat to the ultra-high dose rate of neutrons from the Hiroshima U285 fission bomb [11]. Linear accelerators used in clinical radiotherapy generate neutrons when high-energy X-rays hit the depleted uranium collimator [11]. The measurement of neutron irradiation must now be factored into an analysis of the radiobiology of gamma rays, solar proton events, and GCR. Thus, neutrons represent a fourth source of irradiation exposure to the lunar mission astronauts.

Each of the four components of the radiation that will be sustained by astronauts on any lunar mission must be quantitated and countermeasures must be provided; but first, these countermeasures must be developed. The concept that astronauts on a sortie would have some time to get back to the habitat (assuming that it can be reasonably protected from SPEs and GCR) must be validated to be feasible. If the astronauts are in a vehicle that has been driven/mobilized hundreds of meters from the site of the habitat, and when they are alerted that an SPE is coming, will they have time to drive/walk/run back to the habitat? Walking would be a challenge, but if they have a motorized rover, they could go farther from the habitat on each of these sorties and return fast and safely when instructed to do so.

Will There be a Radiation Safety Officer on the Moon?

There must be available real-time updated calculations for each crew member as to the current cumulative level of exposure, as modified by the higher RBE of protons and GCR. Each of the four radiation sources, inside and outside the habitat, must be monitored, and then the cumulative total made available to each astronaut. A crew member with a high cumulative level might be instructed to stay in the habitat for some period of time and to take medical countermeasures including drugs that are approved as safe radiation mitigators [18, 19, 24].

If there is a habitat constructed of materials that reduce radiation exposure, and if cumulative levels are available for each astronaut in real time, then the data on the capacity of the human body to repair the complex space radiation composite that had been sustained during the time outside the habitat must be known for each person. The individual's time inside the habitat might be dependent on a measure of his/her radiation repair capacity. Not everyone may have the leading to a same "all clear" indicator. Such measures for individuals are not yet validated. Candidate assays might be: (1) level of DNA double-strand breaks measured by H2AX staining in each persons' peripheral blood sample, looking at lymphocytes [23, 24]; (2) plasma level of inflammatory cytokines that are elevated by radiation exposure and fall after a period of time in the shielded area of the habitat; and (3) time after administration of a medical countermeasure. Each individual might be quarantined and remain inside the habitat until a biological measurement indicates that radiation repair has occurred. The policy is currently in effect in hospitals and is applied to all radiation workers. Those with the highest levels based upon quarterly badge readings may be instructed to cease work with radiation equipment or with radioisotopes for several months [45, 46].

There is also information about the capacity of individual humans to repair irradiation damage from current clinical experience, and also information from first responders to radiation accidents.

In clinical radiotherapy, fractionated total body irradiation has been used to prepare patients for bone marrow transplantation. The interval of 4 h between radiation fractions (recently increased to 6 h) has been chosen based on the kinetics of repair of radiation damage in the original cell culture experiments [56]. Waiting 4–6 h between radiation fractions was also chosen as the time for hyperfractionated radiotherapy that was used to treat cancer in protocols that were designed in the 1980s and 1990s [57]. This was a radiobiology approach to better tumor control in which patients received a lower radiation fraction delivered to their tumors, separated by 4 h of "rest." Hyperfractionation experiments were partially successful in control of large tumor volumes providing no additional toxicity to the normal tissues in the radiation beam [57].

Another setting from which some information regarding the capacity of humans to repair radiation damage comes from the emergency responders to radiation accidents. There is one description of a historical "Cold War" monitoring device using radiation to detect the former Soviet Union "backfire" bombers in a military observation site [44]. In this example, the time of exposure is shown to be casual. There was a disaster model that was fashioned in which first responders were tasked with managing a potential disaster. In this case, the monitoring device in the facility was damaged such that large radiation levels were detected in the facility. In this hypothetical scenario, a person was unable to evacuate the site and was still inside. The rescue team was tasked with using a strategy; whereby, individuals in the rotation would go into assemble data on the rescue. The first person would go in and would be tasked with staying in the site for only a limited number of minutes. During that time, the person would gather data on the facility where the injured person, who needed to be evacuated, was located in another observation. This first person would leave the site, give this information to the team, and a second person would go in. This person could gather more information about where the injured person was, and how he/she could be removed, and then, at the same limitation of minutes, would come out and report to the team. A third, fourth, or fifth person would go in for small amounts of time, and then eventually be able to rescue and evacuate the person from the site.

This information led to policies for ambulance facilities that would be used to transport injured persons, who would be evaluated, and the ambulance itself, as well as any materials inside the ambulance (stretcher, medical materials), would be buried or isolated, assuming it contained radioactive materials and/or isotopes of long-lived duration and not practical for decontamination. First responders have learned from these hypothetical scenarios whether the information that is collected by individuals in a radiation-contaminated environment can be reliably used. One responder could not stay in this environment beyond a previously calculated and predetermined time. How does this information potentially have applicability to translate to the exposure of lunar astronauts to continuous low dose rates or sporadic irradiation from the previously described four different radiation sources?

Lunar Missions with Clear Goals: Search for Water and Carrying Out Mining Operations

Two major projects have been described as very relevant to future space missions. A lunar source of water, if found, would facilitate great advances. Mining operations are essential to discover new sources of fuel and materials. It is very difficult to model long-duration missions on the Earth's surface in preparation for such lunar missions. In addition to the sporadic pattern of delivery of each of the four sources of radiation and the need for a personal dosimeter that can measure cumulative levels of each radiation source separately and pool that data from all sources, there is the issue of the reduced one-fifth level of gravity on the lunar surface [50].

An animal model system proves very helpful. Neutron irradiation facilities are available at Columbia University and Colorado State University [12, 13]. Continuous low-dose neutron exposure and fractionated neutron exposure experiments have been published [12, 13]. Neutron irradiation has a high relative biologic effect (RBE), so calculations made on human exposure to gamma rays/X-rays and protons (where there is much available information) must be modified by the available data on neutrons. What materials for the construction of the habitat are susceptible to producing more neutrons? These experiments must be carried out on materials that would be candidates for use in the construction of the habitat. Reducing neutron production by GCR that hits the structure must be minimized. The seasonal variation in the production of SPE can be modeled. The available information from the Curiosity Rover and other unmanned probes provides valuable information on the frequency of GCR. If there are 1000 supernovae per day [9], some occurring hundreds of light years from Earth, and if this has been constant, or is expected to be constant, one can calculate the contribution of GCR to the radiation levels. Furthermore, the relative composition of ions in the GCR can be modeled.

With regard to GCR, there is emerging radiobiology information on Iron59 and mixed beam high linear energy transfer (LET) irradiation from Brookhaven National Laboratory. Using AI algorithms, scientists can model expected radiation exposure of astronauts outside the habitat and can predict the relative accumulation of radiation damage on an hourly basis for people outside the habitat. Then, one can model the attenuation of irradiation when astronauts are inside the habitat (assuming that lightweight irradiation-resistant materials can be used to fashion the structure).

Measuring the response of individual astronauts to individual irradiation would be important to collect during the time of this lunar sortie mission. What are the metrics that can be reliably collected and transmitted to Earth to provide information back to the astronauts?

Some of the monitoring measures for radiation exposure levels can also be applied to determining the overall exposure of each crew member based on a biological parameter. There are techniques available to measure peripheral blood counts, white blood cell phenotypes— lymphocytes, neutrophils, monocytes—as well as platelets and red blood cells. In addition, plasma/serum levels of inflammatory cytokines will be measured if possible [45, 46]. The best measures may be plasma levels of DNA, RNA, and microRNA levels in the circulation can be used [46]. A laboratory to monitor biological dose sustained over time must be contained within the habitat to monitor each of the astronauts.

How frequently should measures of cumulative radiation biological exposure be made? If the first mission would be to reside on the lunar surface for 7–14 days, the frequency of measuring can be modeled by experiments on Earth with animals in a fashioned similar habitat. These habitat models can be exposed to continuing low-level sporadic proton irradiation and gamma irradiation. Constructing such a habitat that would duplicate experimentally the Brookhaven National Laboratory radiation mixed beam (GCR-irradiation beam and receiving sporadic high LET irradiation), adding in protons and X-rays, would be difficult to construct but is possible. Alternatively, animal model data can be bypassed, and rather the first data obtained by collecting actual human astronaut data that would be transmitted to Earth from such a mission. It is possible that one astronaut might sustain high levels of irradiation damage as reflected in the metrics described above, and that person could be told by Earth mission control not to participate in the rotation schedule for activity outside the habitat.

Return to Earth Earlier Due to Radiation Levels

It is unlikely that an early unscheduled return of a subgroup of astronauts from the lunar surface to a vehicle to transport them back to Earth could be possible and associated with a planned return to the Earth's surface. Thus, a highly radiation-exposed individual might be instructed to stay in the habitat. This strategy is that of the plans by radiation safety offices in universities and companies to carry out radiation badge monitoring and ensure that all personnel are closely monitored for ALARA levels. As described in a prior chapter on radiation safety and ALARA ("as low as reasonably achievable") levels [12, 44], physicians working in cardiac catheterization, or with frequent radiation exposure from fluoroscopic devices, or producing PET radioisotopes, can be told to stop work in this area, and if reaching an ALARA level 3, can be taken off the project. The same could follow for astronauts on the lunar surface that are monitored for the biomarkers of radiation exposure. The background information on human genetics is currently not up for discussion.

The availability of these data might allow mission planners to exclude someone, who might be likely to be radiation sensitive. There is no plan to use such information as to exclude individuals from candidacy for a lunar habitat mission based on their genetic profile, which might be interpreted to indicate a higher risk for radiation sensitivity. The concept of genetic engineering for astronaut candidates for prolonged multiyear duration space travel may be part of distant future discussions.

Placing a Lunar Habitat in a Particular Location on the Moon

The greatest shielding for protons SPEs and GCR could be the geology of the moon itself. There is no protective magnetosphere on the moon [58]. Shielding against SPEs could ideally come from placing the habitat between astronauts and the sun. Shielding against GCR can also occur by geology. However, neutron shielding requires an absorber like water or graphite. There is little available data as to the relative contribution of GCR-generated high-charged ions LET (linear energy transfer) comparing one area of the moon to others. If there were differences in the relative contribution of GCR, depending on the geography of the moon, this could also be considered.

All of the above discussions regarding the lunar habitat, duration of sorties, monitoring of astronauts for levels of radiation exposure would be aided by an experiment on the adaptation of humans to each of the four components of space radiation. Two places in previous chapters have discussed the concept of radio accommodation. The experiments at Argonne National Laboratory with out-bred beagle dogs exposed to continuous Cobalt^{60} (Co^{60}) irradiation showed that one-third of the animals did adapt their blood counts and suffered no deleterious effects other than premature aging. How to increase the ability of humans to accommodate to continuously elevated levels of exposure to ionizing irradiation is unknown, but some experiments have yielded useful information [24–49].

References

1. Stevens JC, Hopkins JB. An alternate approach to lunar missions—human sorties at half the price. Space Conference, San Jose, CA. September 19–21, 2006:1–12.
2. Aminalragia-Giamini S, Jiggens P, Anastasiadis A, et al. Prediction of solar proton event fluence spectra from their peak flux spectra. Space Weather Space Clim. 2020;10:1.
3. Chang J, Feng W, Wang Y, et al. Whole-body proton irradiation causes long-term damage to hematopoietic stem cells in mice. Radiat Res. 2015;183(2):240–8. https://doi.org/10.1667/RR13887.1.
4. Brennan L, Slecinski R, Tremayne M, et al. Mechanical design of a lunar habitat structure and deployment mechanism. Acta Astronaut. 2023;213:102–20.
5. Dideikin AT, Vul AY. Graphene oxide and derivatives: the place in graphene family. Front Phys. 2018;6:2018.

6. Burkhardt C. Isotopic composition of the moon and the lunar isotopic crisis. Encyclop Lunar Sci. 2017;23:1–13.
7. Sinha A. First US lunar lander since 1972 launched: the mission, significance. The Indian Express Paper, February 13, 2024.
8. Senesky DG, Lowell S. The right stuff. Scientific American; 2023. p. 42–7.
9. Norbury JW, Schimmerling W, Slaba TC, et al. Galactic cosmic ray simulation at the NASA space radiation laboratory. Life Sci Space Res (Amst). 2016;8:38–51. https://doi.org/10.1016/j.lssr.2015.02.001.
10. Hauri P, Schneider U. Whole-body dose equivalent including neutrons is similar for 6 MV and 15 MV IMRT, VMAT, and 3D conformal radiotherapy. J Appl Clin Med Phys. 2019;20(3):56–70. https://doi.org/10.1002/acm2.12543.
11. Sasaki MS, Endo S, Hoshi M, et al. Neutron relative biological effectiveness in Hiroshima and Nagasaki atomic bomb survivors: a critical review. J Radiat Res. 2016;57(6):583–95. https://doi.org/10.1093/jrr/rrw079.
12. Borak TB, Heilbronn LH, Krumland N, et al. Design and dosimetry of a facility to study health effects following exposures to fission neutrons at low dose rates for long durations. Int J Radiat Biol. 2021;97(8):1063–76. https://doi.org/10.1080/09553002.2019.1588884.
13. Xu Y, Randers-Pehrson G, Turner HC, et al. Accelerator-based biological irradiation facility simulating neutron exposure from an improvised nuclear device. Radiat Res. 2015;184(4):404–10. https://doi.org/10.1667/RR14036.1.
14. AbuAlRoos NJ, Amin NAB, Zainon R. Conventional and new lead-free radiation shielding materials for radiation protection in nuclear medicine: a review. Radiat Phys Chem. 2019;165:108439.
15. Koontz SL, Boeder PA, Pankop C, et al. The ionizing radiation environment on the international space station: performance vs. expectations for avionics and materials. In radiation effects data workshop, IEEE; 2005:110–116.
16. Wilson JW, et al. Galactic and solar cosmic ray shielding in deep space (NASA Technical Paper No. 3682.) NASA, Hampton, VA. 1997.
17. Simonsen LC, Nealy JE. Radiation protection for human missions to the Moon and Mars. NASA Technical Paper 3079. 1991.
18. Singh VK, Newman VL, Romaine PLP, et al. Radiation countermeasure agents: an update (2011–2014). Expert Opin Ther Pat. 2014;24(11):1229–55. https://doi.org/10.1517/13543776.2014.964684.
19. Singh VK, Seed TM. Radiation countermeasures for hematopoietic acute radiation syndrome: growth factors, cytokines, and beyond. Int J Radiat Biol. 2021;97(11):1526–47. https://doi.org/10.1080/09553002.2021.1969054.
20. Carney JP, Maser RS, Olivares H, et al. The hMre11/hRad50 protein complex and Nijmegen breakage syndrome: linkage of double-strand break repair to the cellular DNA damage response. Cell. 1998;93(3):477–86. https://doi.org/10.1016/s0092-8674(00)81175-7.
21. Morgan WF, Day JP, Kaplan MI, et al. Genomic instability induced by ionizing radiation. Radiat Res. 1996;146(3):247–58.
22. Hollander MC, Sheikh MS, Bulavin DV, et al. Genomic instability in Gadd45a-deficient mice. Nat Genet. 1999;23(2):176–84. https://doi.org/10.1038/13802.
23. Olipitz W, Wiktor-Brown D, Shuga J, et al. Integrated molecular analysis indicates undetectable DNA damage in mice after continuous irradiation at −400-fold natural background radiation. Environ Health Perspect. 2012;120(8):1130–6. https://doi.org/10.1289/ehp.1104294.
24. Morgan WF. Non-targeted and delayed effects of exposure to ionizing radiation: II. Radiation-induced genomic instability and bystander effects in vivo, clastogenic factors, and transgenerational effects. Radiat Res. 2003;159(5):581–96. https://doi.org/10.1667/0033-7587(2003)159[0581:nadeoe]2.0.co;2.
25. Cucinotta FA, Schimmerling W, Wilson JW, et al. Space radiation cancer risks and uncertainties for Mars missions. Radiat Res. 2001;156(5 Pt 2):682–8. https://doi.org/10.1667/0033-7587(2001)156[0682:srcrau]2.0.co;2.

26. Cucinotta FA, Durante M. Cancer risk from exposure to galactic cosmic rays: implications for space exploration by human beings. Lancet Oncol. 2006;7(5):431–5. https://doi.org/10.1016/S1470-2045(06)70695-7.
27. Cucinotta FA, Kim M-HY, Chappell LJ, et al. How safe is safe enough? Radiation risk for a human mission to Mars. PLoS One. 2013;8(10):e74988. https://doi.org/10.1371/journal.pone.0074988.
28. Cucinotta FA, Chappell L, Kim MY. Space radiation cancer risk projections and Uncertainties-2012. NASA Technical Paper 2013-217375. 2013.
29. Simonsen LC, Nealy JE. Mars surface radiation exposure for solar maximum conditions and 1989 solar proton events. NASA Technical Paper 3300. 1993.
30. Cucinotta FA, Saganti PB, Wilson JW, et al. Model predictions and visualization of the particle flux on the surface of Mars. J Radiat Res. 2002;43(Suppl):S35–9. https://doi.org/10.1269/jrr.43.235.
31. De Angelis G, Clowdsley MS, Singleterry RC, et al. A new Mars radiation environment model with visualization. Adv Space Res. 2004;34(6):1328–32. https://doi.org/10.1016/j.asr.2003.09.059.
32. Saganti PB, Cucinotta FA, Wilson JW, et al. Radiation climate map for analyzing risks to astronauts on the Mars surface from galactic cosmic rays. Space Sci. 2004;110:143–56.
33. Vacher LG, Fujiya W. Recent advances in our understanding of water and aqueous activity in chondrites. Elements. 2022;18(3):175–80.
34. Greenwood RC, Findlay R, Martins R, et al. The formation and aqueous alteration of CM2 chondrites and their relationship to CO3 chondrites: a fresh isotopic (O, Cd, Cr, Si, Te, Ti, and Zn) perspective from the Winchcombe CM2 fall. Meteorit Planet Sci. 2024;59(5):1170–93. https://doi.org/10.1111/maps.13968.
35. Bates HC, King AJ, Shirley KS, et al. The bulk mineralogy, elemental composition, and water content of the Winchcombe CM chondrite fall. Meteorit Planet Sci. 2024;59(5):1006–28. https://doi.org/10.1111/maps.14043.
36. Vollmer C, Kepaptsoglou D, Leitner J, et al. High-spatial resolution functional chemistry of nitrogen compounds in the observed UK meteorite fall Winchcombe. Nat Commun. 2024;15(1):778. https://doi.org/10.1038/s41467-024-45064-x.
37. Genge MJ, Alesbrook L, Almeida NV, et al. The fusion crust of the Winchcombe meteorite: a preserved record of atmospheric entry processes. Meteorit Planet Sci. 2024;59(5):948–72. https://doi.org/10.1111/maps.13937.
38. Suttle MD, Daly L, Jones RH, et al. The Winchcombe meteorite-A regolith breccia from a rubble pile CM chondrite asteroid. Meteorit Planet Sci. 2024;59(5):1043–67. https://doi.org/10.1111/maps.13938.
39. King AJ, Daly L, Rowe J, et al. The Winchcombe meteorite, a unique and pristine witness from the outer solar system. Sci Adv. 2022;8(46):eabq3925. https://doi.org/10.1126/sciadv.abq3925.
40. Thompson J. Aqua earth. Sci Am. 2023;329(1):8.
41. Freedman WL, Madore BF, Gibson BK, et al. Final results from the Hubble space telescope key project to measure the Hubble constant. The Astrophysical J. 2001;553(1):47.
42. Kalirai J. Scientific discovery with the James Webb space telescope. Contemp Phys. 2018;59(3):251–90.
43. Cucinotta FA, Kim MH, Schneider SI, et al. Description of light ion production cross sections and fluxes on the Mars surface using the QMSFRG model. Radiat Environ Biophys. 2007;46:101–6. https://doi.org/10.1007/s00411-007-0099-y.
44. Dainiak N. Medical management of acute radiation syndrome and associated infections in a high-casualty incident. J Radiat Res. 2018;59(suppl_2):ii54–64. https://doi.org/10.1093/jrr/rry004.
45. Palmans H, Rabus H, Belchior AL, et al. Future development of biologically relevant dosimetry. Br J Radiol. 2015;88(1045):20140392. https://doi.org/10.1259/bjr.20140392.

46. Cui W, Ma J, Wang Y, Biswal S. Plasma miRNA as biomarkers for assessment of total-body radiation exposure dosimetry. PLoS One. 2011;6(8):e22988. https://doi.org/10.1371/journal.pone.0022988.
47. Burrows A. Supernova explosions in the universe. Nature. 2000;403(6771):727–33. https://doi.org/10.1038/35001501.
48. Zeitlin C, Hassler DM, Cucinotta FA, et al. Measurements of energetic particle radiation in transit to Mars on the Mars science laboratory. Science. 2013;340(6136):1080–4. https://doi.org/10.1126/science.1235989.
49. Hassler DM, Zeitlin C, Wimmer-Schweingruber RF, et al. Mars' surface radiation environment measured with the Mars science laboratory's curiosity rover. Science. 2014;343(6169):1244797. https://doi.org/10.1126/science.1244797.
50. Konopliv AS, Park RS, Yuan D-N, et al. High-resolution lunar gravity fields from the GRAIL primary and extended missions. Geophys Res Lett. 2014;41(5):1452–8.
51. Matsumoto SK. Voyager interstellar mission: challenges of flying a very old spacecraft on a very long mission. SpaceOps Conferences, Daejeon, Korea. May 16–20, 2016.
52. Schilling G. Pluto: the planet that never was. Science. 1999;283(5399):157.
53. Salotti J-M, Heidmann R. Roadmap to a human Mars mission. Acta Astronaut. 2014;104(2):558–64.
54. Smith T, Peterman A, Donoviel D. Exponential medicine: challenges of human spaceflight bringing innovations for earth—a case study. In: Friebe M, editor. Novel innovation design for the future of health. Springer Nature; 2022. p. 71–8.
55. Ehresmann B, Hassler DM, Zeitlin C, et al. Charged particle spectra measured during the transit to Mars with the Mars science laboratory radiation assessment detector (MSL/RAD). Life Sci Space Res (Amst). 2016;10:29–37. https://doi.org/10.1016/j.lssr.2016.07.001.
56. Puck TT, Marcus PI. Action of X-rays on mammalian cells. J Exp Med. 1956;103(5):653–66. https://doi.org/10.1084/jem.103.5.653.
57. Withers HR, Horiot J-C. Hyperfractionation. In: Withers HR, Peters LJ, editors. Innovations in radiation oncology. Berlin, Heidelberg: Springer-Verlag; 1988. p. 223–30.
58. Li W, Hudson MK. Earth's Van Allen radiation belts: from discovery to the Van Allen probes era. J Geophys Res Space Physics. 2019;124(11):8319–51.

Chapter 8
The Mars Mission Data from Curiosity Rover Measuring Radiation Exposure

There is much information available about the plans for the Mars mission. The most important information comes from the Curiosity Mission in which the Curiosity Rover robot traveled on the Martian surface [1–13]. The spacecraft to deliver the Martian rover recorded (a one-way mission) radiation levels during the 180-day cruise phase and also radiation levels on the surface of Mars [1–13]. Calculations based on the data from this important mission (involving NASA scientists at all levels including engineers, material scientists, radiation biologists, physicians, and physicists) provided all the information needed to make preliminary plans for this mission. Information on radiation levels and the quality of radiation (protons, X-rays, neutrons, galactic cosmic radiation (GCR)) regarding the cruise phase was not very different from that already known about space irradiation from the Lunar landing missions. The important information from the International Space Station and space shuttle missions also provided data on the radiation levels outside the Earth's protective magnetosphere. What was new was the recording of radiation levels on the Martian surface. Why is the mission to Mars so important?

Space exploration, like any other disciplines of exploration, involves an understanding of the hazards so that one can prepare. Unknown areas of science, whether related to single-cell microbiology, mechanisms of pathophysiology, or approaches to understanding combined sources of stress, lead to questions. With regard to space travel for humans, there is the issue of radiation exposure. From the time the first *Homo sapiens* left their caves or camps and explored neighboring geographic regions, to the time the first mountaineers scaled the highest peaks on Earth, to the first deep dive oceanography missions, there have been risks. However, all of these challenges were those on the planet Earth. Fascination about the number of stars and the possibility of space travel has led humans to reach for higher goals.

There is an added factor regarding space travel and the Mars mission, namely, radiation. The United States launched its response to first Russian Sputnik satellite that circled Earth and released a radio signal in 1958. Television stations and newspapers revealed the United States government's congratulatory message to the

J. Greenberger, *Radiation Oncology and Radiation Biology*,
https://doi.org/10.1007/978-3-031-66300-0_8

Russians. However, there was a clear panic, which led to the premature launching of a Vanguard rocket to deliver a United States satellite and match the Russians. This rocket to deliver the United States satellite crashed and newspaper articles indicated in a joking yet serious and painful message “U.S. Sputnik, Kaput-nik.” In 1958, it was even more embarrassing to the United States, and particularly to its military that we had fallen behind Russia in space travel. By 1969, the United States had caught up and, in fact, had the first Moon landing with the Apollo missions. There was and still is a military justification for the goal of initiating a manned mission to Mars, as well as an obvious scientific justification.

There are many scientific challenges to preparing for the Mars mission, and the prevailing wisdom is that there will be an incremental approach to several additional steps before a mission to Mars is initiated. The greatest challenges now include the issues of budget and finance. Recent reports indicate that the Federal budget in the United States for Defense may be over 50%, while the budget for NASA will be 0.5% or less. While the funding for the Mars mission will be clear enough to keep all of the NASA programs going, it will be inadequate to fund all the meritorious applications for research in the many areas that will be required to generate the necessary data to make the manned Mars mission feasible and safe. Included in the list of needs will be the collection of more data regarding radiation levels, which will be sustained by astronauts during their cruise phases to and from Mars, and on the Martian surface for an estimated 860-day mission. Once radiation levels are known, we must factor in the relative biological effect (RBE) of each physically measured radiation level, and how the RBE will be affected by low gravity and the other conditions of the spacecraft. There are many other challenges.

The choice of a propulsion system/engine for the Mars mission remains a challenge. Private companies are tasked with developing an engine that will use solid fuel rather than a nuclear power system, and the engine must be reliable and functional for over 1000 h of use. The materials scientists developing the structure of the spacecraft and a Martian surface habitat are tasked with finding materials that are lightweight, resistant to corrosion, fatigue, and radiation including having a low probability of producing neutrons from being constantly bombarded by the charged particles of galactic cosmic radiation (GCR) [14–20]. The equipment and materials that will be carried in the spacecraft will be limited. Unlike the Lunar mission and the International Space Station Mission durations, the Mars spacecraft will not be close enough to Earth at all times to make feasible the delivery of extra or replacement materials. There cannot be a timely evacuation of an unexpectedly ill astronaut. Repair and maintenance equipment for the spacecraft and other components of the mission will be limited by weight and space. If there is a Martian rover (vehicle to allow astronauts to travel on the Martian surface), there will be challenges to vehicle maintenance and replacement of parts if necessary. For these and other challenges, it will also be necessary to determine what medical countermeasures including medications, pharmacy agents, and medical and surgical equipment can be fit into the Mars mission spacecraft [21–23]. New pharmaceutical agents are continually being developed including radiation countermeasures, which must be tested for potential toxicity when added to other medications that may be required to treat infections or unexpected conditions of adaptation.

For the Mars mission, a focus on human biology, and particularly radiation biology, will be very important for the planning process [24–31]. While there are specific issues related to the relative biological effect (RBE)00 of the different forms of irradiation that were measured by the Curiosity Rover, there is the important fact that hundreds of space travelers (astronauts) are now being followed for late effects of radiation exposure [24, 25]. These are real data from humans, who have been in space for a prolonged duration including individuals that have been on the International Space Station for periods of over 1 year. It is our understanding that not only the acute effects but also the late effects of various forms of ionizing irradiation are very important. The Mars mission has been estimated to be of 860 days in duration (180 days—6 months of travel to Mars, 500 days on the Martian surface, and 180 days—6 months for the return cruise). This duration is nearly three times longer than the longest duration of residence by an astronaut on the International Space Station. Many publications regarding this length of time for a space mission have addressed issues of psychological isolation, prolonged weightlessness, management of medical conditions, and physiologic changes in astronauts; however, there has been little attention to the expected effects of this length of time of exposure to ionizing irradiation [26]. There is a plethora of data regarding dose–response curves for ionizing irradiation. This comes from tissue culture and experimental animal experiments that date back to the early decades of the twentieth century. However, the majority of these experiments were carried out with X-rays/gamma rays. There is little information on continuous low-dose rate irradiation, even with X-rays. Most importantly, these experiments have not been duplicated with protons, which will be the components of solar proton events, high linear energy transfer (LET) charged particles that comprise galactic cosmic irradiation, and neutron irradiation that will be a component of the complex exposure of astronauts. Neutrons are generated by GCR hitting the spacecraft and components of the habitat.

There is at present robust data on the mixed beam composition of the forms of irradiation that will be hitting the astronauts [9]. Experimental systems on basic radiobiology, including animal experiments, usually focus on one form (quality) of irradiation. The Brookhaven National Laboratories have recently initiated studies with mixed beam irradiation in which charged particles, protons, and X-rays will be combined at varying ratios to simulate space radiation. However, little data is available on the outcomes. There is an assumption that the lack of untoward effects of nearly 1-year exposure to the mixed beam irradiation of space travel, from the residents of the International Space Station, can be translated to expect relative safety of a mission that will be three times that duration (860 days) [1], but this is an expectation not supported by data.

Preparatory Stages for the Mars Mission

The Mars mission will occur, but before the initiation of this mission, there will be incremental steps including a plan for a longer duration mission on the Lunar surface called "Lunar Sorties." This mission will deliver very important data because, as designed, there are plans to transport four astronauts to the Lunar surface, where they will reside in a constructed habitat. Sorties either walking or "moon-buggy" vehicle transport from the habitat will generate valuable information on real issues that will also apply to the Mars landing astronaut party. Much closer to Earth and the cruise phase to get there is much shorter, the critical factor of prolonged residence on the surface of the Moon (or Mars) will have several common factors that will generate important data. Both the Moon and Mars have no magnetosphere to funnel charged particles to the poles. The astronauts will be exposed to continuous GCR from all directions and solar proton events related to storms on the Sun (sunspots), which will be preceded by gamma ray irradiation that will be detected on Earth and reported to the astronauts allowing them time to return to the habitat, where there will, of necessity, be better shielding against protons [17]. For the planned Lunar Sorties mission, there will be a more precise recording of the different forms of irradiation and, particularly, the quantitation of neutrons. Prior to the Lunar Sorties mission, material scientists will have better information on the materials to construct the surface habitat. There is encouraging information from material scientists and engineers that there are lightweight materials that can actually absorb radiation. There is ongoing research to develop the materials for a spacecraft and a habitat that can manage the many forms of irradiation in a fashion that now is only speculative: wouldn't it be amazing if a magnetosphere could be designed to encircle the spacecraft and the habitat so that GCR and protons (with charge) would be funneled/directed toward a specific site in an area not inhabited by the astronauts. The magnetosphere on Earth captures charged particles from GCR and solar proton events and directs these to the polar regions [30]. Construction of a magnetosphere around the spacecraft or habitat would undoubtedly require significant energy to create the magnetic field, and the medical consequences of exposure of the astronauts to this magnetic field must be understood. Penetration of the spacecraft or habitat by X-rays would still occur and a major focus of research now is to minimize X-radiation/gamma radiation exposure to the astronauts. Shielding against non-charged X-rays/gamma rays has been well developed and irradiation machines used to treat cancer have been studied since the turn of the twentieth century [28, 29]. However, the shielding materials are heavy and the cost of fashioning them and transporting them to Mars would be a major issue. Materials scientists are developing x-irradiation resistant materials that are lighter and some have potentially great possibilities for use in the design of spacecrafts and in the Martian habitat. All of these materials must be fashioned to produce the minimal level of neutrons that will be generated by GCR hitting the materials [11, 19, 25]. Those neutrons, which penetrate the artificial magnetosphere, travel through building materials that are effective for X-rays and charged particles.

The significant information on neutron shielding is from work with the construction of nuclear power plants. The fuel rods containing plutonium are balanced by an equal number of graphite-containing shielding rods or control rods that absorb neutrons and regulate the capacity of nuclear reactors to reach critical mass and explode. Is there a graphite-like material that can be used in the construction of the spacecraft and the habitat? Current evidence indicates that there are materials under investigation by material scientists and one or more of these novel materials may be available for testing in the next decade [25].

Medical and radiobiologic experiments on "combined injury" relative to ionizing irradiation are a very important area of research [25]. A dose–response curve for ionizing irradiation injury is shifted to show greater sensitivity to lower cumulative doses, if there is another form of physiologic stress on the system. To prepare for the management of combined injury in astronauts, who will be on an 860-day mission, a major effort is underway in the area of the development of radiation countermeasures. While the radiation dose–response curve can be shifted to show greater sensitivity to lower doses of irradiation by combined injury, the dose–response curve can be shifted in the opposite direction by the presence of a medical countermeasure in the system. Current research continues to focus on pharmaceutical agents that will enhance DNA double-strand break repair that is caused by ionizing irradiation, and enhancement or preservation of antioxidant stores in cells, tissues, and organs. Antioxidant stores are rapidly depleted by ionizing irradiation and restoration of the level of these stores can provide a significant radiation countermeasure [25, 31].

There are new approaches to radiation countermeasures, several of which are particularly exciting. The use of genetically engineered bacteria to reconstitute or shift the balance of microbes in the intestinal microbiome is one area of great interest [21]. For an 860-day mission in which astronauts will be consuming specific forms of liquid and solid nutrition, the intestinal microbiome and, particularly, the balance of different bacterial taxa in the communities of bacteria will change. There are some microbial communities that appear to be radiation protective [21]. There is research underway to determine whether reconstitution of the intestinal microbiome with different communities can be radiation protective [21].

Planned Stages of Space Exploration and Radiobiology

Plans for the Mars mission are well underway, and it is clear that, at some time, this mission will be completed and the astronauts returning from Mars will bring valuable information to scientists at all levels to plan for the next mission of even longer duration. Scientists already have their eyes on the Moon of Jupiter, Europa, and satellite information, including that from the recent Juno Mission, provides exciting evidence that there may be a source of water there. Information from the Hubble and Webb orbiting telescopes has revealed that planets orbiting stars as far away as 180–200 light years may contain water. Just as the Lunar Sorties mission will be an incremental step to Mars, the Mars mission will be an incremental step to space missions of longer duration and to reach more distant targets. The Mars mission will provide yet another very important set of data: namely, how to generate a continuous supply of oxygen and water for the 860 days. The chemistry of the generation of oxygen and generation of water is well established. The plans to implement these technologies on the spacecraft and in the Martian habitat must be designed, with appropriate backup systems and redundant systems to eliminate any potential loss or decrease in the supply of these two critical items. There is suggestive evidence that there may have been water at one point on Mars, and subterranean excavation may reveal a source of ice, potentially an alternative supply of water, but this is speculative. The maintenance of an oxygen system in the spacecraft, in the Martian habitat, and in the spacesuits will also be critical and must have multiple backup systems and redundant systems.

After decades of speculation about the composition of space irradiation and calculations of the estimated risk to humans exposed to such radiation, the data from the Mars Rover Mission (Curiosity Rover) [1] have provided the most up-to-date and potentially valuable information. This mission which was funded by NASA collected data on the Martian surface for 300 days beginning August 7, 2012, and involved a robotic lander on the surface of Mars, which was delivered by a spacecraft, which left Earth in the year 2012 [13, 27]. The published calculations of the cumulative total radiation dose to be expected for a Mars mission was 1.01 sieverts [1]. A sievert is defined as the dose equivalent of the biological effect of ionizing irradiation based on one joule of energy per kilogram of water. The calculation takes into account many factors and estimates based on the best available information that was available.

The Curiosity Robert Mission calculation includes an estimate of 180 travel days for astronauts each way (total 360 days cruising) and 500 days on the planet surface for a total of 860 days of exposure to the conditions in space and on the Martian surface. The number presented, although imperfect, helped to stimulate discussion about the radiobiology. If we assume that the detectors that were on the Curiosity Mission captured all the expected forms of radiation including: (1) gamma rays; (2) solar proton events (SPE); (3) galactic cosmic rays (GCR), also termed galactic cosmic radiation (GCR); and (4) neutrons that were generated by GCR charged particles hitting the spacecraft and the Rover, and if we assume that the RBE (relative biological effect) metrics used were accurate, that is the recorded and the reported number. There is a continuing controversy that number of 1.1 sievert is, perhaps, inaccurate and can only be used as an estimate for all the discussions to follow. The dose of 1.1 sievert is not overwhelming given that 1.1 gray of total body irradiation (TBI), which is all X-rays and is used to prepare patients for a bone marrow transplantation. That clinical TBI dose is acceptably tolerated when delivered in a clinical radiation oncology center and at a dose rate of 3–5 cGy/min in a single exposure, but only if followed by a bone marrow transplant to overcome hematopoietic system failure. If humans tolerate TBI damage to the heart, lungs, intestine, and other organs that is delivered at clinically low dose rate (3–5 cGy/min), and if that 1.1 sievert as reported by the Curiosity Mission is equivalent to 1.1 gray of X-rays, and if that 1.1 sievert is slowly delivered at the very low dose rate, which would be over 860 days, then this estimated radiation damage would be tolerated, correct?

Much additional discussion and generation of new data must precede any answer to the above questions. There is some information about acute radiation effects and how to administer countermeasures [22]. However, radiation late effects are more difficult to predict (Fig. 8.1). The expected 6-month travel duration to and from the Martian surface and the 500 days on the surface is an estimate, so the duration of the mission is not firmly established. The materials used in the design of the spacecraft and the Martian habitat have not yet been established, so calculations of penetration of SPE, GCR, and generated neutrons cannot be reliably estimated [2–11, 14]. Most importantly, the medical and human biological factors (RBE) of the physically measured doses by physical dosimeters [9, 11, 12] have not been considered adequately. Most important are the issues of (1) sporadic GCR and (2) RBE of the radiation sources, which would make that 1.1 sievert number much higher.

The Curiosity Rover took photographs, which were sent back to Earth and led to much excitement and speculation about the Martian surface. The publication in Science in 2014 [1] included an analysis of the data collection with respect to space irradiation. The data are robust and exciting [2–8], and have stimulated much speculation as to the estimated total dose of irradiation that would be sustained by astronauts on the Mars mission. In addition, there is helpful data about human tolerance to space radiation. There have been 260 visitors to the International Space Station [14], including one individual who was there for 370 days (Table 8.1). In addition, there are well over 100 former astronauts, who are being followed for radiation effects.

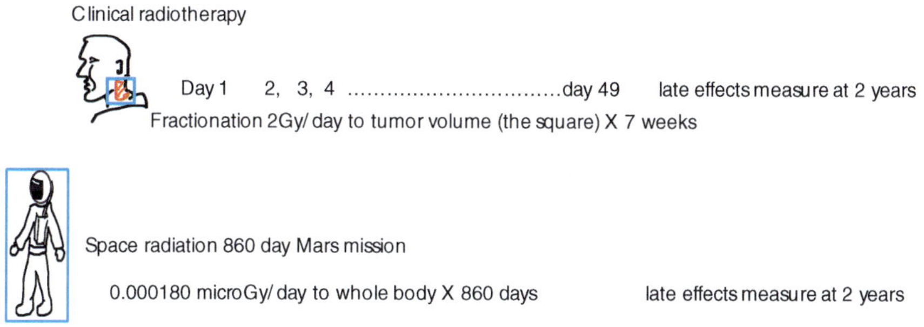

Fig. 8.1 How can data from clinical radiotherapy relate to the potential late effects of space radiation? This figure demonstrates the difference between radiation effects, which would arise from radiotherapy delivered in the clinical treatment of head and neck cancer (top panel) to a comparison of the space radiation, which would be a total body exposure from an 860-day mission on the surface of Mars (bottom panel). The volume of tissue treated is significantly different, which is a head and neck volume in the top panel of clinical radiotherapy compared to total body irradiation for the space radiation (bottom panel). Clinical radiotherapy would be fractionated over 7 weeks or 49 days delivering doses up to 70 Gy, but in a short interval and to a small volume. In contrast, space radiation for an 860-day Mars mission would likely deliver 0.000180 micro Gy per day whole body dose for 860 days. Predicting the late effects at 2 years for each of these exposure situations is very different and is a challenge for scientists and physicians

Table 8.1 The relative timeline for space missions

Date	Mission	Achievements (planned = *)
July 1969	Apollo Moon Landing	Safely landing spacecraft on Moon and safely return to Earth
2014	Curiosity Rover Landing on Mars	Collection of 1 sievert radiation exposure for a planned 380-day mission
200–2028 (2030) International Space Station	260 astronauts from multiple countries, 163 from U.S. visit here	Longest duration occupancy by single astronaut 371 days (Frank Rubio)
2024	Juno the Satellite Discoveries of Jupiter Moons	Possible water on Moon, Europa
2024	Astrobotic Peregrine Moon Lander	Public-Private NASA Partnership
2025	Artemis II	(*) Planned circumnavigate Moon-Landers
2026	Moon landing	(*) Lunar Sorties Mission Construction of habitat
2015 (2019)	Discovery of exoplanet K-2-18b orbiting dwarf star K218	Hubble and Webb telescopes find habitable exoplanet/24 light years from Earth

How Can We Estimate the Biological Effect of Radiation for the Astronauts on the Mars Mission?

Mars has no magnetosphere and a thinner atmosphere, so the measured composition of the radiation exposure that was measured by the Curiosity Rover [1] was quite different. The daily dose measured was predictably higher in the travel vehicle (cruise phase) than on the Martian surface, where the soil surface limited radiation from below and the topography—hills and valleys—limited exposure from lateral/directional SPEs. However, two variables may be very different for the astronauts, who will be involved in the mission. These variables include the composition of the cruise vehicle for optimal shielding and minimal neutron generation, as well as the solar cycle for proton irradiation. The galactic cosmic radiation (GCR) termed GCI elsewhere was estimated at 180–225 micro-gray per day [1]. It was converted to microsieverts, and that was the assumption that charged particles were of equivalent RBE. The variation in RBE, SPE, and neutrons would be taken into account for a modified calculation once the materials that will be used to construct the cruise vehicle and habitat are known. There is much work to be done, but the Curiosity Rover mission gave us a great start.

The radiation biology and radiation medicine issues for the Mars astronauts are now coming into focus. Calculating the level of radiation that will be measured in the spacecraft during the 6-month travel to Mars and doubling this exposure level, anticipating that the return travel would be of equal duration, then we must allow for changes in the relative abundance of each radiation form during the expected 500-day duration that astronauts would spend on the Martian surface. The Curiosity

Mission calculations were reported as a cumulative radiation dose that would be on the borderline of that which could cause the Hematopoietic Syndrome. Thus, the data (even when uncorrected for the RBE of GCR and solar proton events (SPEs) and neutrons) suggest that there will be a measurable risk of bone marrow suppression from radiation. While the data as reported is an estimate, it is, nonetheless, of cancers and valuable for planning what radiation countermeasures to take in the spacecraft. What the data do not report concern the RBE for humans and must be considered.

Space radiation will be sporadic and comprised of multiple different radiation sources, including (as described in previous chapters) solar proton events, X-rays, galactic cosmic irradiation from supernovae that will deliver charged particles in ions of different molecular weights and charges, and neutrons that would be generated by GCR hitting the material elements in the spacecraft [13, 20–25]. The sporadic and unpredictable nature of the GCR and associated neutron production is, perhaps, the most important with respect to RBE. Since the calculation of 1.1 sievert suggests that there is a risk of bone marrow failure, medical countermeasures should be considered [22, 23, 31]. For the administration of medical countermeasures to the Mars mission astronauts, there are two possible administration schedules to consider: (1) continuous administration, as a dietary supplement [31] and (2) that directed by instructions from mission control to prepare for an SPE [16]. Solar proton events (solar storms—sunspots) can be predicted by gamma ray bursts that would be detected on Earth and are related to the appearance of sunspots on the surface of the sun. The SPEs have already been shown to have seasonal variation [17]. However, the detection of a proton event that is "imminent" would not necessarily allow astronauts either in the spacecraft or on the Martian surface to shelter quickly enough to decrease the level of proton irradiation exposures. Given the uncertainty (controversy) about the RBE of each of the charged particles in the compositions of GCR, and the additional controversy about the RBE (relative biological effect) of the mixed beam effect of the combinations of X-rays (gamma rays), solar protons, neutrons, and GCR, these numbers from the Curiosity Rover must be considered estimates. Separation of the composition of the radiation sources that produce the data from the Curiosity Rover is very difficult and even more difficult to relate to the biological effects on humans.

The most interesting and challenging aspect of the calculations of levels of space irradiation is how to relate the data to the RBE, and, most importantly, to the biological mechanisms of continuous repair of low levels of DNA damage, depletion, and replenishment of antioxidant stores [31] and the concept of adaptation to radiation.

Clinical radiation oncology protocols have always included fractionation [18, 30–32], first introduced in the 1970s was the concept of tumor compared to normal tissue adaptation to radiation. The clinical terminology starts with the concept of fractionated radiotherapy to treat cancer patients. Basic radiation biology experiments with animal models and cells in culture preceded by 20 years [18, 31], the design of clinical protocols. These clinical protocols included those for hyperfractionation 2–3 treatments per day with low doses or hypofractionation (larger doses to small volumes with one treatment per day or every other day [31]. The cell culture data first suggested that DNA repair was completed 4 h after the last of several radiation exposures. For hyperfractionation in clinical protocols, radiation oncologists designed ways to deliver a lower dose per treatment (1.5 Gy) to the cancer target volume twice a day separated by 4 h, rather than delivering a single dose fraction of 2.0–3.0 Gy. This number of 4 h between (radiation treatment dose) fractions has now been extended to 6 h between fractions for some current head and neck cancer patient protocols, and the interval between fractions may change for different cancers and different protocols [31]. While these numbers are estimates for the safe delivery of hyperfractionated radiation for head and neck cancer, the concept is that the repair of radiation damage in normal tissues near the cancer, but included in the radiation beam, is different from that of the cells in the cancer, such that the time between exposures would help decrease toxicity. Hyperfractionation was designed to increase the therapeutic ratio (defined as the ratio of tumor cell killing to normal tissue damage). This concept has been present in clinical radiation oncology since the first in vitro radiobiology experiments [18].

What is not known is the time needed for repair of radiation damage from fractionated or low-level continuous GCR. Furthermore, radiation late effects of space irradiation cannot be easily correlated to clinical radiation therapy data (Fig. 8.1). Some fractionation experiments have been performed with protons, charged particles, and neutron irradiation [17, 31]. However, the real challenge is to obtain data with high LET charged particle radiation in the composition of the mixed beam of GCR. The sporadic nature of GCR and the unknown composition of the ions that would hit the astronauts during each GCR exposure are not known. NASA reports that the level of GCR is constant [20]. Some data with carbon ion particle radiotherapy and helium ion (alpha particles) are available [21]. (There is an assumption that all of the elements of GCR would be present with each day of the 860-day mission, and this is a real assumption) (Fig. 8.1). There is little information available on the repair time for this type of radiation damage that would be sustained by the different tissues and organ systems in experimental animals and in astronauts. Therefore, information on the biological effects of the cumulative radiation exposure information from the Curiosity Rover experiments is elusive at present. The fact that the data reported in the recent literature on the Mars mission dosimetry give an estimate that would be in the range for the Hematopoietic Syndrome, and radiobiologists and space radiation physicians have a concern about the need to prepare for preventative countermeasures and for medical management of irradiation-induced bone marrow and other organ system irradiation-induced events in astronauts [1].

For the preparation of a Mars mission, the materials used to produce the spacecraft, as well as any materials that would be used for the Martian lander and the expected sorties on the surface, become a great subject of investigation. Materials that would comprise the cruise-phase Martian spacecraft have led to several investigations. The materials must be light enough, not only to be assembled in space but must be able to withstand significant temperature differences and to provide shielding from some or all forms of space irradiation. The materials must be tested for the generation of neutrons when exposed to charged particles comprising GCR.

Once the materials for the spacecraft have been optimized, there then becomes the issue of the engine propulsion system needed to reach Mars once discharge from the Earth's gravity is obtained. At a recent presentation at the Radiation Research Society in Big Island, Hawaii, a discussion of the power source for the spacecraft was a focus of one presentation. At present, a nuclear-powered engine for the spacecraft has been discarded due to its potential danger of a leakage of radioisotopes for the generation of nuclear power into the Earth's atmosphere at some point during departure or return to Earth. This question about nuclear power is unresolved, but the use of nuclear reactors to power the Mars spacecraft would also pose an additional risk of radiation exposure to the astronauts from inside the vehicle during the 180-day cruise phase to Mars and 180-day cruise phase of return to Earth. Such information on nuclear submarines and aircraft carriers is available to allow measurements of radiation exposure to personnel, but management of leaks could not be essentially carried out in the vehicle.

Calculations are available from military operations in which nuclear weapons are carried in weapon systems. The "broken arrow" drills [32, 33]. are carried out for submarines and ships that have nuclear reactors. A nuclear reactor-powered spacecraft for the Mars mission would necessitate that the astronauts be in close proximity to such a radiation source inside the spacecraft for an estimated 360 days (cruise phase—6 months travel to and 6 months back to Earth).

The available information now is that a solid fuel-powered vehicle would be the engine used to deliver astronauts to the Martian surface. While such a fuel source would be preferable to a nuclear reactor for safety issues, this fuel would be heavy, and that used for the return cruise must be carried to Mars and kept ready for the return trip. The use of solar power for a vehicle has also been discussed, but the inefficiency of collecting solar energy and imperfect battery storage pose challenges. Once, the materials for the spacecraft and the source of power have been established, even more attention will be directed to medical issues, including the health and safety of the astronauts. The issues related to space shuttle missions, the International Space Station, and the Lunar missions would still apply related to radiation exposure, but now with a greater duration including social isolation, weightlessness, and polypharmacy medications including dietary changes and drugs for radiation countermeasures. Even without a nuclear-powered engine, there are many issues involved in how to deal with the health of astronauts during prolonged confinement in a space vehicle.

Preparation for addressing the medical needs of astronauts has thus far focused on physiological conditions that are known, including bone loss associated with weightlessness, stress and psycho-social isolation, viral and bacterial infections, changes in the microbiome, diet-associated changes, and the unavoidable need to prepare for handling physical injury. The "first-aid" kit that would be available on the Mars spacecraft during the cruise phase, as well as in the Martian habitat, would be weight-limited and would also have to prioritize medications for each of these potential conditions. What is not resolved is what, if any, radiation countermeasures should be provided.

NASA has funded research for medical countermeasures and has focused on things that are feasible and practical pharmaceuticals that might be of value in helping astronauts to repair radiation damage or decrease the magnitude of injury from such damage [28].

Radiation countermeasures will be designed to address the feasible approaches, which will include dietary modifications to increase antioxidant stores [31], delivery of pharmaceuticals, potentially a chronic administration of a radiation countermeasure, and a consideration of how to monitor the astronauts for the level of radiation damage—biomarkers [28]. If there are to be additional countermeasures that are developed if there is an impending SPE (proton) from the detection of gamma-ray bursts, what would this "booster" medication be? Would there be a supplement to counteract proton irradiation from SPEs [22]?

Considerations Regarding Travel in a Space Vehicle

The composition of materials to design the space vehicle will be critical to minimize the irradiation penetration of the vehicle and the magnitude of gamma rays, protons, charged particles, and neutrons hitting the astronauts. The last category of neutron irradiation will depend upon the composition of the materials. Neutrons are shielded by water and other materials that can absorb the neutrons. It would be impractical for spacecraft construction using high-volume materials, such as water to shield against neutrons [32, 33]. In addition, the neutrons would be created by solar particles hitting other materials in the spacecraft and generating the neutrons. Therefore, putting a neutron absorber between the outer shell of the spacecraft and the astronauts would not only be impractical, but prohibitive by weight. A shielding mechanism, whereby solar particles from GCR and protons could be deflected from the spacecraft into space by a magnetic field that could be generated to surround the spacecraft, would be ideal, if feasible.

Research in the development of materials for the protection of military personnel has been discussed. Kevlar vests and coverings have greatly decreased fatalities from projectiles including bullets. For military tanks, protection devices for the current generation of military tanks led to the design of materials, whereby an artillery shell hitting the outside of the tank would result in a microsecond-directed outward explosion of a shielding device to deflect the energy outward. Unlike this strategy for deflection of GCR particles on a spacecraft, penetrating anti-tank weapons have been developed to counteract this outward explosion as a novel but effective strategy for a shielding device. Unlike the military approach, the space irradiation approach would have no confusion about the nature of the radiation. It is well known that there will be four sources from outside the spacecraft and shielding devices by which to minimize the penetration of the vehicle from each of these four sources is a clear focus of research in Materials Science and Engineering.

Martian Surface

Mars does not have a magnetosphere and there would be minimal shielding for astronauts on the Martian surface by the deflection and collection of charged particles to the poles [7]. The Martian atmosphere is also significantly thinner. However, there is some component of physical shielding of radiation by the terrain of the Martian surface [19]. The surface does have mountains and valleys and physical shielding of astronauts by physical geographic structures would be possible to calculate. The soil protects from radiation coming from below. The site of the landing of the first Martian manned vehicle would be important to calculate to provide for some shielding of astronauts, who would stay inside the vehicle for different periods of time. Placing the lander in an area shielded by mountainous terrain would protect against protons. However, the galactic cosmic irradiation coming from all directions except from below would be less shielded. Gamma radiation that precedes solar proton events would be partially shielded by the physical nature of the terrain, and the habitat that would be constructed in proximity where the Martin lander resided.

How long would the Martian lander remain on the surface before astronauts returned to the cruise vehicle for the return to Earth? While still a subject of speculation, it is anticipated that astronauts would stay on the Martian surface for some period of time around 500 days [1]. If this were to be weeks–months, then the concept of construction of a habitat is clearly relevant. Depending upon the size of the space vehicle, a component of the Martian lander could serve as a habitat. If there were to be Martian Sorties outside the lander, then the considerations discussed in the previous chapter on Lunar Sorties would be similar. Will there be a "Martian-buggy"? With respect to space radiation, the major difference between the Lunar and Martian Missions is the duration of exposure. The 6-month time of exposure of the astronauts on their way to the Martian surface and 6 months for the return compared to the relatively short time of exposure experienced by astronauts traveling to the Lunar surface. Six months of cumulative radiation exposure during the cruise phase each way = 12 months will factor into the materials used to construct the cruise vehicle, Martian lander, and habitat. The 500 days on the Martian surface may require a different form of protective shielding. Once the anticipated relative accumulation of radiation exposure from protons compared to GCR is better estimated, the components of the shielding can be modified. Data from the Curiosity Rover will be further supplemented by modification for the RBE of each radiation source for humans [1]. The biological effects of the charged particles that will be detected during the 6 months of travel to the Martian surface, compared to the composition of particles detected when the astronauts are on the Martian surface, will be important to know [32, 34]. Can the timing of the intervals between intense GCR be calculated as with SPE events or is GCR consistent? Once these data are obtained, then it must be supplemented by information yet to be published on the composition of materials used to produce the spacecraft. Once the composition of the charged particles (ions) in the GCR can be reliably predicted, then the materials in the spacecraft can be tested for their resistance to penetration, their magnitude of energy levels, and the capacity of each charged particle, when hitting materials in the spacecraft to produce neutrons [9]. Nuclear weapons are known to produce neutrons [33] and some measurements have yielded useful information.

Other Knowns and Unknowns Regarding Space Irradiation During the Mars Mission

There is a high likelihood that the relative contribution and magnitude of irradiation to astronauts that is comprised coming from gamma rays, protons, and neutrons can be reliably estimated. The spectrum of proton energies has been derived from Lunar missions [14–17] and this composition will be compared to be relations the same for the Mars mission. Until there is more information on the composition of GCR, the ion composition of GCR, and the RBE of each element in the composition, more reliable information on this form of irradiation will not be available. Using available estimates from the data so far obtained, one can estimate the composition of ions in the GCR and use known materials, such as stainless steel, titanium, carbon fiber, aluminum, and other novel materials to estimate the magnitude, spectrum, and energy levels from the production of neutrons by GCR [9].

NASA and other international space agencies are working on these calculations and radiation biologists will continue to work on designing radiation countermeasures for each radiation source.

The spacesuit worn by current astronauts has been designed with the primary goal of stabilizing temperature, delivering oxygen, absorbing carbon dioxide, and being of light enough weight to allow mobility and functioning of astronauts during extra-vehicular activities [20]. Spacesuit design has not had as a primary goal the minimizing of radiation exposure to the astronauts. For the Mars mission, the design of the spacesuit may well incorporate a consideration of radiation absorbing or reflecting materials and it must be tested for the level of generation of neutrons. If materials in the spacesuit are hit by GCR ions, it will not simply be the composition of the irradiation but the dose, the dose rate, the spectrum of energies of the particles, and the frequency of irradiation (sporadic or continuous). The baseline health and physiology of the astronauts will be a major consideration for spacesuit design.

Will astronauts for the Mars mission be screened using more restrictive criteria than those currently used for those being considered for the Lunar Sorties mission? Will cancer risk be considered? Will genetic screening be carried out including a family history of cancer [26]? Until more information is available about the capacity of humans to sustain and continually repair radiation damage from each of the forms of space irradiation in the mixed beam irradiation and under conditions of zero gravity, this question cannot be reliably answered.

References

1. Hassler DM, Zeitlin C, Wimmer RF, et al. Mars' surface radiation environment measured with the Mars science laboratory's curiosity rover. Science. 2014;343(6169):1244797. https://doi.org/10.1126/science.1244797.
2. Farley KA, Malespin C, Mahaffy P, et al. In situ radiometric and exposure age dating of the Martian surface. Science. 2014;343(6169):1247166. https://doi.org/10.1126/science.1247166.
3. Vaniman DT, Bish DL, Ming DW, et al. Mineralogy of a mudstone at Yellowknife Bay, Gale Crater. Mar Sci. 2014;343(6169):1243480. https://doi.org/10.1126/science.1243480.
4. Grotzinger JP, Sumner DY, Kah LC, et al. A habitable fluvio-lacustrine environment at Yellowknife Gay, Gale Crater. Mar Sci. 2014;343(6169):1242777. https://doi.org/10.1126/science.1242777.
5. Grotzinger JP. Exploring martian habitability. Habitability, taphonomy, and the search for organic carbon on Mars. Introduction. Science. 2014;343(6169):386–7. https://doi.org/10.1126/science.1249944.
6. Ming DW, Archer PD Jr, Glavin DP, et al. Volatile and organic compositions of sedimentary rocks in Yellowknife Bay, Gale Crater. Mar Sci. 2014;343(6169):1245267. https://doi.org/10.1126/science.1245267.
7. Cucinotta F, Smirnova O. Astronaut safety in Mars exploration missions: dynamical modeling approach to the radiogenic leukemia risk assessment. 43rd COSPAR Scientific Assembly, January 28, 2021—February 4, 2021.
8. Webster CR, Mahaffy PR, Atreya SK, et al. Background levels of methane in Mars' atmosphere show strong seasonal variations. Science. 2018;360(6393):1093–6. https://doi.org/10.1126/science.aaq0131.
9. Kohler J, Ehresmann B, Zeitlin C, et al. Measurements of the neutron spectrum in transit to Mars on the Mars science laboratory. Life Sci Space Res (Amst). 2015;5:6–12. https://doi.org/10.1016/j.lssr.2015.03.001.
10. Zeitlin C, Hassler DM, Wilmmer-Schweingruber RF, et al. Calibration and characterization of the radiation assessment detector (RAD) on curiosity. Space Sci Rev. 2016;201:201–33.
11. Ehresmann B, Hassler DM, Zeitlin C, et al. Charged particle spectra measured during the transit to Mars with the Mars science laboratory radiation assessment detector (MSL/RAD). Life Sci Space Res (Amst). 2016;10:29–37. https://doi.org/10.1016/j.lssr.2016.07.001.
12. Ehresmann B, Zeitlin CJ, Hassler DM, et al. The charged particle radiation environment on Mars measured by MSL/RAD from November 15, 2015 to January 15, 2016. Life Sci Space Res (Amst). 2017;14:3–11. https://doi.org/10.1016/j.lssr.2017.07.004.
13. Simonsen LC, Wilson JW, Kim MH, et al. Radiation exposure for human Mars exploration. Health Phys. 2000;79(5):515–25. https://doi.org/10.1097/00004032-200011000-00008.
14. Thirsk R, Kuipers A, Mukai C, et al. The space-flight environment: the international space station and beyond. CMAJ. 2009;180(12):1216–20. https://doi.org/10.1503/cmaj.081125.
15. Alperin N, Bagci AM, Lee SH. Spaceflight-induced changes in white matter hyperintensity burden in astronauts. Neurology. 2017;89(21):2187–91. https://doi.org/10.1212/WNL.0000000000004475.
16. Liu B, Gu Y, Liu Y, et al. Space neutron radiation shielding property of continuous fiber and functional filler reinforced polymer composite using Monte Carlo simulation. Compos A: Appl Sci Manuf. 2023;168:107483.
17. Ali A, Sadykov V, Kosovichev A, et al. Predicting solar proton events of solar cycles 22-24 using GOES proton and soft-X-ray flux features. ApJS. 2024;270:15.
18. Yan W, Khan MK, Wu X, et al. Spatially fractionated radiation therapy: history, present and the future. Clin Transl Radiat Oncol. 2019;20:30–8. https://doi.org/10.1016/j.ctro.2019.10.004.
19. Simonsen LC, Nealy JE, Townsend LW, et al. Space radiation shielding for a Martian habitat. SAE Trans. 1990;99(1):972–9.

20. Paige C, Newman D, Lombardo SJH, et al (2020) An integrated innovative 3D radiation protection fabric for advanced spacesuits and systems. 2020 IEEE Aerospace Conference, March 7, 2020 – March 14, 2020.
21. Li K, Epperly M, Greenberger J, et al. Longitudinal fecal microbiome study of total body irradiated mice treated with radiation mitigators identify bacterial associations with survival. Front Cell Infect Microbiol. 2021;11:715396. https://doi.org/10.3389/fcimb.2021.715396.
22. Greenberger JS. Radioprotection. In Vivo. 2009;23(2):323–36.
23. Carnell LS, Homer M, Hoots K, et al. Medical countermeasures for radiation induced health effects: report of an interagency panel session held at the NASA human research program Investigator's workshop. Int J Radiat Biol. 2021;97(sup1):S117–24. https://doi.org/10.1080/09553002.2019.1665214.
24. Parihar VK, Allen B, Tran KK, et al. What happens to your brain on the way to Mars. Sci Adv. 2015;1(4):e1400256. https://doi.org/10.1126/sciadv.1400256.
25. Cacao E, Cucinotta FA. Modeling heavy-ion impairment of hippocampal neurogenesis after acute and fractionated irradiation. Radiat Res. 2016;186(6):624–37. https://doi.org/10.1667/RR14569.1.
26. Cucinotta FA, Durante M. Cancer risk from exposure to galactic cosmic rays: implications for space exploration by human beings. Lancet Oncol. 2006;7(5):431–5. https://doi.org/10.1016/S1470-2045(06)70695-7.
27. Cucinotta FA. Review of NASA approach to space radiation risk assessments for Mars exploration. Health Phys. 2015;108(2):131–42. https://doi.org/10.1097/HP.0000000000000255.
28. Hada M, Ikeda H, Rhone JR, et al. Increased chromosome aberrations in cells exposed simultaneously to simulated microgravity and radiation. Int J Mol Sci. 2018;20(1):43. https://doi.org/10.3390/ijms20010043.
29. Kleiman NJ, Hall E, Weil MM, et al. Radiation cataract in an outbred population of mice following gamma or high-LET irradiation. Invest Ophthalmol Vis Sci. 2016;57:2509.
30. Montesinos CA, Khalid R, Cristea O, et al. Space radiation protection countermeasures in microgravity and planetary exploration. Life (Basel). 2021;11(8):829. https://doi.org/10.3390/life11080829.
31. Epperly MW, Wang H, Jones J, et al. Antioxidant-chemoprevention diet ameliorates late effects of total body irradiation and supplements radioprotection by MnSOD-plasmid liposome administration. Radiat Res. 2011;175(6):759–65. https://doi.org/10.1667/RR2398.1.
32. Jones B, Dale RG. Estimation of optimum dose per fraction for high LET radiations: implications for proton radiotherapy. Int J Radiat Oncol Biol Phys. 2000;48(5):1549–57. https://doi.org/10.1016/s0360-3015(00)00781-1.
33. Liolios T. Broken arrows: radiological hazards from nuclear warhead accidents (the Minot USAF base nuclear weapons incident). Med Phys. 2009;15:39.
34. Zeller EJ, Ronca LB, Levy PW. Proton-induced hydroxyl formation on the lunar surface. J Geophys Res. 1966;71(20):4855–60.

Chapter 9
Challenges with Spacecraft Design to Deal with Ionizing Irradiation: Solar Proton Events, Galactic Cosmic Irradiation, and Neutron Irradiation from Interaction with Components of the Spacecraft

Problems with Spacecraft Design to Deal with Ionizing Irradiation: Solar Proton Events, Galactic Cosmic Radiation (GCR), Secondary Neutrons That Are Generated by GCR Interaction with Components of the Spacecraft

The data obtained from the unmanned missions to Mars and simulations of space irradiation have been provocative and exciting [1–4]. While the actual manned mission to Mars may be planned in the future, scientists have now focused on the critical items that must be addressed before any such mission can be realistically planned.

Engine for the Spacecraft and Its Fuel Supply

Fission reactors provide the variable source of energy now used in nuclear submarines, aircraft carriers, and in the generation of electric power [5]. The discussion about the use of a fission reactor to power a spacecraft to and from Mars led to the conclusion that there is a danger of contamination of the Earth's atmosphere by radioisotopes in the event of an accident. If the nuclear reactor would be powered by Plutonium 239, contamination of the atmosphere with this isotope would lead to a global catastrophe. Accordingly, a fission reactor for powering the spacecraft has not been a primary alternative. Fusion power will be daunting to achieve for a spacecraft engine given the state of physics research to produce nuclear fusion [6].

What about a fusion reactor? The first description of the Tokamak Fusion Reactor has been much interest in developing this source of generation of electricity. This fusion reactor is, in principle, a genius design. There are four states of matter, solid, water, gas, and ionic. Extremely high heat is required to generate fusion on the order

J. Greenberger, *Radiation Oncology and Radiation Biology*,
https://doi.org/10.1007/978-3-031-66300-0_9

of 1.5 billion degrees centigrade. This temperature is higher than that on the surface of the sun, which generates its power by fusion reactions converting hydrogen isotopes into helium. The Tokamak Fusion Reactor concept is based on the ability to heat gases to these temperatures citing circular or donut-shaped series of magnets that keep the plasma (ionic state of matter) internally within the reactor [6]. The fusion reaction, which would come from the introduction of deuterium and tritium into the plasma, would generate fusion at these high temperatures and could be a source of tremendous power including the generation of electricity. Problems with the design of these fusion reactors include handling the neutrons that are produced by the fusion reaction, and keeping these neutrons separated from the walls of the reactor, where they can cause damage and, ultimately, the destruction of the reactor. Different shapes and strategies for modifying the Tokamak design have been put forward and several recent private companies are working on the source of power. The energy required to generate the heat for the fusion reaction is not trivial. The materials for the design of the fusion reactor are still being developed (Philip Ball Star Power "Does Fusion Have a Future After All? [6]). Given that fission reactor power has its dangers and safety concerns, and that fusion reactors are not yet ready for installation in a spacecraft, let alone in an Earth-resident power station, the focus has continued to rely on solid fuel rockets. Transport of the components of a Mars spaceship including its fuel supply could be lifted into the Earth's orbit at a space station, and then assembled in space. As with the other sources of power, there is always the concern about the repair of a damaged power source, spare parts, and maintenance. Given the inefficient state of battery power and difficulty with amplifying solar power, the focus on the engine for the Mars mission continues to be a solid fuel component.

Components of the Spacecraft and Spacesuits for the Astronauts

Shielding against neutrons has been studied [7–14]. High-dose rate photons/X-rays present a different challenge [15]. Shielding against protons presents yet another challenge [16–20]. Charged particles from GCR present yet another challenge for shielding [21–23]. Complex radiation beams and low dose rates further complicate the design of appropriate shielding [24–28]. In clinical radiotherapy, nuclear power stations, and in uranium mining, the lowest possible radiation dose sustained by personnel applies [29–34]. There is acceptance of the concept that galactic cosmic irradiation will be constant and continuous during the entire transit phase from Earth to Mars (approximately 180 days) and will be an issue for the Martian residency phase, projected to be around 500–600 days. The high LET (Linear Energy

Transfer) ionic particles comprise galactic cosmic irradiation and generated neutrons when they hit various materials are a concern the relative biological effect (RBE) of neutrons has been estimated to be around 10 (10 × greater than that for X-rays), and the RBE number is even higher for the different types of ions (silicon, carbon, iron), and other high energy particles. Nevertheless, there is concern about the exposure of the astronauts to both GCR and the neutrons that are generated when these particles hit materials. Spacecraft materials the Martian habitat for residents on the Martian surface, and spacesuits have been designed with a focus on radiation shielding [16]. Boron capture has been a strategy for stopping neutron penetration through materials and to the astronauts. However, this design strategy has not proven to be effective, and the issue of weight of materials and the amount of material required is still an issue. Complex mixtures of charged particles from GCR are difficult to shield [35].

Spacecraft and Martian Habitat Design

Any materials that will be involved in the design implementation of both the spacecraft and the Martian habitat have to be delivered to an assembly site. Clearly, the construction of a habitat for the astronauts on the Martian surface must involve materials that are brought from Earth. The issue of weight is always a concern. Getting the materials from the surface of the Earth to assembly or storage in the spacecraft will require huge amounts of energy and multiple missions to get to an assembly site. Once the crew arrives at Mars, the delivery of materials to the Martian surface will require multiple "soft" landings and, of course, assembly. Materials scientists and engineers are working on the major challenge, which is to achieve all the necessary requirements of the materials, but to minimize weight. Protection from x-irradiation requires high-*Z* (large molecular weight) compounds, which are heavy. Protection from protons from solar proton events, galactic cosmic irradiation, and neutrons will require different classes of materials [16–20]. Radiation protection is a major concern, but there are other issues as well including flexibility of materials, size of habitat, and other factors, which may be limiting. When one looks at the history of exploration, explorers have used materials found at the site of their arrival to construct habitats and to provide for their needs, whether it be a food supply, water supply, shelters or other factors. Until it is clear what materials are available on the Martian surface, let us assume that everything that will be needed for the Martian residence time will be materials that must be brought from Earth. This, of course, is limited by the weight and space on the spacecraft that will deliver the materials to the Martian surface.

Water and Oxygen Requirements and Weight of the Spacecraft

Until it is certain that there is a source of water on Mars, either in frozen areas that have not been confirmed to exist yet, or through the discovery of materials that may contain water for extraction, the astronauts on the Martian surface will be required to generate water from chemistry that they will bring with them. The same principles will be applied to the need for oxygen. An estimate of the first Mars mission has been around 869 days alone for the transit to and from Mars, and the approximate 500 days on the Martian surface. The ability to generate a stable supply of water and oxygen is currently a paramount concern. Experience from the International Space Station missions including those of greater than 1 year duration have encouraged the strategy of generating both water and oxygen from chemical reactions. Clearly transporting liquid oxygen from Earth to Mars would not be practical, particularly, if available back-up systems (chemical reactions) were possible. With such a primary focus on the need for continuous supplies of water and oxygen, it is not surprising that radiation protection has not been the top priority. However, radiation protection must be addressed.

Radiation Exposure of Astronauts from Multiple Sources During the Mars Mission

The basics of radiation biology on space travel are issues applied to all aspects of radiation biology. These are radiation dose, fraction size (or dose rate if this is continuous irradiation), the volume of tissue treated (one would assume this would be total body irradiation for space travel), and time of exposure. With regard to space irradiation, one must assume for the entire 860 days of a Mars mission there will be radiation exposure. The fluctuations that are known to occur are those associated with solar proton events (sunspots), and there is a consensus that galactic cosmic irradiation will be constant as will be gamma irradiation (X-rays).

What will be the consequences of an 860-day exposure to these levels of irradiation? Data from the Curiosity Rover experiments on the Martian surface and from the radiation dose estimates from space travel to Mars have led to a general calculation of the total amount of radiation exposure. What types/quality and levels of radiation will come from the core of Mars compared to levels from the atmosphere? Publications that show that the exposure would be 1 Sievert have led many scientists to conclude that this will be a "manageable" exposure. The word "safe" has not been used to describe this level of radiation exposure because the RBE stipulations must be refined [26, 29]. Radiation measurements that were made by the Curiosity mission were those with physical radiation detectors rather than biological measures. Until astronauts sustain these levels of irradiation during the Mars mission, it will not be possible to exactly predict the consequences of such exposure. However, certain principles have been suggested. Continuous radiation exposure during the 860 days will lead to accelerated aging, increased risk of carcinogenesis, increased decline of neurocognitive functions, and potentially other physiologic accelerated processes. Combining these physiologic changes with the other phenomenon of weightlessness during space travel, reduced gravity on the Martian surface, and other sources of stress on the astronauts, we must conclude that there will be biological consequences of this radiation exposure.

NASA and other scientific funding agencies have been interested in developing radiation countermeasures. Given that the level of radiation exposure will be constant and continuous, and that the radiation exposure will be complex including several forms of irradiation including gamma rays, neutrons, galactic cosmic radiation, and protons, radiation countermeasures are being developed that would apply to all forms of these radiation exposures. The astronauts will be on a specific diet, such as an antioxidant/chemopreventive diet or another diet supplemented with a radiation-protective drug, and drugs or components of a diet that would be expected to decrease the consequences of continuous radiation exposure. One question that has been asked is whether astronauts for the Mars Mission will be screened for genetic risk factors that might increase the level of irradiation-induced carcinogenesis, neurocognitive decline, aging, and other physiologic changes. It is not clear that astronauts for a long Mars Mission would be screened for these genetic factors. However, based on the clear knowledge that specific genetic components do influence the onset and severity of these consequences of continuous radiation, the question must be continually asked.

If one looks at the history of radiation safety policies in the United States for clinical radiotherapy and in developed countries, there has been a primary focus on the issue of shielding [1]. In the case of known high levels of irradiation such as that found in and around nuclear power stations, installations in which nuclear weapons and nuclear weapons grade Plutonium 239 and Uranium 235 are being produced and purified to produce fission or fusion weapons [14], there is an ongoing analysis to improve shielding to both protect workers and prevent contamination. The best ionizing irradiation shielding is to increase one's distance from the radiation-emitting source, whether from a device or from radioisotope [1]. A second approach to shielding is to analyze the quality of the irradiation, the energy of X-rays, gamma rays, or charged particles, and then implement shielding using materials that reduce the levels of exposure to each form of irradiation as much as possible [14]. Irradiation shielding materials vary with the quality/type of irradiation. For example, X-rays/gamma rays are shielded by high atomic weight (Z) atoms in the shield including lead. In contrast, neutrons pass through many high-Z materials and are best shielded by absorption into water or a neutron contour material such as graphite, which is used in the control rods in nuclear power stations. The concept of ALARA (as low as reasonably achievable) seeks to lower the radiation exposure level by humans to a level as low as reasonably possible. The ALARA concept [29] is the basis for radiation safety policies in nearly all hospitals and medical care facilities in the United States. In addition, the ALARA principle has been applied to nearly all places in which radiation detectors are used to monitor and record radiation levels. Hospitals and medical care facilities, where X-ray equipment is routinely used, have notices posted on doors and walls to advise patients and their families to refrain from entering these areas containing radiation equipment if they are pregnant or think they might be pregnant. There are warnings everywhere about the hazards of ionizing irradiation.

Given the concern about radiation levels, the need for shielding and the requirements for radiation protection of hospital workers and patients (lead aprons), there is a continuing need to understand the nervousness of the general population. In contrast, hospital and industrial workers, who choose employment in a location, where there is an irradiation-hazardous environment will have required training [29–34]. Radiation workers are advised of the increased risks of working in an irradiation-intense environment. These radiation workers choose to accept a higher level of exposure compared to that of the general population. These workers willingly exceed the ALARA levels for the general population, but there are maximum levels monitored for these individuals. Radiation workers wear radiation film dosimetry badges that are quantitated regularly. They are monitored to not exceed their accepted level of quarterly and yearly exposure levels. Radiation workers include hospital personnel including radiologists, cardiologists, and physicians, who carry out fluoroscopy. Also, technicians who work with positron emission tomography (PET) scan isotopes and other healthcare professions willingly accept higher levels of radiation exposure [31]. Based on the reported increased incidence of cancer, in Uranium, and in other miners who have been exposed to higher levels of radiation, recommended maximum levels of exposure have been advised about the hazards of irradiation. There have been multiple publications of their higher incidence of cancer and other medical conditions and other biomarkers of premature aging [32, 33].

All of these historical considerations, which are relative to radiation safety hospitals and nuclear power station workers, have contributed to the planned design of shielding of spacecraft for the Lunar-Sortie Mission, and ultimately the Mars Mission. Given all the published information about shielding based on decades of research on Earth, it is clear that the materials used to design a spacecraft and a lunar or Martian habitat must take into account the challenging requirements for a light-weight material that can also provide effective shielding against gamma rays/X--rays, protons, neutrons, and GCR. The design of such materials, their current availability, cost, weight, and practicality present a huge challenge to NASA and to all space programs.

Shielding Requirements for a Spacecraft or Extra-Terrestrial Habitat: What Is Achievable, Reasonable and Practical?

Engineering, materials science, and physics research have provided valuable information on the requirements for shielding of each of the forms of ionizing irradiation that will be encountered during space travel. X-rays and gamma rays require shielding using materials that have a high Z or high molecular weight. The Z of a material includes the atomic number of the chemical elements in the shield. Each element has a *Z* value, which is measured by the number of protons and neutrons in the nucleus of that particular elemental atom. Accordingly, high-*Z* materials that are used to shield X-rays include lead, depleted Uranium 238, and other very heavy materials. Lead for a space vehicle is impractical due to its weight and cost of assembly. X-rays and gamma rays penetrate materials of low *Z*, and the depth of penetration is directly related to the energy of the photons (nonparticle) radiation. When X-rays/gamma rays hit a high molecular weight (high *Z*) material, they produce secondary effects. Low-energy X-rays produce the photoelectric effect in which visible light is generated. This is the basis for diagnostic X-rays in which high *Z* biological materials such as the calcium apatite in bone appear white and low *Z* materials, such as the oxygen, nitrogen, and carbon dioxide in air in the lungs appear black. The film in the X-ray readout records the level of penetration of the X-rays into the chemicals in the film, which is developed much the same as a photograph. Higher energy X-rays/gamma rays produce the physical effect of Compton scattering [25], and the highest energy X-rays produce the physical effect called pair-production (creation of electron and positron particles in positron pairs). The three physical effects of X-rays/gamma rays are secondary events that occur in all materials that are hit with X-rays. The easiest and most understandable shielding for all the forms of space irradiation is that for X-rays/gamma rays. However, the problem is the need for high molecular weight materials (high *Z*). The feasibility of designing a spacecraft with several inches of lead shielding would be impractical. In addition, the cost and assembly of this heavy structure in space. Getting the lead into space would require large rocket-powered shuttles to deliver the lead to the assembly site at a space station or on the Moon. Is there an alternative to avoid the use of high-*Z* materials? Is there another way to attenuate the X-rays in the beam that penetrate the spacecraft materials? The highest molecular weight materials are still used in shielding in hospitals and in clinical medicine, but what about space irradiation? A solution would be a material that absorbs X-rays/gamma rays much like graphite or water absorbs neutrons.

Radiation of one quality can produce radiation of another quality. For example, electron beam radiation is useful to treat skin cancer due to the low level of tissue protection. Machines that generate an electron beam cause Bremstrahlung and/or "breaking irradiation" [27]. As electrons hit high-*Z* materials that are used in the collimator head of linear accelerators, they generate X-rays, which must be shielded or quantitated in the dosimeters as part of the treatment delivered [28]. There is another challenge for Radiation Oncology departments on the use of high-*Z* shielding materials. High-energy X-ray beams are used to treat patients with tumors that are deep in tissues. Linear accelerators delivering high-energy X-rays above 10 MV shape the beams using collimators so as to treat only the tumors and avoid normal tissues. To achieve this goal multileaf collimators have been fashioned, but the materials in the collimators generate neutrons. When the X-rays above 10 MV hit the high *Z* metals in the collimators they produce neutrons. The linear accelerator collimators are composites of very thick strips/leaves of high-*Z* material that move and produce a shape in the collimator head of the radiation machine, such that the beam that enters the patient is precisely fashioned/shaped. There are new micro-multileaf collimators, which are now routinely used for stereotactic radiosurgery and stereotactic ablative radiosurgery. It is these collimators that are state-of-the-art for delivering high radiation dose fractions to very small volumes (several millimeters in diameter) [28]. For example, to treat primary tumors in the brain and brain metastasis from other organs these small fields are used. The target might be close to a critical structure, which should not be irradiated. The precision of the field treated with the use of multileaf collimators and immobilization of patients allows a high radiation dose (15–18 Gy) to be delivered to target volumes of 1 cm diameter or less, but some are within millimeters of a critical structure such as the brainstem or the spinal cord [28]. The thickness of the shielding in the leaves of the multileaf collimators (usually is lead or another high-*Z* material) which is indeed, etc. very thick. The thickness of the leaves in the collimator leaf is quantitated by "half-value-layers." A half-value layer reduces the radiation beam by ½ so multiple half value layers, reducing that ½ Gy ½ or ¼ the dose is delivered. Ten half-value layers are the sought-after value. The half-value layer metric refers back to the original lead or Sarabande (metal) blocks that were placed on a lucite tray that was attached to the collimators of the earliest linear accelerators in the 1970s. These shielding devices were composed of molded heavy lead or other high-*Z* material blocks that were individually designed for each patient and were fixed to the linear accelerator to shield the normal tissue from the radiation beam [28].

These heavy blocks that shielded normal tissues in the 1970s were difficult for radiation therapists (technicians) to lift and attach to the treatment device for each individual patient on a daily basis for each fraction (40-day) treatment course. Multileaf collimators were designed to fit into the linear accelerator and replaced the block trays and heavy blocks. The data on both block trays and multileaf collimators provided strong evidence that the shielding materials for X-rays (and gamma rays) required material that was very heavy (high *Z*). When high-energy X-rays hit the collimator leaves they produced neutrons.

To shield a spacecraft or habitat against x-irradiation would be clearly impractical to carry tons of lead, depleted uranium, or other high *Z* material into space to assemble the vehicle. Therefore, research on X-ray shielding is a top priority. A clever but impractical solution would be to create a magnetosphere around the spacecraft. Materials scientists have developed ways to assemble building materials in a zero gravity atmosphere to allow molecular alignment in different configurations so that relatively lighter weight materials can also shield against X-rays and produce fewer neutrons. This materials science research is in the early developmental stages and not yet ready for application to designing a spacecraft [7]. Therefore, one must return to the basics of X-rays/gamma rays physics and study the phenomenon of energy of the X-rays.

X-rays/gamma rays are not the only problem. In the case of spacecraft design, X-rays will be penetrating the spacecraft from their role as precursors to protons from SPEs (solar proton events) (there is an X-ray/gamma ray burst preceeding solar protons), there is also the challenge of shielding against the high LET (linear energy transfer) charged particles from supernovae (galactic cosmic irradiation). There is an entire spectra of charged particles for supernovae, and these represent many elements including iron, silicon, and carbon [35]. These particles will hit the spacecraft, and they will produce secondary events including X-rays and neutrons. The energy of the X-rays is directly related to their depth of penetration into low *Z* materials. Thus, low-energy X-rays, similar to those found in the earliest orthovoltage radiation machines, or with low-energy gamma rays, can be used to shield by several millimeters rather than centimeters of lead. This phenomenon is readily demonstrable in the lead aprons that radiation workers may use when carrying out fluoroscopy or using C-arm radiation machines in the operating room. Also, lead shielding is placed over patients' genital areas if they are having X-rays of the upper body. Low-energy X-rays can be easily shielded. It is the high-energy X-rays that will be a problem for the spacecraft and for the Lunar and Martian habitats.

Shielding Against Protons

For both the Lunar and Mars Missions, solar proton events (SPEs) will be a real issue. Sunspots and SPEs can be predicted and are seasonal. However, they cannot be entirely prevented. Our sun creates energy through the process of fusion and conversion of hydrogen to helium. This is associated with the explosion of gamma rays from the radiochemical interactions, which precede the release of protons. Proton energies and X-ray energies from SPE have been calculated, and estimated and also known as the predicted levels and energies of protons that will hit the spacecraft, as well as, the Lunar and Martian habitats [35]. All have been measured and can be predicted. In the data that were collected with the Curiosity Rover experiments, the levels of protons and X-rays have been measured.

Shielding against protons follows the same physical principles as shielding against X-rays, but like GCR, the protons are charged and could be channeled by a magnetic field to a receptacle in a theoretical spacecraft or habitat (Fig. 9.1). It is highly speculative that one could create a magnetosphere around the spacecraft to simulate the magnetosphere on Earth (Fig. 9.1). The energy of protons is directly associated with the depth of penetration into shielding materials and into human tissues. Protons produce the same forms of radiation damage to cells, tissues, organs, and organ systems as do X-rays, but with a high level of deposition of energy at the end of their travel course called the Bragg peak [14]. After this depth of penetration and energy deposition, the protons cause less tissue damage. The Bragg peak can be adjusted to occur at any desired level of penetration by tuning the energy of the protons. This tuning constitutes the basis of precision radiotherapy of patients using protons [18].

The relative biological effect of protons is higher than that of X-rays, and data from cell culture experiments and with experimental animal studies of exposure to protons have confirmed the higher RBE (relative biological effects) of protons [18]. There is much information available on the radiobiology of protons because proton irradiation is currently used in the treatment of cancer worldwide. The availability of complex proton delivery systems include multiple gantry facilities, where the

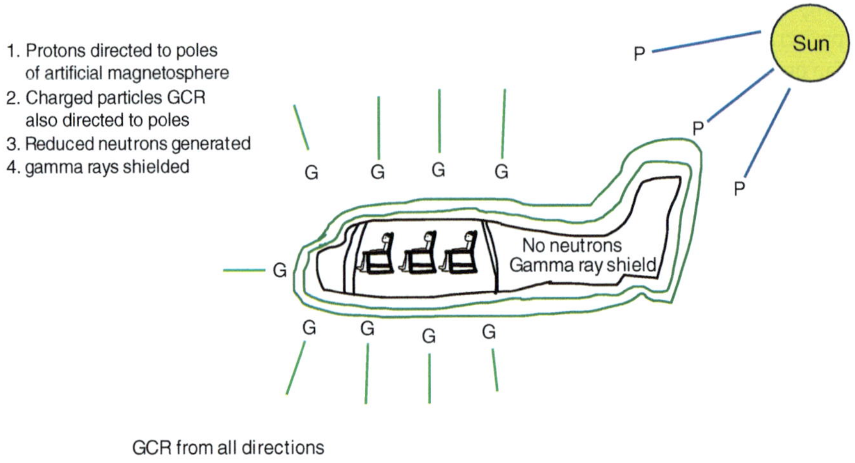

Fig. 9.1 Theoretical construction of a charge particle shielding of a space vehicle. The Magnetosphere of the Earth channels charged particles including protons and galactic cosmic irradiation to the poles. Constructing a Magnetosphere (wavey green lines) around a spacecraft during the 860+ day Mars Mission or beyond would be a challenge and would require significant energy. However, as shown in this figure, protons or charged particles hitting the spacecraft would be directed by the Magnetosphere around the craft to the charged particle collection device at both ends of the spacecraft. This would limit a radiation exposure from solar protons or GCR. The GCR being channeled to the receptacles on the end of the spacecraft would generate neutrons only in those areas, and these could be collected and neutralized. This is theoretical and would require huge amounts of energy to construct the magnetic device

proton beam is created by a cyclotron, and then channeled down tubes to each of several treatment rooms [17]. The proton energies are tuned to the desired levels, and the beam is funneled through delivery system tunnels to deliver the beam to multiple clinical treatment tables for each patient in each multiple rooms. These therapy machines that deliver cyclotron-generated protons have been studied in great detail. Shielding against protons also requires high-*Z* materials. The generation of secondary particles (neutrons) and by X-rays by protons hitting high *Z* materials is of great interest, particularly, with the current emphasis on the quantitation of neutron production. Measurement of neutrons that are secondarily produced by high-energy X-ray machines and by proton machines has not been exhaustedly studied, nor have the data on biological effects been extensively reported.

The design of a space vehicle and a Lunar and Martian space habitat and spacesuits for astronauts carrying out extravehicular activities, such as the “space walks,” has yielded valuable information about proton levels that penetrate spacesuits [16]. The design of spacesuits space vehicles, and habitats will require the evaluation of energy levels of protons, the materials used to make the shielding devices, whether the layers of shielding material used in the spacesuit contain metals, carbon fibers, or other silicon materials used in the space vehicle and habitat will be important. These must be designed to minimize penetration by protons but also must be lightweight and flexible to allow mobility of the wearer. Spacesuits must deliver oxygen and keep the astronauts warm within a range of body temperatures. As these material research programs continue, there will be increasing emphasis on measuring neutron production by the materials that block or absorb proton transit.

There will be competing priorities for research being carried out to optimize spacesuits, the space vehicle, and both the lunar and Martian habitats. The optimal shielding materials will require a balance between physical comfort, oxygen, temperature control, and the degree of the completeness of attenuation of the radiation components hitting the astronauts. Materials that will be transported from the surface of the Earth to a space station or habitat and in the cruise vehicle will require the analysis of the “transport expense.” Heavier materials will require more fuel to get out of the Earth’s atmosphere. Light-weight materials will be easier to transport and manage, but the materials must still provide effective radiation shielding against X-rays, solar protons, and GCR, and not generate neutrons, all of which might enter the bodies of the astronauts. Since the RBE of neutrons is important to consider, the materials must also create the lowest possible levels of neutrons.

Shielding Against Galactic Cosmic Radiation (GCR)

The most challenging part of spacecraft and habitat design will be considerations for shielding against GCR. There is valuable information from the Curiosity Rover experiments and a plethora of data from the measurement of high LET particles that have penetrated the space shuttle, International Space Station, and the robot spacecraft, including that which delivered the Curiosity Rover to the Martian surface [35]. The relative compositions of different charged particles within GCI have been measured and constitute many different elements ranging from carbon ions, silicone, iron, and others.

There is some valuable information on carbon ion radiobiology, which has been provided from the recent development and the use of carbon ion linear accelerators [21]. To treat cancer patients, the carbon iron radiotherapy machines that have been in use in Germany and other treatment facilities have provided information on necessary shielding. In addition, experiments with cells in culture and in animal model systems at the Brookhaven Laboratories have studied Iron 59 particles and carbon high LET irradiation [2]. Current experiments use a “mixed beam” containing multiple different ion compositions designed to mimic the irradiation that would be experienced by galactic cosmic irradiation events.

The shielding for these high LET particles has the same principles as those for SPE. The higher the LET and the higher the energy of the particles, the greater the requirement for shielding. The data from the Curiosity Rover experiments [23] provided cumulative evidence and daily measurements over 300 days of the frequency of detection of these high LET radiation events. What is not known is the optimal way to shield against GCI. Therefore, the research focus again must return to materials design. The primary concern for shielding materials used to attenuate the charged ions in galactic cosmic irradiation, SPE, and high-energy X-rays must consider the relative levels of the creation of neutron irradiation.

The issue of dose rate must be considered for the analysis of the RBE of each form of irradiation. The ultrahigh dose rates of a nuclear bomb detonation have been shown to produce more damage than that of clinical radiotherapy dose rates [14]. Dose–response curves are difficult to derive since the data from the atmospheric tests of nuclear weapons in the 1950s at the Nevada test sites are limited. The experimental animal data from these tests in the 1950s are limited [14] and the new FLASH radiotherapy machines are just coming into use [15]. New experimental data are being generated with animal models of FLASH irradiation with X-rays and protons [15]. These are early limited clinical trials of FLASH irradiation. These early clinical studies suggest that there is more (RBE) causing more tissue damage with these ultrahigh dose rates of FLASH (FLASH dose rates deliver thousands of Gray irradiation in a fraction of a second). Given the relative newness of FLASH irradiation, there is no published study of the late effects of experimental FLASH irradiation with animal models. Most importantly, for the issue of space radiation, there is little analysis of whether such ultrahigh dose rate events would occur during space travel for the Lunar sortie or Mars Missions [15].

Shielding Against Neutrons

The most challenging question related to shielding against space irradiation focuses on the issues of neutrons. Neutron irradiation has been studied in many settings. It is known that the Nagasaki bomb, "Fat-man," which contained a fissionable Plutonium 239 core generated relatively fewer neutrons in the fission reaction than did the Hiroshima bomb containing Uranium 235 [23]. Production of neutrons from nuclear fission and from thermonuclear bomb detonation (nuclear fusion) has been measured. The RBE of neutrons has been studied and is significantly higher than that of protons or of X-rays [10–12]. Cell culture experiments and small animal radiation studies have been carried out with two currently available experimental neutron radiation sources (Colorado State University and Columbia University) and shielded valuable information on the RBE of neutrons. The neutron is of greater molecular weight than protons and causes more nuclear DNA damage [10]. While having no charge, the penetration of animal tissue by neutrons is similarly determined by the energy of the neutron beam and to determine the depth of penetration of the tissue. Shielding for neutrons is much more difficult than that for protons or X-rays because neutrons pass through nearly all materials regardless of Z. The best shielding for neutrons is water. Water has been used to attenuate neutron production in nuclear reactors that are used for nuclear power stations [11]. Shielding of the radiation reactions in the nuclear power station reactor is achieved by graphite rods that absorb neutrons to limit the atomic pile. The nuclear fuel rods contain plutonium and are limited from reaching critical mass by graphite control rods [5]. Graphite rods are inserted into the core of the machine and also neutrons are controlled by water surrounding the reactor. The radiobiology of neutrons reveals that there is significant tissue damage, which is greater than that detected by similar energy levels of protons or X-rays. All of this information is valuable and important, but the most critical information is missing [7]. That is the determination of the level of neutron production, frequency of production, and the energy of neutrons produced by the GCR space irradiation hitting the spacecraft, habitat, and spacesuits. Neutron therapeutic radiation was tested at the University of Washington-Seattle in a series of clinical studies [8]. These have been calculations of the RBE of neutrons compared to X-rays or photons [10]. Therefore, the creation of neutrons when the charged particles of GCR hit the space vehicle or habitat structures must be considered to be a potential hazard to the health and safety of the astronauts.

Summary and Conclusions

Irradiation of astronauts will be unavoidable. The available information from measuring instruments on space probes indicates the dose levels and contributions of various forms of irradiation to be expected for the exposure levels of a Mars Mission compared to the Lunar Missions to date. The design of materials for space vehicles and habitats must take into account radiation safety. However, limiting steps include the composition of shielding materials and then weight. Current research is focused on the RBE (relative biological effects), which will follow radiation penetration of the astronauts' bodies and the best shielding levels that can be practically achieved. Thus, the radiobiology of space travel must entail a collaboration with the research of materials scientists, engineers, physicists and radiobiologists. These collaborators must work together design the best ionizing irradiation shielding materials for space travel [36].

References

1. Berger T, Matthia D, Burmeister S, et al. Long term variations of galactic cosmic radiation on board the international Space Station, on the moon, and on the surface of Mars. J Space Weather Space Clim. 2020;10:article 34.
2. Brown K, Ahrens L, Chiang IH, et al. The NASA space radiation laboratory at Brookhaven national laboratory: preparation and delivery of ion beams for space radiation research. In: Joram C, editor. Nuclear instruments and methods in physics research section a: accelerators, spectrometers, detectors, and associated equipment, vol. 618. Science Direct; 2010. p. 97–107.
3. Hassler DM, Zeitlin C, Wimmer-Schweingruber RF, et al. Mars' surface radiation environment measured with the Mars science laboratory's curiosity rover. Science. 2014;343(6169):1244797. https://doi.org/10.1126/science.1244797.
4. Zhang S, Wimmer-Schweingruber RF, Yu J, et al. First measurements of the radiation dose on the lunar surface. Sci Adv. 2020;6(39):eaaz1334. https://doi.org/10.1126/sciadv.aaz1334.
5. Kaneko Y, Akino F, Kitadate K, et al. Measurements of multiple control rods effect in graphite moderated reactors. J Nucl Sci Technol. 1971;8(10):569–87.

6. Seo J, Kim SK, Jalalvand A, et al. Avoiding fusion plasma tearing instability with deep reinforcement learning. Nature. 2024;626(8000):746–51. https://doi.org/10.1038/s41586-024-07024-9.
7. Barabash V, Federici G, Linke J, et al. Material/plasma surface interaction issues following neutron damage. J Nucl Mater. 2003;313–316:42–51.
8. Stelzer KJ, Laramore GE, Griffin TW, et al. Fast neutron radiotherapy: the University of Washington experience. Acta Oncol. 1994;33(3):275–80. https://doi.org/10.3109/02841869409098417.
9. Blue TE, Gupta N, Woollard JE. A calculation of the energy dependence of the RBE of neutrons. Phys Med Biol. 1993;38:1693. https://doi.org/10.1088/0031-9155/38/12/002.
10. Hall EJ, Novak JK, Kellerer AM, et al. RBE as a function of neutron energy: I. Experimental observations. Radiat Res. 1975;64(2):245–55.
11. Dunning JR, Pegram GB, Fink GA, et al. Interaction of neutrons with matter. Phys Rev J. 1935;48:265.
12. Zhang W, Feng Y, Althakafy JT, et al. Ultrahigh molecular weight polyethylene fiber/boron nitride composites with high neutron shielding efficiency and mechanical performance. Adv Compos Hybrid Mater. 2022;5:2012–20.
13. Douple EB, Mabuchi K, Cullings HM, et al. Long-term radiation-related health effects in a unique human population: lessons learned from the atomic bomb survivors of Hiroshima and Nagasaki. Disaster Med Public Health Prep. 2011;5 Suppl(01):S122–33. https://doi.org/10.1001/dmp.2011.21.
14. Hashizume T, Maruyama T, Shiragai A, et al. Estimation of the air dose from the atomic bombs in Hiroshima and Nagasaki. Health Phys. 1967;13(2):149–61. https://doi.org/10.1097/00004032-196702000-00004.
15. Esplen N, Mendonca MS, Bazalova-Carter M. Physics and biology of ultrahigh dose-rate (FLASH) radiotherapy: a topical review. Phys Med Biol. 2020;65(23):23TR03. https://doi.org/10.1088/1361-6560/abaa28.
16. Kuess P, Sejkora N, Klampfer A, et al. Characterising potential space suit textiles in proton beams using radiotherapy-based dosimetry. Adv Space Res. 2022;70(7):1925–34.
17. Shang C, Evans G, Rahman M, et al. Beam characteristics of the first clinical 360° rotational single gantry room scanning pencil beam proton treatment system and comparisons against a multi-room system. J Appl Clin Med Phys. 2020;21(9):266–71. https://doi.org/10.1002/acm2.12984.
18. Quinn TJ, Ding X, Li X, et al. Amelioration of mucositis in proton therapy of Fanconi anemia Fanca−/− mice by JP4-039. In Vivo. 2019;33(6):1757–66. https://doi.org/10.21873/invivo.11666.
19. Ilicic K, Combs SE, Schmid TE. New insights in the relative radiobiological effectiveness of proton irradiation. Radiat Oncol. 2018;13(1):6. https://doi.org/10.1186/s13014-018-0954-9.
20. Xapsos MA, Barth JL, Stassinopoulos EG, et al. Characterizing solar proton energy spectra for radiation effects applications. IEEE Trans Nucl Sci. 2000;47(6):2218–23.
21. Tsujii H, Kameda T. A review of update clinical results of carbon ion radiotherapy. Jpn J Clin Oncol. 2012;42(8):670–85. https://doi.org/10.1093/jjco/hys104.
22. Ratliff HN, Smith MBR, Heilbronn L. Simulation of the GCR spectrum in the Mars curiosity rover's RAD detector using MCNP6. Life Sci Space Res (Amst). 2017;14:43–50. https://doi.org/10.1016/j.lssr.2017.07.003.
23. Wilson JW, Thibeault SA, Cucinotta FA, et al. Issues in protection from galactic cosmic rays. Radiat Environ Biophys. 1995;34(4):217–22. https://doi.org/10.1007/BF01209745.
24. Tang FR, Loganovsky K. Low dose or low dose rate ionizing radiation-induced health effect in the human. J Environ Radioact. 2018;192:32–47. https://doi.org/10.1016/j.jenvrad.2018.05.018.
25. Pratt RH, LaJohn LA, Florescu V, et al. Compton scattering revisited. Radiat Phys Chem. 2010;79(2):124–31.
26. Okafor CE, Okonkwo UC, Okokpujie IP. Trends in reinforced composite design for ionizing radiation shielding applications: a review. J Mater Sci. 2021;56:11631–55.

27. Nakel W. The elementary process of bremsstrahlung. Phys Rep. 1994;243(6):317–53.
28. Cosgrove VP, Jahn U, Pfaender M, et al. Commissioning of a micro multi-leaf collimator and planning system for stereotactic radiosurgery. Radiother Oncol. 1999;50(3):325–36. https://doi.org/10.1016/s0167-8140(99)00020-1.
29. Hendee WR, Edwards FM. ALARA and an integrated approach to radiation protection. Semin Nucl Med. 1986;16(2):142–50. https://doi.org/10.1016/s0001-2998(86)80027-7.
30. Greenberg MR. The United States nuclear factories. In: Nuclear waste management, nuclear power, and energy choices. London: Springer-Verlag; 2013. https://doi.org/10.1007/978-1-4471-4231-7.
31. Connolly B, Racadio J, Towbin R. Practice of ALARA in the pediatric interventional suite. Pediatr Radiol. 2006;36(Suppl 2):163–7. https://doi.org/10.1007/s00247-006-0192-4.
32. Brugge D, Buchner V. Health effects of uranium: new research findings. Rev Environ Health. 2011;26(4):231–49. https://doi.org/10.1515/reveh.2011.032.
33. Brugge D, deLemos JL, Oldmixon B. Exposure pathways and health effects associated with chemical and radiological toxicity of natural uranium: a review. Rev Environ Health. 2005;20(3):177–93. https://doi.org/10.1515/reveh.2005.20.3.177.
34. Jones BA. What are the health costs of uranium mining? A case study of miners in Grants, New Mexico. Int J Occup Environ Health. 2014;20(4):289–300. https://doi.org/10.1179/2049396714Y.0000000077.
35. Mewaldt RA. Galactic cosmic ray composition and energy spectra. Adv Space Res. 1994;14(10):737–47. https://doi.org/10.1016/0273-1177(94)90536-3.
36. Hashemi SA, Mousavi SM, Faghihi R, et al. Lead oxide-decorated graphene oxide/epoxy composite towards X-ray radiation shielding. Radiat Phys Chem. 2018;146:77–85.

Chapter 10
Rationale for the Opinion that Humans Can Never Live Outside the Earth

There are polar opposite opinions about the capacity of humans to live outside of Earth [1–3]. One group of scientists argues from a positive perspective that humans have virtually infinite and unlimited capacity to adapt to new environments [4–6]. This side bases the argument on the capacity to adapt that is in the genome of *Homo sapiens* [6]. Support for this opinion includes evidence of the migration of primitive humans from areas in Africa northward and in multiple directions over millennia and into extreme climates [4]. There is evidence that has been well documented in the archeologic record. The adaptation of humans to extreme temperature, altitude, and different environments was shared with other predatory species during the Pleistocene epoch of the Cenozoic Era [4, 5]. The evolution of humans, including their migration and adaptation from hunter-gatherers to farming and harvesting, has been well documented [6].

In contrast, with respect to the limits to human adaptability, there is evidence that *Homo sapiens* can adapt to life only outside of the Earth when there is oxygen, water, and adequate gravity [7–11]. This more negative view is based on real impediments to human existence outside of Earth, namely, finding rather than synthesizing oxygen and water. Solable problems include zero or decreased gravity environments, which can be facilitated. However, the lack of oxygen and the need for water are real challenges, and we must add to this list. Increased irradiation exposure to levels to which humans may not easily adapt.

The problems of reduced gravity and a lack of oxygen and water are being solved by technology; however, the problem of elevated levels of ionizing irradiation cannot be rapidly solved and supports the position that humans cannot survive in space or outside the Earth. The record for survival is over a year at the International Space Station (Table 10.1). The Mars mission will require 870+ days, which is over 2 years, and a trip to Europa will be 11+ years.

Overwhelming importance of gravity and an oxygen-rich environment cannot be solved but technology will facilitate these solutions. The ability to provide continuous permanent availability of an oxygen environment can be solved by chemistry to

J. Greenberger, *Radiation Oncology and Radiation Biology*,
https://doi.org/10.1007/978-3-031-66300-0_10

Table 10.1 Challenges in establishing that humans can live outside the Earth

Requirements	Oxygen Water Temperature control Radiation countermeasures Radiation shielding Physiologic adaptation to the environment Weightlessness—artificial gravity	
Milestones		**Duration**
1965	Low-orbit travel capsules (hours)	Hours
1967	Low-orbit travel (longer hours) space walk (hours)	Hours
1967	Moon landing (days)	Days
1969	Space travel cruise and lander (weeks)	Weeks
1980	Space shuttle (weeks)	Weeks
2006	International Space Station (over 1 year)	>1 year
2026	Lunar sorties from habitat (months)	>1 year
2036	Mars Mission (year)	>1.5 years
.		
.		
.		
?	Mission to Europa (years)	4–5 years
?	Mission to outer solar system	>10 years
?	Colonization of a distant planet/moon	?

produce oxygen [7]. The stresses on the human body from zero gravity can be solved by artificial gravity. Water can be produced by chemistry, provided the reagents are available [10–13]. These negative conclusions point to the effect of continuous exposure to ionizing irradiation on the human body outside the protective magnetosphere. There are currently no available physical shielding materials that are adequate to address the problem of continuous irradiation exposure. Data from the International Space Station, shuttle, and other astronauts are being collated and will likely show some toxic late effects, such as neurodegenerative disease, higher instances of cancer, and premature aging; however, will these data be enough to stall or delay the push by NASA and other nation's space programs to push toward and beyond a Mars Mission? To become radioresistant requires genetic changes in humans [14–19] and drugs to prevent DNA damage [20–22] or to prevent antioxidant depletion [21, 22]. Genetic changes take generations and can introduce deleterious consequences [23–26].

Science writers have argued that resolving these two extreme opinions requires innovative solutions. The identification of a place where humans can relocate after a journey to a safe Earth-like alternative environment must be a priority. Where is this other planet or moon that has gravity, an oxygen-rich environment, and water? The speed of travel is currently limited [27]. The lifespan of humans limits travel, and space radiation accelerates aging [28–32]. Another strategy is to transplant tissues into humans to alter radioresistance [31–33]. There is currently no way to prevent the late effects of cumulative radiation doses [34–41].

How Can Humans Be Prepared for Long-Distance Space Travel?

Once established as a place for relocation, a plan for the relocation of humans to this site can be designed. Current discussions have focused on the moon of Jupiter, Europa, and possibly the moons of Saturn [10]. Water can possibly be identified as ice on planets in our own solar system [9]. The astrological studies that have identified potentially habitable new planets that orbit distant stars [10] have not addressed how humans can get there. There are astrophysical and astrochemical analyses leading to conclude that there is theoretical potential for these target locations to contain water- and oxygen-bearing environments. The analysis of such speculative data also requires an understanding of the magnitude of the distance of these potential habitable sites from our solar system and the means of travel to such locations. If a potential planet with moons orbiting the planet is "only" several hundred light-years away [12, 27], how is that fact encouraging unless travel to it can be facilitated? The literature on such scientific discoveries suggests that we do not yet have the technological means for travel in excess of light speed, so the concept of travel to such sites remains, at best, speculative.

Incremental Approaches to Establish that Humans Can Live Outside of Earth

The two polar extremes of opinion regarding the ability of humans to live outside of Earth do not take into account the important factor of adaptation to galactic cosmic irradiation and solar proton events during travel to such a location. The best strategy appears to take an incremental approach. The feasibility of plans for intergalactic space travel or even the Mars Mission is currently based on the assumption that radiation exposure levels will not limit safety. The data or radiologic exposure is described in a previous chapter on the Mars Mission and the Curiosity Rover relative biological effects (RBE) measurements. Is the current data from physical measurements of space radiation to and from Mars accurate? Is the data biologically relevant? Can the data be reliably used for planning space missions?

One additional question is: Can humans adapt to the radiation levels of space travel? The ability of cells in culture and experimental animals to adapt to low-dose-rate irradiation is provocative [14] but does not take into account the composition and relative levels of the different forms of space irradiation. The sporadic nature of SPE and GCR irradiation is a concern. The molecular mechanisms of radiation damage repair have evolved in humans. The adaptation to continuous "low-dose irradiation" has evolved over billions of years in life form on Earth [14]. Bacteria can adapt to radiation by rapid doubling and rapid natural selection. The discovery and isolation of the bacterium *Deinococcus radiodurans* is a perfect example [15].

The number of bacterial doublings required for the generation of a radiation-resistant bacterium has been calculated to be several thousand [16]. The purpose of the experiment was to deliver several thousand Gy of radiation to meat products to sterilize the food and make it safe. Unexpectedly, a radioresistant bacterial strain that grew in the irradiated meat was recovered. How could this have occurred? The irradiation-resistant bacterium was of the taxon *Deinococcus*, and the resistant mutant was termed *radiodurans*. The selection of this new bacterium, its natural selection, and its very existence were based on the assumption that at least 10, and likely more, mutations in radiation repair and antioxidant genes occurred and were selected forms in radiation resistance. Furthermore, each mutation must have been stably selected and remained stable in the many generations of progeny of that mutant bacterium. Then, the next mutation occurred, conferring further radiation resistance, was selected and was stable [17]. The process continued up to and past a tenth mutation until a mutant strain that was stable and grew in the radiation beam was selected.

Bacteria can double every 4 h, so such a natural selection process and accumulation of 10 or more advantageous mutations could have occurred in a realistic experimental time frame over a measurable time interval of weeks to months [18].

Could such adaptation to radiation in single-celled bacteria be extrapolated to be likely in multicellular organisms?

How Do Organisms Become Radioresistant?

Both plants and animals have been studied for their ability to adapt to ionizing irradiation [19, 30]. For studies with the flatworm (Phylum Platyhelminthes), *C. elegans*, there was also some evidence of a requirement for multiple generations of mutation and selection for adaptation [29]. With the more complex animal phylum Arthropoda, the fruit fly *Drosophila melanogaster*, lower doses of X-rays have been delivered for the selection of larvae with radioresistance to ionizing irradiation, and several mutations have been discovered [28]. To accumulate multiple mutations during ongoing irradiation, such as in the high-dose and high-dose rates of meat products, as well as in the setting of a continuous low-dose rate and sporadic radiation in space travel, mutations that produce resistance to ionizing irradiation would be conserved in either case through the process of natural selection. To achieve accumulation of the appropriate number of mutations to provide biological radioresistance in a complex organism, several assumptions must be made. The number of mutations in genes in *Deinococcus radiodurans* that lead to its phenotype of radioresistance is different from that in the original bacterial taxon [23]. The cumulative genetic changes in *D. radiodurans* include the duplication of radiation resistance and antioxidant genes. Thus, gene duplication is another way to become radioresistant, indicating another dynamic in the selection process. Can one then extrapolate the potential for the selection of a radioresistant mammalian species or humans? Such an experiment could not be done given the current limitations of laboratory research and the mammalian life cycle.

Even inbred strains of the laboratory mouse could be used to carry out such an experiment of adaptation to continuous irradiation, but the doses and quality of irradiation would have to be scaled down to allow survival of enough animals to continue the expansion of a colony of radioresistant mice. One generation of mice was 21 days. Several generations that would be required to select a radioresistant mouse by natural selection would be required. There would be a need for 150 or more new generations.

Natural selection did occur with Homo-Neanderthal, which lived from 300,000 to 30,000 years ago. Neanderthals selected several genes that have been associated with adaptation to cold weather [25]. Some of these genes of Neanderthal origin are present in modern humans and are associated with the pleiotropic effects of mental illness [25].

There are recent data about one generation of radiation adaptation in dogs. The experiments with continuous irradiation of beagle outbred dogs [22] in one generation of approximately 100 adult dogs. This experimental model delivered 3–5 Roentgens in air = 3–5 centigray (cGy) per day over 2 years of total body irradiation (TBI) delivered 20 h per day. Four hours was required to clean the cages, feed and water the animals, and collect blood and bone marrow samples. The data revealed that two-thirds of the animals died of either bone marrow failure (1/3) or leukemia (1/3). The final third of dogs comprised a fascinating subset that had radioaccommodated and survived for 2 years [22]. However, even these animals demonstrated significant medical problems, including premature aging. Fertility was not reported, nor were other late effects beyond the two-year study. These animals received 3–5 Roentgens of Cobalt60 gamma irradiation in the air (potentially 3–5 cGy per day) and total body irradiation. Therefore, the irradiation was of one gamma ray X-ray quality provided by Cobalt60 gamma rays with RBE = 1. There was no component of protons or no high LET irradiation from ionized atoms, such as those found in the GCR, and no neutrons generated by the high LET particles hitting the cage materials or the dogs themselves.

Relating these data to the Mars Mission, if one assumes that the RBE of solar protons and galactic cosmic irradiation would be higher than the 1 Sievert (1 Gy) that was the expected cumulative radiation dose as calculated from the Curiosity Rover experiments [9], then it must be concluded that the effect of such a radiation dose on humans or even on experimental animals, such as rodents, would be much higher than 1 Sievert of gamma rays. The Curiosity Rover experimental calculations do not separate the quality of irradiation sustained (gamma rays, protons, and galactic cosmic irradiation), nor do they account for neutron irradiation, which is generated by secondary effects in the spacecraft. Neutrons are generated by GCR hitting materials, including bones and other tissues of the astronauts themselves). Therefore, even if scientists and engineers can provide a continuous source of gravity, water, and an oxygenated atmosphere, they cannot reliably provide physical and biological protection from continuous space radiation (Table 10.1). If space irradiation is the limiting factor for human existence outside of the Earth, then the conclusion of the naysayer (humans can never live outside the Earth) will have merit at present. However, things will change, so the word "never" is inappropriate.

Challenges for Humans Living Outside of Earth

To attempt to solve the potential problem of humans leaving Earth, the prevailing approach has been to carry out incremental experiments and monitor biological, as well as physical, levels of ionizing irradiation at each step (Table 10.1).

The Lunar Sortie Mission and the construction of a lunar habitat appear to be a good first step. If humans can live on the moon with reduced (but not absent) gravity and provide an oxygen-rich environment, they can be constructed inside a habitat or spacesuit and allow astronauts to safely exist for months or years. The measurement of physical parameters of radiation levels and simultaneous measurement of biological effects over time would be a logical next step to determination the feasibility of each strategy for radiation protection. The effects of reduced gravity and an artificial oxygen-containing environment must also be studied as a "combined injury" to understand space radiation. The physiology of human adaptation to radiation in the current realistic environment of limited space travel is yielding truly valuable data to collect. The experiments with humans living at the International Space Station for up to 1 year and soon during ship cruising to and from the moon and in the Lunar Habitat for over 1 year should be valuable. These data should include a search for radiation-induced genetic changes in easily accessible peripheral blood cells, such as lymphocytes and monocytes, which are derived from the irradiated bone marrow [31, 32]. These data could then be extrapolated to other stem cell populations in other organs and could be appropriately studied. This strategy of incremental steps for the duration of space travel and an increase in cumulative radiation dose effects provides a blueprint for expectations regarding longer-duration Mars Mission.

The next incremental step after the Lunar Sorties Mission, as defined by NASA, would logically be the Mars Mission. There are other challenges to completing the Mars Mission besides the issue of radiation protection. The challenge of selecting an engine propulsion system (engine) for the 6-month cruise to Mars and the 6-month return cruise must be met. Another challenge of spacecraft design is that it must include materials that are sufficiently light for assembly and the Earth's temperature during reentry and that decrease the radiation exposure to astronauts. The materials must minimize the generation of neutrons in the materials as they are continuously hit with the GCR. Biology experiments must be continually carried out during the mission.

After a Lunar Sortie Mission, will NASA go directly to a human mission to Mars? Unlike the multiple-stage experiments that preceded the 1969 lunar landing, including all the experiments with rodents, nonhuman primates, and other species, there is the question of whether such preliminary experiments could be carried out relative to a Mars Mission. The isolation of experimental animals in an environment of zero gravity with an artificial oxygen environment with an artificial oxygen atmosphere could be easily carried out to simulate a space journey to and from Mars. Even with a 500-day simulated surface landing, what results would this experiment deliver that could guide the preparation of humans for a Martian landing and return to Earth? For animals maintained in this environment for months to years, the interaction of animals with command control and the ability of animals to manage events that would occur on the spacecraft or on the Mars surface could not be simulated. Therefore, it is likely that the first Mars Mission involved humans. The first Mars Mission provided the ultimate information on both the effects of long-duration exposure to low-dose sporadic space irradiation in the setting of an artificial oxygen environment and reduced gravity. Risks of complex space irradiation can then be established. It is essential that the astronauts be continuously monitored during both the 6-month outbound leg of travel, the time on the Martian surface (previously calculated to be 500 days by the Curiosity Rover Mission), and the 6 months (180 days) for the inbound/return trip.

What Data from the Mars Mission Would Lead to a Conclusion that (At the Present Time) Humans Cannot Or Should Not Exist Outside of the Earth?

Finally, the Mars Mission should not be contemplated if a possible outcome is to conclude that humans cannot live in space. The biology of adaptation to space irradiation is very important to document. A possible result would be that the RBE of space irradiation was indeed higher than that predicted by the physical radiation dosimetry from monitors in the robotic Curiosity Rover experiments. The best evidence of such an underestimate would be the finding that peripheral blood counts decreased more than expected and that the administration of available radiation countermeasures did not correct the drop in blood counts and provide strong evidence of the mitigation of damage to the most sensitive stem cell population in humans (in the bone marrow). These data suggest that humans cannot adapt to space irradiation. However, before an 18-month Mars Mission, incremental experiments ensure the quantitation of RBE. In contrast, if peripheral blood counts do not significantly drop and recover to normal levels with help from the administration of radiation countermeasures periodically, then the data will be encouraging. Astronauts can treat blood count drops by administering treatments of G-CSF or another countermeasure. There may be delivery of a continuous bone marrow stem cell radiation mitigator, such as JP4–039 [21], GS-nitroxide, or other antioxidants [20], or a cytokine or biological countermeasure [27]. Successful results would relieve some of the concerns that space irradiation could be reduced.

If the first astronauts returning from a Mars Mission showed that they were adaptable to the conditions of space irradiation, as well as the other conditions of 18–24 months of experience in zero gravity or reduced gravity and in an artificial oxygen environment, and if no significant physiological or other biological effects were detectable, this result would add further support to the feasibility of humans living outside the Earth. The returning astronauts are closely watched, as are all International Space Stations, and shuttle astronauts for the development of radiation late effects in the more controllable research setting of back on Earth. The issue of radiation late effects may be significant and will be documented.

Late Effects of Continuous Low Dose Rate/Sporadic Irradiation Could Be Expected in Individuals, Who Show No Deleterious Early/Acute Effects

For weeks/months/years after return to Earth from the Mars Mission, astronauts would be observed for evidence of genetic alterations in stem cell populations within their bodies. The most obvious target for such analysis would be peripheral blood cells as an indication of late effects on the bone marrow. The continuous appearance of chromosome aberrations in peripheral blood lymphocytes suggests evidence of alterations in the bone marrow microenvironment caused by prior long-term radiation exposure.

Animal studies have shown that prolonged radiation exposure affects not only stem cell populations but also the microenvironment in which stem cells reside [13]. Radiation late effects on stem cell populations in the bone marrow, intestine, and other rapidly proliferating tissues can be monitored using techniques that have been used to follow patients who have received total body irradiation in preparation for a bone marrow transplant.

Bone marrow transplantation has been carried out not only in patients with cancer but also in other noncancer patients who received a bone marrow transplant to correct a "genetic abnormality" of the hematopoietic system (bone marrow). These categories of patients include those with Fanconi anemia [31] and other disorders of DNA repair of bone marrow stem cells; other patients with a genetic etiology of an enzyme deficiency [32]; patients with a disorder of hematopoiesis (chronic granulomatous disease, sickle cell anemia, and others); patients with a lipid-storage disease of bone marrow origin (Gaucher Syndrome); and others with a genetic disorder of metabolism. These patients, who were prepared for marrow transplantation using total body irradiation, provide valuable information on the late effects of irradiation. These patients received gamma irradiation or X-ray exposure only, so the results should be interpreted with caution and of limited extrapolation to the late effects of space radiation.

Caution should be applied when using clinical data to speculate on its relevance to space radiation. There was no combination of reduced or zero gravity, nor was there an artificial oxygen-containing environment for clinical BMT patients. The late effects that are observed in the subset of patients with each of these categories of disease, who receive total body irradiation and bone marrow transplantation can be used as a guide for physicians monitoring astronauts on the Martian research team upon their return to Earth. Organ systems likely to express radiation late effects include (in addition to the bone marrow and intestine) the lungs [34], the liver, and the brain [1, 38, 39]. One recent study carried out by NASA scientists suggested that the exposure of experimental animals to space irradiation may lead to significant neurocognitive deficits [35, 36]. How does the human central nervous system respond to continuous low-dose/sporadic space irradiation? The answer is not yet known.

The information coming from studies with airline pilots and crews and from frequent flier passengers and other personnel, who have long experience in time spent at high altitudes, is of interest but does not take into account the GCR or SPEs that would be experienced outside the Earth magnetosphere [37]. Those astronauts who have spent time in shuttle missions, such as the International Space Station, provide some evidence for the effects of GCR and SPE, and neutron exposure comprises a valuable cohort to follow; however, the calculations of neutrons generated have been incomplete. These individuals, who have prolonged experience with lunar landings or lunar orbit missions, can be added to the groups of individuals on the International Space Station and shuttle missions and provide more data on the late effects of space radiation. The current cohort of astronauts is known to have displayed some late effects of radiation that appear earlier or at an increased frequency [38]. Astronauts have been developing cataracts at an earlier age and of a more serious magnitude [39]. Neurocognitive studies are being carried out on individuals in astronaut cohorts to obtain information likely to apply to managing the Mars Mission.

What Scientific Rationale Can Be Used to Overcome the Concern About Space Radiation as a Potential Roadblock to Human Space Travel?

Perhaps the most compelling evidence that biological systems can adapt to irradiation comes from experiments with *Deinococcus radiodurans* [15, 16]. All organisms must have water [41], so the search for water [9, 10] or the ability to produce it must be solved [41]. While single-cell bacteria may appear to be unrelated to humans, there is interesting information that must be considered. The number of generations required for adaptation in bacteria can be achieved by an organism that can resist irradiation and live in a high-irradiation environment. The complexity of multicellular organisms in humans cannot be assumed to adapt in the same way as bacteria do. The number of humans that would be exposed to radiation to generate the first generation of mutants that are radioresistant can be compared to the calculated number that occurred in the bacteria experiment. However, one lesson to be learned is that the genes for radiation resistance are in the categories of DNA repair, antioxidant, and accumulation in resistant bacterial strains at the expense of the elimination of other genes.

Can this be done with a multicellular organism? Can this be done with a mammalian experimental system? How could this be done with humans? Genetic change is not the only way to adjust to space radiation. The genes are present, and transcription and translation can be increased. Epigenetic regulation can increase the action without the need for natural selection. Finally, radiation countermeasures can be administered to "create" a genetic adaptation to space radiation. Other chapters in this book dealing with genetic engineering and cryopreservation will address this.

References

1. Szocik K. Human place in the outer space: skeptical remarks. In: Szocik K, editor. The human factor in a mission to Mars. Switzerland: Springer Nature; 2019. p. 233–52.
2. Heyl JS. The long-term future of space travel. Phys Rev. 2005;72:107302.
3. Von Hoerner S. The general limits of space travel: we may never visit our neighbors in space, but we should start listening and talking to them. Science. 1962;137(3523):18–23. https://doi.org/10.1126/science.137.3523.18.
4. Rito T, Vieira D, Silva M, et al. A dispersal of *Homo sapiens* from southern to eastern Africa immediately preceded the out-of-Africa migration. Sci Rep. 2019;9(1):4728. https://doi.org/10.1038/s41598-019-41176-3.
5. Vermeij GJ. The limits of adaptation: humans and the predator—prey arms race. Evolution. 2012;66(7):2007–14. https://doi.org/10.1111/j.1558-5646.2012.01592.x.
6. Hervella M, Izagirre N, Alonso S, et al. Ancient DNA from hunter-gatherer and farmer groups from Northern Spain supports a random dispersion model for the neolithic expansion into Europe. PLoS One. 2012;7(4):e34417. https://doi.org/10.1371/journal.pone.0034417.
7. Hendrickx L, De Wever H, Hermans V, et al. Microbial ecology of the closed artificial ecosystem MELISSA (micro-ecological life support system alternative): reinventing and compartmentalizing the Earth's food and oxygen regeneration system for long-haul space exploration missions. Res Microbiol. 2006;157(1):77–86. https://doi.org/10.1016/j.resmic.2005.06.014.
8. Clement GR, Bukley AP, Paloski WH. Artificial gravity as a countermeasure for mitigating physiological deconditioning during long-duration space missions. Front Syst Neurosci. 2015;9:92. https://doi.org/10.3389/fnsys.2015.00092.
9. Nazari-Sharabian M, Aghababaei M, Karakouzian M, et al. Water on Mars—A literature review. Galaxies. 2020;8(2):40. https://doi.org/10.3390/galaxies8020040.
10. Khurana KK, Kivelson MG, Russell CT. Searching for liquid water in Europa by using surface observations. Astrobiology. 2002;2(1):93–103. https://doi.org/10.1089/153110702753621376.
11. Brown L, Peick J, Pickett M, et al. Aquatic invertebrate protein sources for long-duration space travel. Life Sci Space Res (Asmt). 2021;28:1–10. https://doi.org/10.1016/j.lssr.2020.10.002.
12. Webb S. Space travel. In: All the wonder that would be: exploring past notions of the future (science and fiction). Springer; 2017. p. 67–94.
13. Sivananthan A, Shields D, Fisher R, et al. Continuous 1 year oral administration of the radiation mitigator, MMS350, after total body irradiation restores bone marrow stromal cell proliferative

capacity and reduces age-related senescence in Fanconi anemia (Fanca−/−) mice. Radiat Res. 2019;191(2):139–53. https://doi.org/10.1667/RR15199.1.
14. Olipitz W, Wiktor-Brown D, Shuga J, et al. Integrated molecular analysis indicates undetectable DNA damage in mice after continuous irradiation at −400-fold natural background radiation. Environ Health Perspect. 2012;120(8):1130–6. https://doi.org/10.1289/ehp.1104294.
15. Krisko A, Radman M. Biology of extreme radiation resistance: the way of Deinococcus radiodurans. Cold Spring Harb Perspect Biol. 2013;5(7):a012765. https://doi.org/10.1101/cshperspect.a012765.
16. Mennecier S, Servant P, Coste G, et al. Mutagenesis via IS transposition in Deinococcus radiodurans. Mol Microbiol. 2006;59(1):317–25. https://doi.org/10.1111/j.1365-2958.2005.04936.x.
17. Cox MM, Battista JR. Deinococcus radiodurans—the consummate survivor. Nat Rev Microbiol. 2005;3(11):882–92. PMID: 16261171
18. Harris DR, Tanaka M, Saveliev SV, et al. Preserving genome integrity: the DdrA protein of Deinococcus radiodurans R1. PLoS Biol. 2004;2(10):e304. https://doi.org/10.1371/journal.pbio.0020304.
19. Maurya GK, Kota S, Misra HS. Characterisation of ParB encoded on multipartite genome in Deinococcus radiodurans and their roles in radioresistance. Microbiol Res. 2019;223-225:22–32. https://doi.org/10.1016/j.micres.2019.03.005.
20. Epperly MW, Wang H, Jones J, et al. Antioxidant-chemopreventive diet ameliorates late effects of total body irradiation and supplements radioprotection by MnSOD-plasmid liposome administration. Radiat Res. 2011;175(6):759–65. https://doi.org/10.1667/RR2398.1.
21. Rwigema J-CM, Beck B, Wang W, et al. Two strategies for the development of mitochondrial-targeted small molecule radiation damage mitigators. Int J Radiat Oncol Biol Phys. 2011;80(3):860–8. https://doi.org/10.1016/j.ijrobp.2011.01.059.
22. Singh VK, Romaine PLP, Seed TM. Medical countermeasures for radiation exposure and related injuries: characterization of medicines, FDA-approval status and inclusion into the strategic National Stockpile. Health Phys. 2015;108(6):607–30. https://doi.org/10.2097/HP.0000000000000279.
23. Slade D, Lindner AB, Paul G, et al. Recombination and replication in DNA repair of heavily irradiated Deinococcus radiodurans. Cell. 2009;136(6):1044–55. https://doi.org/10.1016/j.cell.2009.01.018.
24. White O, Eisen JA, Heidelberg JF, et al. Genome sequence of the radioresistant bacterium Deinococcus radiodurans R1. Science. 1999;286(5444):1571–7. https://doi.org/10.1126/science.286.5444.1571.
25. Nowak MP, Pawelczyk T. Is Neanderthal gene introgression into Homo sapiens genome an adaptive anti-inflammatory phenomenon that increases depression risk? J Psychiatry Clin Psychol. 2023;23(1):27–33.
26. Reed DH, Frankham R. How closely correlated are molecular and quantitative measures of genetic variation? A meta-analysis. Evolution. 2001;55(6):1095–103. https://doi.org/10.1111/j.0014-3820.2001.tb00629.x.
27. Hamade DF, Epperly MW, Fisher R, et al. Release of interferon-β (IFN-β) from probiotic Limosolactobacillus reuteri-IFN-β (LR-IFN-β) mitigates gastrointestinal acute radiation syndrome (GI-ARS) following whole abdominal irradiation. Cancers (Basel). 2023;15(6):1670. https://doi.org/10.3390/cancers15061670.
28. Parashar V, Frankel S, Lurie AG, et al. The effects of age on radiation resistance and oxidative stress in adult Drosophila melanogaster. Radiat Res. 2008;169(6):707–11. https://doi.org/10.1667/RR12225.1.
29. Kuzmic M, Galas S, Lecomte-Pradines C, et al. Interplay between ionizing radiation effects and aging in C. elegans. Free Radic Biol Med. 2019;134:657–65. https://doi.org/10.1016/j.freeradbiomed.2019.02.002.

30. Volkova PY, Duarte GT, Kazakova EA, et al. Radiosensitivity of herbaceous plants to chronic radiation-exposure: field study in the Chernobyl exclusion zone. Sci Total Environ J. 2021;777:146206.
31. Ebens CL, MacMillan ML, Wagner JG. Hematopoietic cell transplantation in Fanconi anemia: current evidence, challenges, and recommendations. Expert Rev Hematol. 2017;10(1):81–97. https://doi.org/10.1080/17474086.2016.1268048.
32. Peters C, Steward CG. Hematopoietic cell transplantation for inherited metabolic diseases: an overview of outcomes and practice guidelines. Bone Marrow Transplant. 2003;31(4):229–39. https://doi.org/10.1038/sj.bmt.1703839.
33. Ringden O, Growth CG, Erikson A, et al (1995) Ten years' experience of bone marrow transplantation for Gaucher disease: transplantation. Transplantation 59(6): 864–870.
34. Mukherjee A, Olson JD, Schaaf GW, et al. Radiation-induced pulmonary fibrosis in non-human primates (NHPs) is preceded by cellular senescence and upregulation of tyrosine kinase Fgr, which is detectable by bronchial alveolar (BAL) gavage. Radiat Res. 2024; (in press)
35. Andrews RN, Bloomer EG, Olson JD, et al. Non-human primates receiving high-dose total-body irradiation are at risk of developing cerebrovascular injury years postirradiation. Radiat Res. 2020;194(3):277–87. https://doi.org/10.1667/RADE-20-00051.1.
36. Cucinotta FA, Alp M, Sulzman FM, et al. Space radiation risks to the central nervous system. Life Sci Space Res. 2014;2:54–69.
37. Rafnsson V, Hrafnkelsson J, Tulinius H. Incidence of cancer among commercial airline pilots. Occup Environ Med. 2000;57(3):175–9. https://doi.org/10.1136/oem.57.3.175.
38. Cucinotta FA, Schimmerling W, Wilson JW, et al. Uncertainties in estimates of the risks of late effects from space radiation. Adv Space Res. 2004;34(6):1383–9. https://doi.org/10.1016/j.asr.2003.10.053.
39. Cucinotta FA, Manuel FK, Jones J, et al. Space radiation and cataracts in astronauts. Radiat Res. 2001;156(5 Pt 1):460–6. https://doi.org/10.1667/0033-7587(2001)156[0460:sracia]2.0.co:2.
40. Meholic G. Beyond the light barrier: A concept for superluminal travel. 1998. https://doi.org/10.2514/6.1998-3410.
41. Ma B, Bai Y, Hu C, et al. Space aquatic chemistry: a roadmap for drinking water treatment in microgravity. Environ Sci Ecotechnol. 2024;19:100344. https://doi.org/10.1016/j.ese.2023.100344.

Chapter 11
Genetic Engineering of Radioresistant Organisms

One of the most exciting advances in biology has been the discovery of the CRISPR/CAS-9 system for gene editing [1–14]. According to this technology, scientists have taken advantage of a biological process by which an interaction between bacteria and plasmids (small circles of DNA that live as independent organisms in the bacterial cytoplasm) interacts with each other to preserve both biological entities. The CRISPR/CAS-9 construct cuts the DNA of the chromosome in the bacteria and replaces genetic sequences with those that are carried in as part of the cutting process. By using a genetic sequence that is homologous with that which is desired to be corrected, the CAS-9 targets a specific gene sequence, cuts it out, and replaces it with the desired sequence. This is a revolutionary technology and paves the way for gene editing. Theoretically, one can remove a defective gene and replace it with the correct gene. While this process naturally has been carried out for millennia involving the interaction between bacteria and plasmids, now there is much theoretical speculation as to how the components of the process could be adapted to human genetic engineering. What is genetic engineering?

The modern definition of the term "genetic engineering" is to use biological engineering concepts to remove, replace, duplicate, or silence specific genes. In practice, this phenomenon has been carried out for years since the first generation of knockout mice (homologous recombinant deletion) or transgenic mice [15] in which a gene has been either removed or inserted into the genome. The first knockout mice were generated decades ago. The first transgenic mice, as well, appeared in the scientific literature decades ago [16, 17].

The next stage of research leading to the current concept of "genetic engineering" was the development of gene therapy. The definition of this term, which originated in the 1980s, was to deliver a genetic sequence in a virus, a plasmid, or even as naked DNA, into cells or tissues such that the DNA would produce RNA, and protein, and, thus, provide a source of an intracellular molecule [18–36]. These two precursor technologies while, both predecessors of genetic engineering, are very different. The former creation of knockout or transgenic mice is a genetic

J. Greenberger, *Radiation Oncology and Radiation Biology*,
https://doi.org/10.1007/978-3-031-66300-0_11

manipulation of the chromosome [15]. The latter is an introduction of a foreign genetic sequence transiently into cells. If the transient introduction is by a virus or a plasmid, this is cleared, and it does not become a part of the germ line of the animals to be passed on to progeny. The former condition of knockout or transgenic mice does produce a germ line change, which is apparent, not only in the generation in which the gene change was introduced, but also in subsequent generations. In both of these predecessor technologies, there were problems. With knockout mice or transgenic mice, there were problems with the first progeny. In some cases, the knockout animal did not survive and died during gestation [15]. In other cases, there was compensation for the absence of the gene (knocked-out) in which the animal during gestation in order to promote its survival made other genetic changes that balanced the deletion in the knockout or balanced the overproduction in the transgenic animal by decreasing another gene expression [15]. Similarly, in gene therapy, there were problems. The overproduction of a specific protein could cause unexpected toxicity in a tissue, the appearance of a "foreign" protein also could produce an antibody response and, in some cases, the experiment did not work at all. Examples of problems of each of these predecessor technologies [37–39] highlight the anticipated problems with the CRISPR/CAS-9 genetic engineering.

In the case of knockout mice, there is a vivid example of how removal of a gene, its associated RNA, and protein can lead to a phenotypic change. The recent discovery of the Fgr tyrosine kinase, which is a regulator of the downstream transcription of many profibrotic genes that lead to the late effect of radiation damage, radiation-initiated pulmonary fibrosis (RIPF), proved to be complex in its function. The Fgr−/− (knockout) mice when receiving thoracic irradiation did not develop pulmonary fibrosis and survived longer than control mice, which had an intact Fgr gene. This was the expected result. However, the survival was not perfect and some animals did develop fibrosis [40]. This result suggested that during gestation the Fgr−/− mouse made corrections to its own genetic programming and may have overexpressed other genes that led to fibrosis, or shutoff other genes that facilitated survival in the absence of the Fgr gene. The proof of this hypothesis was that a drug (TL02–59), which was a specific inhibitor of Fgr kinase, when given to animals by continuous perfusion, allowed all animals to survive and acute radiation exposure. And while the Fgr−/− mice were not completely protected from radiation-induced death [40] they showed intrinsic upregulation of levels of radiation protection proteins. Thus, medical removal/pharmacologic removal of the function of the gene by the drug TL02-59 in a control animal mouse was able to neutralize all the effects in the absence of any genetic changes that may have occurred during gestation to produce the Fgr−/− mouse.

What was learned from the Fgr−/− mouse experiment is that sometimes it is better to deliver a pharmacologic agent [40] to treat a specific condition, rather than attempt to eliminate the condition completely by removing a gene, which has been hypothesized to cause the condition. In the case of gene therapy, there are many examples from the past two decades of research in this area, which prove that simple addition of a gene product may not solve the problem in those particular individuals. In the case of gene therapy for the blood clotting disorder, Hemophilia, decades of research led to molecular cloning of the gene for Factor VIII and the ability to insert it into a vector (virus or plasmid), where it could be delivered in patients, who had the absence of this clotting factor [19–21]. The theory was that by replacing this protein, which is in the cascade of the factors leading to platelet activation and clotting, Hemophilia could be cured. The experiments worked in animal models, but as was the case with delivering recombinant protein for Factor VIII, the gene therapy delivery of the gene product resulted in the generation of antibodies in the patients, which blocked the functioning of this gene product [20].

Both of these examples highlight a problem, which will be encountered, very likely, in the process of modern genetic engineering. The biggest problems are that the host, whether during embryonic gestation, or after experience of the gene product in an adult, who had not seen this gene product for decades, will compensate for the new balance in its system [41–44]. The compensation could be in the form of upregulation of other genes that neutralize the effect of the knockout or transgenic process in a fetus or could be in the form of generation of a neutralizing antibody for upregulation of other genes that would block the effect of the new gene therapy-mediated introduction of the product [15].

There are potential pitfalls and unresolvable problems with use of the CRISPR/CAS-9 or other technique of editing a gene to produce radiation resistance or remove a process that resulted in cell death from radiation? To answer this question, we must go back to the principles that were discussed in Chap. 1; namely, the evolution of radiation resistance on the planet Earth. Natural selection occurred during the production of the Deinococcus radiodurans bacteria by the continued generation of new clones of bacteria that were bombarded by high-dose irradiation in the attempt to sterilize meat products [45]. The generation of Deinococcus radiodurans took hundreds if not thousands of generations of cell doubling with elimination of progeny of some cell doublings that resulted in cell death. Finally, after hundreds, if not thousands of generations of bacterial cell doubling, a clone of bacteria was generated that was radiation-resistant. Analysis of the genome of Deinococcus radiodurans revealed duplication, selection of genes for DNA repair, and antioxidants. The selection of progeny during the generations of bacterial cell doublings allowed bacteria to survive that had multiple copies of specific genes, or stable production of the products of DNA repair enzymes and antioxidants. How does this phenomenon relate to the evolution of life on Earth? The Deinococcus radiodurans was selected over weeks–months, because of the rapid selection pressures of having been required to survive and double in the presence of high doses of irradiation. The evolution of life on Earth occurred during continuous low-dose irradiation, which penetrated the Magnetosphere. One cannot determine how many generations of single-cell organisms had to occur over hundreds, or thousands, or even millions of years on the early Earth environment until one was selected that had the first enzymes for repairing DNA double-strand breaks. Then, after the generation of eukaryotes that had mitochondria resulting from the cellular presence of archeobacteria in the cytoplasm of nucleated cells, there arose a "marriage" of two different genetic elements, the cells with the nuclear DNA that had been experiencing adaptation to radiation, and now the archeobacteria, which became intracellular organelles in these first eukaryotes

(An eukaryote is a cell that has mitochondria and undergoes oxidative metabolism, as opposed to a prokaryote, which does not have mitochondria.) [16, 17]. Over millions of years, single-cell organisms to evolved and became multicellular (flatworms, roundworms, segmented worms, and then leading to more advanced forms of invertebrates, then eventually to mammals and to humans), and during every one of these speciation, evolutionary trends, the radiation resistance genes were carried forward and remained a stable part of the genome. Every human contains these radiation repair genes and antioxidant genes, which are similar in construction, DNA sequence, and function to those in the most primitive organisms.

How can a process, which resulted in stable response to ionizing irradiation over millions of years, be duplicated by a technique of genetic engineering in one generation; namely, to protect the astronauts that would board a space vehicle for a long trip through the environment in which there was no protective Magnetosphere? Basic first experiments for gene editing are in process, but the challenge for creating a genetically engineered organism, that is, a human, is daunting.

There are other fundamental problems with using a CRISPR/CAS-9 gene-editing approach for human genetic engineering. The change in a gene would have to occur in embryonic stem cells and be stably introduced such that all differentiated cells during growth and development of the organism would express that genetic change [46]. The basic lesson from developmental biology is that the change of a specific gene, which was engineered to produce a specific outcome, could result in an untoward unexpected consequence, particularly, during gestation.

An example of a failed attempt to fix a gene defect by genetic engineering was made using knockout mice (homologous deletion recombinant) to correct a defect in the Fanconi Anemia mouse strain Fancd2−/− mice [15]. The experiment was designed to test the hypothesis that the anemia of this disease was caused by the bone marrow cells in the Fancd2−/− mouse having an overly intense response to an inhibitory growth factor, TGF-β. Since there was another mouse strain known to resist TGF-β by having a homologous deletion recombinant negative (knockout), of the signaling pathway for TGF-β, it was hypothesized that making a double knockout mouse (Fancd2−/− SMAD3−/−) animal would correct the defect in Fanconi Anemia. What was discovered was that the animals were very severely compromised during development in utero, and only a very small number of animals survived with the genotype of having deletion of both genes [15]. The majority of the animals died during mid-gestation at around day 13 (the mouse gestation interval is 21 days), and analysis of the defective embryo showed that they were dying, because of the inability to repair DNA [15]. The unexpected and untoward consequence of attempting to use a knockout of another gene to correct the defect was that the signaling pathway for TGF-β was also required in utero for animals to be able to repair their DNA by the process of non-homologous end-joining. The Fancd2-/- mice having already lost the ability to repair DNA by homologous recombination (the absence of the Fancd2 gene). Now needed the NHEJ pathway to survive.

A possible similar unexpected result could occur if CRISPR/CAS-9 genetic engineering was used to correct a defective gene for radiation repair or for production of an antioxidant [47]. During gestation in order for the embryonic stem cell that was corrected, to be able to differentiate to all tissues in an adult animal, that corrected gene could produce a condition in which during gestation required the embryo to upregulate or downregulate other genes that could be lethal and result in embryonic death, or could also result in an animal that had a different genetic defect.

While genetic engineering is not yet ready for application to produce radiation resistance and certainly not to facilitate any helpful approach to astronaut responses to continuous low level of irradiation, there is a lesson to be learned from these previous examples. It may be advantageous at the present time to deliver a pharmaceutical agent (radiation countermeasure) in the form of a drug, cytokine, or even dietary supplement that could produce a situation similar to that in a desired genetically engineered organism or human to make that person radiation-resistant.

Genetic engineering has become a realistic phenomenon in the scientific community [1]. With the recent discovery of the CRISPR/CAS9 technique [2] of using a specific transposon to target genetic sequences in the chromosome can now be used to excise a specific genetic sequence [3] and replace it with an altered sequence, the possibility of genetic engineering for humans has become a reality [3]. The phenomenon of changing a gene within embryonic cells leading to altered somatic cells has become a theoretical method that can be tested in experimental animals. This technique is now highly experimental and the adaptation of the technique to genetically altering organisms has led to publications in multiple scientific journals [5–10]. With the recognition that genes can be edited/changed, the possibility of enhancing radiation resistance by altering or duplicating genes is real.

There was a prior approach to genetic engineering that was based upon a technique called "gene therapy" [36–39]. In gene therapy, a genetic vector or infectious agent such as a virus was used to deliver an inserted gene into cells or tissues. The gene therapy vector was administered to target the host [37]. However, in contrast to the potential of modern genetic engineering, there was a limited vista in gene therapy for scientific approaches to alter the host response to a particular disease or environmental condition [27, 36–39]. When applied to radiation sensitivity, gene therapy might deliver a transgene in a vector to make a product that enhanced radiation resistance, such as the gene for manganese superoxide dismutase (MnSOD) [18]. The expression of MnSOD would be transient and would be inherited by future generations since the vector may not integrate with the germ line with genetic engineering. With MnSOD, one could replace or "fix" a defective gene in the host animal with a corrected gene for that host and for future generations. It then becomes theoretically possible to correct radiation sensitivity and actually produce a radiation-resistant replacement gene [15].

Gene therapy has not been previously considered to be a method to alter radiation sensitivity. However, the technique has been used successfully with cells in culture and altered a phenotype [11] and also in experimental animals [19]. In contrast, gene therapy has been used in humans and clinical trials have been published. Disease states that have been corrected or modulated by gene therapy include blindness caused by a missing gene product in retinal blindness [19]. Blindness has been corrected by use of an intraocular injected vector carrying the missing gene. Gene therapy has been effective for Hemophilia B [21] and Hemophilia A [20], blood clotting disorders are caused by the absence of clotting factors IX or VIII, respectfully; and deficiency of liver enzymes that are required for effective metabolism [22]. Initially, in the first experiments of gene therapy, genes were inserted into cells by using an infectious agent (virus) or a vector (plasmid liposome) [16]. The vector was designed to enter the cells or into tissues in an organism and the inserted gene would produce a product to correct a genetic deficiency. The inserted gene sequence was to place a new gene into the nucleus of cells in culture. The technique was applied to small organisms, such as bacteria, yeast cells, or larvae of a flatworm or insect [41]. The first gene therapy techniques used viruses [16]. Studies were published using the large adenovirus [16], smaller adeno-associated virus [19], and also plasmids [42] (which are small circles of DNA that are naturally found in bacteria). Plasmids were delivered in liposome formulations [18]. Gene therapy techniques also used other viruses including herpes viruses and retroviruses including lentivirus [12].

The technique of gene therapy is being utilized in clinical protocols and clinical trials are underway [27]. The adeno-associated virus (AAV) has been most effectively used to deliver Factor IX to correct Hemophilia B in experimental animals and recently in clinical trials has shown effectiveness in humans [19]. The larger clotting factor, Factor VIII, which is responsible for the defects leading to Hemophilia A, which is the most common form of clinical Hemophilia, and the cause of most of the morbidity and mortality in patients with this disease, has also been adapted for gene therapy delivering a smaller sequence of the large Factor VIII gene given to experimental animals in the AAV vector and now to humans [22]. While the AAV virus is smaller than adenovirus and has limited capacity to carry a large inserted gene (called a transgene), the AAV is relatively safe in humans and has become an accepted technique for using gene therapy in clinical trials [19].

The more recent use of a retrovirus (lentivirus) has gained great acceptance for gene therapy, because of its recent use now with the technique of immunotherapy [14]. There were initial and in retrospect quite realistic fears of the use of lentivirus, which is in the same category of viruses as the retroviruses and, specifically, the human immunodeficiency virus (HIV) that causes AIDS [43]. Retroviruses also include those that cause leukemia in animals and in lymphomas in the HTLV-1 and HTLV-2 in humans in Japan [40], and the human immunodeficiency HIV viruses. The idea of using a closely related lentivirus to deliver genes for therapeutic application to humans first appeared to be dangerous.

To use a lentivirus for gene therapy was initially rejected, because of early failures of gene therapy clinical trials using other viral vectors. There were problems using retrovirus to deliver genes for a clinical trial in children with the disease called subacute combined immunodeficiency syndrome (SCID) [14]. There was one form of SCID in which the patients T lymphocytes were missing an enzyme called adenosine deaminase leading to failure of T-cell function. The correction of this form of immunodeficiency in SCID children seemed to be a perfect place for a clinical trial of delivering the gene for the enzyme using an infectious retrovirus that would target T cells [14]. The first studies using retrovirus to deliver a missing gene in T cells led to the unexpected integration of the retrovirus into the nuclear DNA near an oncogene in the bone marrow site of hematopoietic stem cells [14]. Bone marrow hematopoietic stem cells are precursors of the T cells that were deficient in SCID children and were expected to correct the genetic defect by supplying the ADA gene to all T cells that developed/differentiated from the stem cells and thus would normalize and correct the immune deficiency in these children. These SCID children lived in biological containment rooms or "bubbles" and were called "bubble children," because they could not fight infections [39]. They lived in containment rooms, because they lacked a functioning immune system and could not survive in the outside world due to susceptibility to common infectious agents. The first clinical trial was stopped, because the retrovirus vector had caused leukemia in several of the children in the first treated cohort [39]. The retrovirus integrated into the bone marrow stem cells at a site next to an oncogene for leukemia [36–39]. The therapeutic trial to correct SCID lead to cases of acute leukemia [14]. This "accident" of clinical gene therapy was not the first. The retrovirus that induced leukemia followed a clinical trial using adenovirus to carry a missing gene into the liver of a patient with another enzyme deficiency.

In a clinical trial at the University of Pennsylvania, a lentivirus was used to deliver a gene to the liver of a patient with a missing tyrosine deaminase gene. This was a severe case of infection caused by the adenovirus itself. The use of adenovirus to deliver a missing gene to the liver of a patient with a protein enzyme deficiency (Jesse Gelsinger) [37] in a clinical trial at the University of Pennsylvania was widely publicized and stalled the research into gene therapy quite abruptly. These two "failures" of clinical trials of gene therapy delayed progress in the emerging field of Gene Therapy for many years until the recent advent of the successes with adeno-associated virus (AAV) [19] and lentivirus [26].

The use of lentivirus in the therapeutic approach to immunotherapy for cancer has been called CAR-T cell therapy (chimeric antigen recombinant-T) cell therapy [36]. This technique using lentivirus provided some renewed optimism about using gene therapy to treat patients with specific deficiencies in the production of a critical protein. CAR-T cell therapy is now used to treat cancers in which the gene for and antigenic surface components of the patient's cancer is inserted into lentivirus and then is amplified by growing the individual patients explanted T cells in culture. The transfected and transduced T cells are amplified in tissue culture and then infused back into the individual patient. These T cells are, thus, "trained" in vitro by the inserted gene to attack the tumor antigens and thus kill the tumor. The lentivirus used to transfect the T cells proved to be safe and successfully produced a chimeric antigen that proved to be effective for the expanded T cells to now have a target to attack the cancer when infused back in vivo. This technique of gene therapy is currently used to treat several forms of human cancers including B-cell lymphomas [38].

The leap from gene therapy to genetic engineering, however, will require overcoming a major hurdle.

Genetic engineering to correct a defect—in this case radiation sensitivity—or induce radiation resistance must be approached in sequential steps. Genetic engineering can first be targeted to one organ or cell type or can be targeted to all cells in an organism. The latter approach requires stable expression of the corrected gene in all cells, organs, and organ systems starting with embryonic stem cells [46]. The problem of correction of a gene in all cells and organs requires stable gene expression of the corrected gene in embryonic stem cells, and then, all differentiated cells in all organs as the embryo grows and develops into a full organism. The correction of defects in embryos is a technique that is being developed in animal models at present and has uncovered several problems [35]. There are many problems that have already been detected in experiments that have been associated with changing genes that are correcting a mutation either by the use of CRISPR/CAS-9 in specific T cells, or inserting a missing gene into embryonic cells [46]. The gene can be methylated and shut off (or somatic change) (Fig. 11.1, Table 11.1). Once the technique has been effective at targeting the appropriate location in a specific chromosome on a specific chromosome and in specific cells the challenge of the response of all the other genes and gene pathways to this new gene becomes a potentially neutralizing event. There has been the detection of "side effects" or untoward consequences of introducing a new gene, which occurs due to the host reaction to the new gene in vivo.

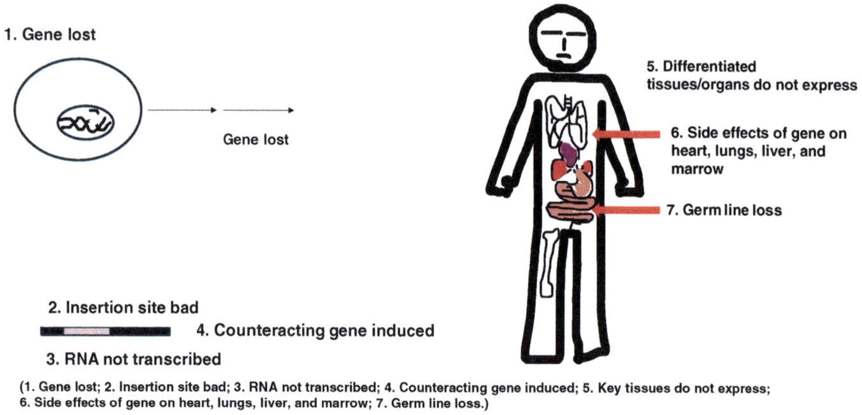

Fig. 11.1 Challenges of genetic engineering by inserting a gene for radiation resistance. Methods by which to make a radioresistant human would require insertion or modification of genes in the fertilized ovum. Shown at the top is the condition in which a gene is lost, a new gene is inserted, or there is a modification of a gene. Problems include possibilities that during implantation of the genetically engineered embryo the gene is lost (1), the insertion site in the chromosome or in the specific arm of a chromosome is a bad site (2), the RNA is not transcribed (3), there is a counteracting gene induced (4), or there are key tissue expression restraints that do now allow the gene modifications to be present in all tissues, particularly, radiosensitive key tissues, such as the intestine or bone marrow (5). There are other problems, such as there could be side effects of the gene—a pleotropic effect on the heart, lungs, liver, or bone marrow (6). There is a possibility that there could be no germ line expression such that the progeny of such engineered humans would not be radioresistant (7). The bottom panel demonstrates the chromosome site in which the radiation resistance gene was inserted and how the events described above could occur

Table 11.1 Targets for genetic engineering a radiation-resistant organism

Major strategies	
Genetic	Gene insertion
	Gene duplication
	Translation enhancement
Epigenetic	Remove methylation sites that inhibit transcription and translation
	Methylate genetic sites that counteract specific genes
Specific targets	
Specific genes	DNA repair genes
	Antioxidant genes
	Inflammatory cytokine genes
	Bone marrow stem cell enhancement
	Intestinal stem cell targets

Precedents for Genetic Engineering

Animal model systems have provided great insight into methods by which a successful correction of a gene defect can be accomplished. Several lessons, but also cautions have been presented from the phenomenon of genetic engineering.

Systems in which a missing gene or mutated gene results in a profound clinical change have been available for study of the effect of adding a new gene for decades. Animal model systems have been used to remove or correct a gene that associated with increase in the incidence of cancer [35]. This has been the case with oncogenes including K-RAS, C-MYC, and, most recently, the BRACA1, and BRACA2 genes that have been associated with animal models of breast cancer [32]. This is a place, where genetic corrections have been introduced by genetic engineering of embryos is that with missing or altered genes. The example cited above for gene therapy for Hemophilia, which was successfully approached with gene therapy, is an example of how an animal model system for a clotting deficiency can also be used as a way to test the phenomenon of genetic engineering.

Several experiments revealed problems that were associated with correcting a gene rather than supplying a missing gene product. Inserting the gene by "gene therapy" into tissues of an adult organisms using a vector was shown with Hemophilia B or retinal disease to deliver a new corrected gene and was successful [19]. However, correcting the intrinsic gene by genetic engineering is a different challenge. This experiment produced a different and inefficient result [30] than that seen with inserting another missing gene for Factor IX in Hemophilia B. Correcting a mutant or defective gene by a technique of CRISPR/CA-S9 was not directly successful and was not trivial. The technique was also tested in other diseases.

The disease in which there are mutations that are associated with Fanconi anemia (FA) is an example. The Fanconi anemia example is relevant to radiation biology, because of the radiosensitivity of animals and humans who have specific forms of FA [15]. Correction of a genetic defect in two of the genes in the FA pathway, Fancd2, and Fanci has not been successfully carried out yet with CRISPR/CAS9 technique [47]. The FA example is a good one because there are 26 different genes in the FA pathway leading to repair of DNA double-strand breaks. Fixing one gene led to alterations in other FA pathway genes and also in non-FA pathways [15]. These results uncovered a phenomenon of adaptation of the developing organism during embryogenesis and during gestation the corrected defective or missing gene by can result in alterations that will do other things and may not alter the organism to survive. Thus, the defective gene if replaced or fixed may disrupt the process by which the organism adapted to the absence of that gene and its product (Table 11.1, Fig. 11.1). The adaptation of the developing organism to the insertion of a new gene may work against the goal of the original genetic engineering to correct a gene defect. The developing organism may reject the gene, shut down its function, or invoke other gene functions to neutralize its planned therapeutic outcome.

Most of the successful experiments with genetic engineering have been carried out in single-cell organisms such as bacteria or more complex animal models [6–9]. Genetic engineering has the theoretical advantage of correcting a gene defect by inserting a gene into the present and immediate generation. However, there are challenges of genetic engineering that cannot be compared to the process of natural selection, which requires many generations of reproduction and elimination of many progeny until the desired phenotype is achieved. The alternative process of natural selection will alter radiation sensitivity, as in the case of Deinococcus radiodurans [45]. A radioresistant organisms was derived and achievable, but this required 100 s of generations in organisms that has a doubling time of 4 h. Bacteria facilitate the selection of a radioresistant subline in weeks to months, but during the selection process hundreds of generations of bacteria died from radiation.

Could natural selection be applied to generate a radioresistant mouse, non-human primate, or human? The ethical consensus is prohibitive. Genetic engineering is the preferred approach. Theoretically, mouse embryos could be generated in vitro and irradiated in vitro until one was observed to survive radiation and implantation into a surrogate mother and survive a live birth but the adaptation of such a fetal mouse to survive all of the events leading to live birth would undoubtedly require multiple unexpected genetic pathway alterations. At present, it is impractical for using natural selection to produce radioresistance in a higher organism not possible as with Deinococcus radiodurans.

Other Major Obstacles to Be Overcome for the Use of Genetic Engineering to Alter Radiosensitivity

The most problematic issue with genetic engineering is the side effects or untoward consequences (Table 11.1, Fig. 11.1). Inserting a gene in the appropriate place can be achieved with cells in culture, but is much more difficult with embryos. In a hypothetical situation, in vitro fertilization can be carried out producing a multicellular zygote. Demonstrating that every cell within the zygote had the corrected gene in the appropriate place in the genome, on the correct chromosome, and correct site would be necessary to prove. Then, implantation of engineered embryos into a surrogate female would be carried out. The developmental stages of an embryo, in the mouse model (which has a 21-day gestation), would require experiments in which embryos were removed at serial times after implantation of the genetically engineered embryo and demonstration that the developing organs had the gene correction in all relevant tissues.

In experiments with transfection of embryos using viral vectors, it has been demonstrated that successful introduction of a gene (or theoretically correction of a gene with CRISPR/CAS-9) in a multicellular zygote does not necessarily lead to stable maintenance of the corrected gene in all forming tissues and organs (Table 11.1, Fig. 11.1). For example, the technique of overexpressing the gene for radioresistance (manganese superoxide dismutase (MnSOD)) in embryos, led to a generation of mice that had varying levels of overexpression of MnSOD in different tissues [33]. This study was carried out with vector transfer, and the technique of gene therapy of embryos, but would also apply to a CRISPR/CAS-9 corrected embryo. The phenomenon of tissue-specific levels of expression of an altered gene relates to the levels of expression of associated genetic pathways in the developing embryo. For example, the rapidly proliferating organ such as the bone marrow or intestine during the 21-day gestation of mice is associated with tissue-specific levels of genes that we associated with production of the RNA and protein from the altered gene.

An example of von Willebrand factor (vWF) [47] shows the relevance of tissue-specific alterations in an inserted gene expression level during gestation. Jarhoudi, et al. showed the observation in mice that the altered gene was expressed at high levels in the adult mouse brain but not in other tissues [48]. There were high levels of expression of the altered gene in the embryo, but the only expression in the adult was in the brain endothelium [48]. The vWF gene is expressed in endothelial cells, and in the embryo, all endothelial cells in all organs could activate the vWF promotor and express the inserted attached gene, but at the time of birth only brain endothelial cells still expressed the attached gene. Would this happen to a genetically engineered radiation resistance gene as well, and what will be required to genetically engineer multiple genes to derive a radioresistant animal?

What specific factors turned off or neutralize the expression of an engineered new gene? In the vWF experiment [48], the result showed that expression of the new gene was specific for brain and only in endothelial cells [48]. The studies on vWF [48] demonstrated that as organs develop and distinguish specific functions in the adult animal, there are organ-specific differences in that cell phenotype. The conclusion from this study was that all endothelial cells are not the same. Endothelial cells in the mouse brain, but not other organs shared characteristics with embryonic endothelial cells, such that the inserted gene for vWF was maintained in the blood vessels in the brain [48]. The development of other organ systems during gestation resulted in the need for endothelial cells to provide circulation for those organs, but the biology and control of gene expression in endothelial cells in other organs were not the same. This organ-specific phenomenon may well extend to CRISPR/CAS-9 genetic engineering in which correction of a gene defect in the embryo may not extend to correction in all organs in the developing fetus. As applied to engineering a gene for radiation resistance, in embryonic stem cells, the adult organisms might have expression in several organs, but not in bone marrow, or have expression everywhere [46], but show induction of other genes that neutralized the new gene. In both cases, the adult organism would be susceptible to ionizing irradiation and unaltered in resistance.

Embryogenesis and Alteration of Genetically Engineered Genes

In addition to the different levels of expression of an inserted gene (gene therapy), or theoretically altered gene (genetically engineered gene) is a real phenomenon of tissue-specific alteration of levels of expression. Furthermore, the presence of an altered or corrected protein in embryonic cells and in the embryo may not extend to similar levels of expression in each tissue as the embryo develops into a fetus and then into a newborn. Embryogenesis is a very complex phenomenon, which is only recently been partially elucidated. One principle derived from early experiments in this area is that the attempts of a developing embryo to survive in the presence of an altered gene often lead to other genetic alterations. An example of this phenomenon is the recent demonstration of attempted correction of gene defect in Fanconi Anemia (Fancd2−/−) mice by genetically engineering a second gene, which would block the deleterious effects of the original Fancd2−/− gene [15].

The recent publication revealed a result, which urges caution in any attempt at genetic engineering of an embryo to generate a radioresistant animal [15]. In these experiments, an attempt was made to correct the Fanconi Anemia associated sensitivity of bone marrow stem cells to the negative regulatory growth factor of hematopoiesis, TGF-β. It was demonstrated in animal models, as well as, in humans that the defect in Fanconi Anemia leading to lack of production of stem cells and the paucity of erythroid progenitors, which causes anemia in an attempt to overcome this phenomenon, Fancd2−/− were bred to mice with a block in the TGF-β signaling pathway, namely, by elimination of the SMAD3 gene [15]. It was discovered that during embryonic development, these mice with both lack of the Fancd2 gene and the SMAD3 gene led to embryonic lethality at mid-gestation. In the mid-gestation at day 13 (mouse gestation is 21 days), a number of expected double heterozygous recombinant negative (double knockout) mice was consistent with the number expected based on the breeding of double heterozygote animals. However, by 21 days, the number of live births was significantly decreased [15]. It was discovered that during embryogenesis, embryos required naturally occurring alternate pathway for repairing DNA double-strand breaks that occurred during all cell doublings.

A previous chapter in this book has described the calculation of around 1000 DNA double-strand breaks with every cell division. Cells have two mechanisms by which to repair such breaks. One is homologous recombination (HR) and a second non-homologous end-joining (NHEJ). It was discovered from these experiments with DKO mice that Fancd2−/− mice with the defect in HR required non-homologous-end-joining (NHEJ) to survive embryogenesis. The secondary effect of deletion of the SMAD3 gene (in addition to its blocking of TGF-β signaling) was to alter NHEJ [15]. Developing embryos could not survive without NHEJ as the alternative mechanism for DNA double-strand break repair. The few animals that survived the DKO genotype bypassed the lack of NHEJ and survived 21-day gestation, but the number was very low. In four different combinations of breeding double knockout (DKO) mice, the low, but detectable number of DKO animals was mouse strain specific. Thus, there were other genetic factors associated with the inbred mouse strains that modulated the adaptation of embryos to the lack of both HR and NHEJ. How would this phenomenon relate to the discussion of genetic engineering for radiation resistance? Even if it were possible to insert multiple genes into an embryo prior to implantation into a surrogate host, the control of each inserted gene or genetically engineered gene would not necessarily be regulated to express in all organs such that its absence would create a significant problem. That neutralized organ or organs would not be altered in its response to ionizing irradiation and the organism might not survive.

There is another potential problem with genetic engineering, namely, adaptation of every organ and organ system to the corrected/engineered and thus altered gene. The developing embryo might reject the genetically engineered change (Table 11.1, Fig. 11.1), or to switch on or switch off other genetic pathways that will in effect neutralize the engineered gene.

In Deinococcus radiodurans, the process of the selection of the radiation-resistant bacterium with multiple amplifications of radiation repair genes and antioxidant genes and the 4-h life cycle of bacteria leading to cell doublings every 4 h was not closely monitored [45]. Thus, the events over many bacterial generations (doubling) that occurred in bacteria during selection of those with radiation resistance were not described in detail. Based upon other data with gene therapy models and also with CRISPR/CAS-9 models, many generations of bacteria were rejected, did not survive, and did not undergo further cell doublings. Many were lost during the process of natural selection. This phenomenon could occur in bacteria with rapid proliferation and multiple generations allowed one to be selected for the desired phenotypes over weeks of exposure to high-dose irradiation. The phenomenon could clearly not be used to generate radioresistance in more complex animals and certainly not in non-human primates or human embryos. Thus, genetic engineering to facilitate radiation resistance for prolonged exposure to space irradiation is at present feasible and, thus, impractical. Genetic engineering in one generation not only may not work, it may result in activation of competing and/or neutralizing gene pathways that produce other serious medical problems in the germ line and affect subsequent generations.

What Would Be the Theoretical Use of Genetic Engineering to Facilitate Long-Term Exposure to Galactic Cosmic Irradiation?

All of the literature on the effects of continuous non-lethal ionizing irradiation to date describes the phenomenon of adaptation [49–51]. The capacity of complex organisms to adapt to an environmental challenge is well known. However, along the way multiple members of a population may be lost due to the inability to adapt. In the example cited previously of the Argonne Laboratories experiments with outbred beagle dogs, exposed to 3–5 Roentgens in air of Cobalt60 irradiation [50], continuously for 2 years, one-third of the animals died of anemia, another third died of erythroleukemia, and the one-third, which radio-accommodated and survived, suggests that the phenomenon of adaptation is highly inefficient. Furthermore, the one-third that did survive had multiple other associated defects including rapid aging and abnormalities of hematopoiesis, thus using adaptation to this level of irradiation in a complex animal such as the dog cannot be compared to the phenomenon of the adaptation of bacteria to much higher levels of continuous radiation, as in the case of Deinococcus radiodurans. In the latter example, rapid proliferation and loss of bacteria along the way was not calculated, but must be assumed to be very high until a colony was selected with the adapted radiation resistance genes and antioxidant genes. In the absence of an approach to genetic engineering, other strategies must be sought. Adaptation is the only practical phenomenon that can now be considered to be practical and a potentially reasonable approach. Humans that live for decades at sea level will adapt to living in the lower oxygen concentrations in the air at Leadville, Colorado, which is two miles above sea level [51, 52]. Initially, people have increased breathing rate due to the reduced oxygen level, but within months, they produce more red blood cells and increase their hematocrit and carry more oxygen [51, 52]. Their breathing rate normalizes. Can this adaptation occur in the environment of space radiation? What will the adaptations be? Will this be detectable genetic changes that can be observed over months? Will epigenetic changes occur in levels of existing gene expression for antioxidant genes, or could this ever be duplications, enhanced transcription or elevated levels of gene product production? Research in using genetic engineering to create radioresistant organisms and eventually humans will be important to NASA and to the general scientific community to consider if we are to achieve the reality of space travel.

References

1. Mukhopadhyay S. CRISPR-Cas-9: a recent tool for gene editing a review on discovery and application. Am J Appl Bio-Technol Res. 2023;4(2):28–33.
2. Sorgner SL, Viafora C, Kremer A, et al. Chapter 1. Genes, CRISPR/Cas 9, and Posthumans. In: Sinaci M, Sorgner SL, editors. General ethical challenges of emerging (bio) technologies. Trivent Publishing; 2018.
3. Sharma RK, Santiago-Sanchez GS, Rabelo-Fernandez RJ, et al. Abstract 2503: Crispr/cas-9-mediated genome editing reveals that RBPMS acts as a tumor suppressor in ovarian cancer. Cancer Res. 2021;81(13 supplement):2503.
4. Mehmood S, Syed A, Rafique F, et al. Applications of CRISPR Cas-9 in ovarian cancer research. Protein Pept Lett. 2023;30(8):653–67. https://doi.org/10.2174/0929866530666230607104453.
5. Wang X. A review on the molecular mechanism, superiorities, applications, limitations, and experimental workflow of CRISPR/Cas-9 system, and the future of gene engineering. Mater Sci Eng. 2020;729:012044.
6. Coogan M, Alston V, Su B, et al. CRISPR/Cas-9 induced knockout of myostatin gene improves growth and disease resistance in channel catfish (*Ictalurus punctatus*). Aquaculture. 2022;557:738290.
7. Bhagwat AC, Patil AM, Saroj SD. CRISPR/Cas 9-based editing in the production of bioactive molecules. Mol Biotechnol. 2022;64(3):245–51. https://doi.org/10.1007/s12033-021-00418-4.
8. Alagoz Y, Gurkok T, Zhang B, et al. Manipulating the biosynthesis of bioactive compound alkaloids for next-generation metabolic engineering in opium poppy using CRISPR-Cas 9 genome editing technology. Sci Rep. 2016;6:30910. https://doi.org/10.1038/srep30910.
9. Khurana A, Sayed N, Singh V, et al. A comprehensive overview of CRISPR/Cas 9 technology and application thereof in drug discovery. J Cell Biochem. 2022;123(10):1674–98. https://doi.org/10.1002/jcb.30329.
10. Driehuis E, Clevers H. CRISPR/Cas 9 genome editing and its applications in organoids. Am J Physiol Gastrointest Liver Physiol. 2017;312(3):G257–65. https://doi.org/10.1152/ajpgi.00410.2016.
11. Zhu G-D, Yu J, Sun Z-Y, et al. Genome-wide CRISPR/Cas9 screening identifies CARHSP1 responsible for radiation resistance in glioblastoma. Cell Death Dis. 2021;12(8):724. https://doi.org/10.1038/s41419-021-04000-3.
12. Shrock E, Guell M. Chapter 6—CRISPR in animals and animal models. In: Torres-Ruiz R, Rodriguez-Perales S (eds) Progress in molecular biology and translational science (book series). Sci Direct. 2017;52:1–138.
13. Yao S, He Z, Chen C. CRISPR/Cas9-mediated genome editing of epigenetic factors for cancer therapy. Hum Gene Ther. 2015;26(7):463–71. https://doi.org/10.1089/hum.2015.067.
14. Howe SJ, Mansour MR, Schwarzwaelder K, et al. Insertional mutagenesis combined with acquired somatic mutations causes leukemogenesis following gene therapy of SCID-X1 patients. J Clin Invest. 2008;118(9):3143–50. https://doi.org/10.1172/JCI35798.
15. Rodriguez A, Epperly M, Filiatrault J, et al. TGFβ pathway is required for viable gestation of Fanconi anemia embryos. PLoS Genet. 2022;18(11):e1010459. https://doi.org/10.1371/journal.pgen.1010459.
16. Greenberger JS, Epperly MW. Radioprotective antioxidant gene therapy: potential mechanisms of action. Gene Ther Mol Biol. 2004;8:31–44.
17. Greenberger JS, Epperly M. Pleiotropic stem cell and tissue effects of ionizing irradiation protection by MnSOD-plasmid liposome gene therapy. In: Columbus F, editor. Progress in gene therapy. Nova Science Publications; 2005. p. 110–8.
18. Epperly MW, Guo HL, Bernarding M, et al. Delayed intratracheal injection of manganese superoxide dismutase (MnSOD)-plasmid liposomes provides suboptimal protection against irradiation-induced pulmonary injury compared to treatment before irradiation. Gene Ther Mol Biol. 2003;7:61–8.

19. Stieger K, Lheriteau W, Moullier P, et al. AAV-mediated gene therapy for retinal disorders in large animal models. ILAR J. 2009;50(2):206–24. https://doi.org/10.1093/ilar.50.2.206.
20. Chiang GG, Rubin HL, Cherington V, et al. Bone marrow stromal cell-mediated gene therapy for hemophilia a: in vitro expression of human factor VIII with high biological activity requires the inclusion of the proteolytic site at amino acid 1648. Hum Gene Ther. 1999;10(1):61–76. https://doi.org/10.1089/10430349950019192.
21. Cherington V, Chiang GG, McGrath CA, et al. Retroviral vector modified bone marrow stromal cells secrete biologically active factor IX in vitro and transiently deliver therapeutic levels of human factor IX to the plasma of dogs after reinfusion. Hum Gene Ther. 1998;9(10):1397–407. https://doi.org/10.1089/hum.1998.9.10-1397.
22. Baruteau J, Waddington SN, Alexander IE, et al. Gene therapy for monogenic liver diseases: clinical successes, current challenges, and future prospects. J Inherit Metab Dis. 2017;40(4):497–517. https://doi.org/10.1007/s10545-017-0053-3.
23. Zwacka RM, Dudus L, Epperly MW, et al. Redox gene therapy protects human IB-3 lung epithelial cells against ionizing radiation-induced apoptosis. Hum Gene Ther. 1998;9(9):1381–6. https://doi.org/10.1089/hum.1998.9.9-1381.
24. Colella P, Ronzitti G, Mingozzi F. Emerging issues in AAV-mediated in vivo gene therapy. Mol Ther Methods Clin Dev. 2017;8:87–104. https://doi.org/10.1016/j.omtm.2017.11.007.
25. Stickle RL, Epperly MW, Klein E, et al. Prevention of irradiation-induced esophagitis by plasmid/liposome delivery of the human manganese superoxide dismutase (MnSOD) transgene. Radiat Oncol Investig. 1999;7(4):204–17. https://doi.org/10.1002/(SICI)1520-6823(1999)7:4<204::AID-RO12>3.0.CO;2-S.
26. Connolly JB. Lentiviruses in gene therapy clinical research. Gene Ther. 2002;9(24):1730–4. https://doi.org/10.1038/sj.gt.3301893.
27. Tarhini AA, Belani C, Luketich JD, et al. A phase I study of concurrent chemotherapy (paclitaxel and carboplatin) and thoracic radiotherapy with swallowed manganese superoxide dismutase (MnSOD) plasmid liposome (PL) protection in patients with locally advanced stage III non-small cell lung cancer. Hum Gene Ther. 2011;22(3):336–42. https://doi.org/10.1089/hum.2010.078.
28. George LA, Sullivan SK, Giermasz A, et al. Hemophilia B gene therapy with a high-specific-activity factor IX variant. N Engl J Med. 2017;377(23):2215–27. https://doi.org/10.1056/NEJMoa1708538.
29. Pipe SW, Gonen-Yaacovi G, Segurado OG. Hemophilia A gene therapy: current and next-generation approaches. Expert Opin Biol Ther. 2022;22(9):1099–115. https://doi.org/10.1080/14712598.2022.2002842.
30. Greenberger JS. Gene therapy approaches for stem cell protection. Gene Ther. 2008;15(2):100–8. https://doi.org/10.1038/nature03445.
31. Tachibana M, Amato P, Sparman M, et al. Towards germline gene therapy of inherited mitochondrial diseases. Nature. 2013;493(7434):627–31. https://doi.org/10.1038/nature11647.
32. Farmer H, McCabe H, Lord CJ, et al. Targeting the DNA repair defect in BRCA mutant cells as a therapeutic strategy. Nature. 2005;434(7035):917–21. https://doi.org/10.1038/nature03445.
33. Rhieu BH, Shinde A, Epperly MW, et al. Organ-specific responses of total body irradiated doxycycline-inducible manganese superoxide dismutase Tet/Tet mice. In Vivo. 2014;28(6):1033–43.
34. Greenberger JS, Epperly MW, Gretton J, et al. Radioprotective gene therapy. Curr Gene Ther. 2003;3(3):183–95. https://doi.org/10.2174/1566523034578384.
35. Morgan RA, Gray D, Lomova A, et al. Hematopoietic stem cell gene therapy: progress and lessons learned. Cell Stem Cell. 2017;21(5):574–90. https://doi.org/10.1016/j.stem.2017.10.010.
36. Das SK, Menezes ME, Bhatia S, et al. Gene therapies for cancer: strategies, challenges, and successes. J Cell Physiol. 2015;230(2):259–71. https://doi.org/10.1002/jcp.24791.
37. Smith L, Byers JF. Gene therapy in the post-Gelsinger era: JONA's healthcare law, ethics, and regulation. JONAS Health Law Ethics Regul. 2002;4(4):104–10. https://doi.org/10.1097/00128488-200212000-00004.

38. Jogalekar MP, Rajendran RL, Khan F, et al. CAR T-cell-based gene therapy for cancers: new perspectives, challenges, and clinical development. Front Immunol. 2022;13:925985. https://doi.org/10.3389/fimmu.2022.925985.
39. Blaese RM, Culver KW, Miller AD, et al. T lymphocyte-directed gene therapy for ADA-SCID: initial trial results after 4 years. Science. 1995;270(5235):475–80. https://doi.org/10.1126/science.270.5235.475.
40. Mukherjee A, Epperly M, Shields D, et al. Ionizing irradiation induced Fgr in senescent cells mediates fibrosis. Cell Death Discov. 2021;7(1):349. https://doi.org/10.1038/s41420-021-00741-4.
41. Jain R, Rivera MC, Moore JE, et al. Horizontal gene transfer in microbial genome evolution. Theor Popul Biol. 2002;61(4):489–95. https://doi.org/10.1006/tpbi.2002.1596.
42. Pardridge WM. Brain delivery of nanomedicines: Trojan horse liposomes for plasmid DNA gene therapy of the brain. Front Med Technol. 2020;2:602236. https://doi.org/10.3389/fmedt.2020.602236.
43. Rodriguez-Penney AT, Ludicello JE, Riggs PK, et al. Co-morbidities in persons infected with HIV: increased burden with older age and negative effects on health-related quality of life. AIDS Patient Care STDs. 2013;27(1):5–16. https://doi.org/10.1089/apc.2012.0329.
44. Proietti FA, Carneiro-Proietti ABF, Catalan-Soares BC, et al. Global epidemiology of HTLV-1 infection and associated diseases. Oncogene. 2005;24(39):6058–68. https://doi.org/10.1038/sj.onc.1208968.
45. Blasius M, Hubscher U, Sommer S. Deinococcus radiodurans: what belongs to the survival kit? Crit Rev Biochem Mol Biol. 2008;43(3):221–38. https://doi.org/10.1080/10409230802122274.
46. Rathjen PD, Lake J, Whyatt LM, et al. Properties and uses of embryonic stem cells: prospects for application to human biology and gene therapy. Reprod Fertil Dev. 1998;10(1):31–47. https://doi.org/10.1071/r98041.
47. Greenberger JS, Berhane H, Shinde A, et al. Can radiosensitivity associated with defects in DNA repair be overcome by mitochondrial-targeted antioxidant radioprotectors? Front Oncol. 2014;4:24. https://doi.org/10.3389/fonc.2014.00024.
48. Jahroudi N, Ardekani AM, Greenberger JS. An NF1-like protein functions as repressor of vWf promoter. J Biol Chem. 1996;271(35):21413–21. https://doi.org/10.1074/jbc.271.35.21413.
49. Jonsson KI, Levine EB, Wojcik A, et al. Environmental adaptations: radiation tolerance. In: Schill RO, editor. Water bears: the biology of tardigrades, vol. 2. Springer; 2018.
50. Seed TM, Carnes BA, Tolle DV, et al. Blood responses under chronic low daily dose gamma irradiation: I. Differential preclinical responses of irradiated male dogs in progression to either aplastic anemia or myeloproliferative disease. Leuk Res. 1989;13(12):1069–84. https://doi.org/10.1016/0145-2126(89)90152-5.
51. Moeller D, Sun L-S. Comparison of natural background dose rates for residents of the Amargosa Valley, NV, to those in Leadville, CO, and the states of Colorado and Nevada. Health Phys. 2006;91(4):338–53. https://doi.org/10.1097/01.HP.0000218426.41326.6d.
52. Mhaidly R, Verhoeyen E. The future: in vivo CAR T cell gene therapy. Mol Ther. 2019;27(4):707–9. https://doi.org/10.1016/j.ymthe.2019.03.012.

Chapter 12
Other Strategies in Genetic Engineering and Genetic Alterations for Ionizing Irradiation Adaptation

Genetic Engineering: Genetic Alterations for Radiation Adaptation

The U.S. Space Agency with a budget of $2.6 billion in contracts available through 2028 has partnered with private companies to place payloads on robotic landers and this process has achieved recently a successful landing of the Odysseus System on the lunar surface [1–3]. The private company "Intuitive Machines" based in Houston, Texas, was paid $118 million dollars to safely land scientific payloads on the Moon. While this success is impressive, the Artemis II Human Mission for a 10-day circumnavigation of the Moon, will be a challenge and is to be followed by a Moon landing a year later by Artemis III. Even further delayed is the plan to have a permanent human presence on and around the Moon ahead of an even further delayed Mars Mission. This recent information highlights the importance of collaboration between the United States Space Agency, NASA, and commercial companies [1–3].

Unfortunately, all planned missions do not always work. The prior landing by a collaboration of the agency with the company Astrobotic of Pittsburgh, Pennsylvania, and its failed Perrigrine lander was a setback. The current success of Odysseus helps to place the trajectory of successful space missions back on target. This is the first successful Moon landing by the United States in 52 years. There is, therefore, renewed and aggressive activity with space agencies from Japan, India, and China.

With all of the enthusiasm and excitement about successful incremental advances with respect to Lunar landings and development of resident structures on the Moon, there is still a need for effects of radiation on the humans, who will inhabit the habitat structures on the Moon and Mars. Exploration and mining operations on the Moon will undoubtedly follow, and there will be information about ionizing irradiation effects on these individuals.

As materials scientists and engineers approach the daunting problem of generating power sources and engines to transport astronauts to Mars and beyond, there are

J. Greenberger, *Radiation Oncology and Radiation Biology*, https://doi.org/10.1007/978-3-031-66300-0_12

discussions about fusion reactors to generate power and even matter-antimatter power sources. There are discussions about concentrating anti-protons to produce antimatter and discussions about purification of positrons, which are the antimatter equivalent of electrons. The amount of energy that can be generated by controlled fusion reactions is huge, and several orders of magnitude even greater if one could control antimatter engine power. These are speculations that can involve huge investments by government collaboration with private companies and many articles have been written suggesting that these engine devices are not limited by science, but rather by finance, and amounts of money that must be invested. However, all of these hurdles are surmountable.

Not yet surmountable is the hurdle with respect to use genetic engineering as a possible strategy to be able to protect astronauts from effects of space radiation. Such scientific considerations must also involve the discipline of "ethics" as it applies to structuring the human genome. The previous chapter focused on the specific experiments that can be done now with bacteria, yeast, small multicellular organisms, small mammals, and even non-human primates to alter radioprotection genes. This chapter will deal with an alternative strategy, but also poses targeting genetic radiation-induced inflammation, the significant challenges of translating such advances into physical approaches for humans.

The Situation Regarding Human Genetic Engineering

The past decades have seen tremendous advances leading up to what some day can be genetic engineering of astronauts. Gene therapy for diseases was thought to be an ethical dilemma. Experiments carried out decades ago led to an approach to use a retrovirus to insert the correct hemoglobin gene into the cells of a patient with thalassemia. Genetic engineering of human cells in culture is routinely being carried out and clinical trials using lentivirus or adeno-associated virus as vectors to transfer genes are being used in new clinical trials [4]. The use of AAV to treat a congenital disease of the retina has led to improvement in vision for patients in clinical trials. Similarly, the use of lentivirus to deliver chimeric genes to explanted individual patient T-cells has led to a now common practice of CAR-T cell immunotherapy for cancer patients. In a third example, the severe blood clotting abnormality found in patients with Hemophilia A has been the subject of clinical trials using AAV (adeno-associated virus) to deliver a corrected form of the gene to patients with this disease. Gene therapy is the first step in genetic engineering as reviewed in the previous chapter.

A second step in genetic engineering has been the gene correction technique of gene editing. Rather than inserting the correct gene into cells, this technology uses CAS9/CRISPR [4] technology to use specific gene sequences to enter cells, cut a specific spot in a defective gene, and replace it with correct sequences. This more precise technology enables gene correction in individuals and eliminates the concern for the use of a virus vector to carry a new gene into cells. Limited success with the CRISPR-CAS9 technique has been published, and this approach appears to be the next step for clinical trials in humans with specific diseases.

Genetic Engineering for Radiation Protection and Radiation Resistance

There is a definite possibility that humans exposed to continuous low-level space radiation, whether it be solar protons, galactic cosmic irradiation, neutrons generated by GCR hitting components of the spacecraft, and/or gamma irradiation will adapt. There will be little tolerance for a risk of any increases in carcinogenesis, neurocognitive defects, and other varied consequences of the irradiation of space travel. The adaptation of humans to continuous irradiation will require continuous modification of those processes, which are known to be required for survival in a radiation environment, namely, repair of DNA damage and replenishment of antioxidant stores [5–15], and more recently using small molecules to enhance antioxidant neutralization of radiation effects [16–20]. Research in aging has revealed similarity to ionizing irradiation-induced damage [21–23]. Enhancing the capacity of humans (or experimental animals) to survive in a continuous irradiation environment will involve the understanding of the mechanism of ionizing irradiation-induced aging. Therefore, one approach to a potential genetic engineering of radiation-resistant humans might also apply to genetic engineering approaches to prevent or delay aging. The ethics that are associated with carrying out such experiments in humans will involve ethics discussions that will be based on new evolving experimental data. The experiments to produce data to support genetic engineering to prevent aging are in progress in experimental animals.

The previous chapter described experimental systems for genetic engineering. Animal models of progeria (premature aging) have been an excellent place to start. Correcting the defective genes in animal models of progeria will lead to valuable information that can be used in dealing with the ethics of human genetic engineering. These experiments are in progress and probably useful data will be decades away. What will be necessary is data showing that genetic engineering of animals with the condition of progeria including the animal model systems that can be applied to create genetically normalized mice that might have a restored normal lifespan and do not have a higher incidence of background carcinogenesis [24], neurocognitive defects [25–27], or other components of genes other than those that had been targeted as phenotypic evidence of rapid aging. Steroids are used to limit inflammation [28–30] and do alter irradiation-induced inflammation response; however, there is little effect of steroids on permanently changing the radiation-induced late effects [31, 32]. There is much evidence that targeting the genes for inflammation rather than DNA damage may be a better strategy for genetic engineering [33–35].

Ethical Considerations in Genetic Engineering of Humans

Consider a situation in which a group of physicians in a modern hospital care system were reviewing data leading to approval of a clinical trial for genetic engineering of human embryos. The political landscape in the United States right now has continued controversy about what constitutes a child. Is it a frozen embryo? The other extreme of human gestation is the controversy about termination of pregnancy in the third trimester and whether this constitutes abortion or murder. The political landscape in the future when ethics in hospital protocol committees are reviewing data for genetic engineering of a human embryo, undoubtedly, reflects the political landscape in the country. If it is determined that insertion of multiple copies of radiation resistance genes into human embryos is ethical and is approved by protocol committees to allow the first clinical trials, one can envision an experimental model system for the first test.

Genetic Engineering of Radiation-Resistant Astronauts

Much information will be obtained from the returning astronauts after the planned Mars Mission. It may be that supplement of the diet of these astronauts with antioxidants and chemopreventive agents will increase their capacity for repairing ionizing irradiation damage and follow-up of these individuals after return to Earth will show that their health and well-being over the next decades shows no deleterious effects of the anticipated 880-day Mars Mission. If this is the case, and if further information about successful supplement of these individuals with radiation mitigator or radiation protector drugs, then the need for genetic engineering to produce radiation resistance may not be a critical consideration. However, if returning astronauts from a Mars Mission show significant effects of radiation exposure and countermeasures, which are then available appear to be inadequate, there may be a return to the discussion about genetic engineering. A discussion of genetic engineering for producing radiation-resistant astronauts will undoubtedly occur in an environment where genetic engineering is being considered for correction of other human conditions including human diseases. As time goes on, advances in multiple scientific disciplines occur in parallel. By the time that there is a discussion about human genetic engineering, there will be a plethora of new data from experimental model systems that have successfully used genetic engineering (insertion or duplication of new genes) into animal embryos correction of multiple diseases. Removal or neutralization of genes that are associated with carcinogenesis in animal models will lead to data indicating that derivative mouse strains that have had these genes removed or replaced with other genes that neutralize the effects of such genes (e.g., oncogenes like K-RAS, C-MYC, or others) have been successful. At the time when discussions about genetic engineering of human embryos become a reality, there will be much information about safety in animal models. One of the first consequences of genetic engineering of animal embryos will be the data on the occurrence of other untoward events. For example, if inserting genes into embryos corrects defects in progeria or premature aging, but also induces genetic translocations, or alterations in epigenetic control [36, 37] of other gene expression patterns, there will be a delay in any potential translation of such technology to humans.

What Would the Theoretical Genetic Engineering Approach to Create a Radiation-Resistant Human Be?

If the safety and efficacy of genetic engineering of radiation-resistant rodents and non-human primates becomes a reality, there will be initial examples of genetic engineering to correct human diseases. If there are data to support a successful experiment in which human embryos have been created which contain new genes for resistance to pandemic viral pathogens, such as which produced COVID-19, and this experiment was to be carried out at a time when a new pandemic of a viral disease is a reality, and if such successful generation of a cohort of humans that are resistant to this pandemic virus and other similar viruses and live normal lives, no untoward effects, then these data can be used to support techniques for genetic engineering of radioresistant humans.

All of this theoretical mental exercise will be unnecessary, if those astronauts returning from prolonged space missions show capacity to adapt to space irradiation and once return to Earth show no deleterious effects of the prolonged exposure to space irradiation. Then, the necessary experiments regarding safety and efficacy of genetic engineering of a class of astronauts will be unnecessary.

Theoretical Requirements for Safety and Efficacy of Genetic Engineering of Radioresistant Humans

What would such experimental data look like? The most important considerations for safety and efficacy will involve dose response curves of inserting genes or duplicated genes into human embryos. Current research has demonstrated that genetic defects, which occur spontaneously including chromosome duplications, chromosome deletions, and other imbalances that occur during fertilization, zygote formation, embryo implantation, and development, usually will lead to spontaneous death of the embryo. Those individuals, who are born with a genetic defect, such as Trisomy 21, X0 (Turner's syndrome), or triple X chromosome (Klinefelter's syndrome) should display phenotypic differences from fertilized normal human birth. Genetically engineered embryos will have to show evidence of deleterious chromosome duplication or loss and absence of deleterious phenotypic changes in the surviving children. This will be a component of safety.

Efficacy will probably follow current policies and practice for in vitro fertilization. Efficient in vitro fertilization is that which leads to the generation of viable embryos. The percentage of embryos that will successfully implant will lead to a viable fetus and normal birth is not 100%. Implantation of multiple embryos that are the result of in vitro fertilization may lead to a non-viable fetus and spontaneous abortion, or the other extreme multiple live births. Genetically engineered humans that are radioresistant will be the subject of efficacy studies that follow successful gene insertion or duplication.

Genetic Engineering is a term that defines a process by which to change the genome of an organisms. This is the most complete way to correct or change an organism [4]. The assumption is that the change will be either permanent or inducible by applying a drug or molecule that induces the change and that it will be stable and passed on to future generations by the germ cell. It is also the most difficult task to achieve. However, this process has been achieved in mice with deleted genes that breed true (or added genes that breed true (MnSOD transgenic mice) [13]. There are conditional deleted (knockout) genes as in the Cre/Flox [13] mice and conditional knockout mice, as well [13]. But to be a genetic engineering result, the genetic change must be permanent. This goal would be difficult to achieve to produce a radioresistant human.

Inserting or amplifying the levels of expression of DNA repair genes or knocking out a gene that blocked DNA repair is not the only way to increase radioresistance to ionizing irradiation. There are more ways to facilitate a genetic approach adaptation to the ionizing irradiation of space travel, including inhibiting that damage that would be sustained by periodic sporadic and unpredictable exposure to each of the several forms of irradiation that would be experienced by astronauts. These forms of irradiation include (1) gamma radiation of varying dose rates and energies; (2) solar proton events; (3) galactic cosmic irradiation (GCR), which is also termed high LET (linear energy transfer) irradiation [24]. High LET irradiation includes that delivered by charged particles and (4) neutrons that would be created by the high LET particles (ions) hitting the materials in space vehicle and the Martian habitat. The charged particles from GCR include ions of silicon, iron, and other elements [24] that are expelled into space by supernovae (the death of distant stars). The neutron irradiation is not trivial and would be generated by GCR hitting the spacecraft, spacesuits, and other materials in the space vehicle, as well as those generated by GCR hitting the Martian surface habitat would contribute to the cellular, tissue, and organ damage experienced by the astronauts. How can one possibly use genetic engineering to make humans resistant to all these forms of radiation?

There are multiple ways to develop a way to apply genetic engineering techniques for radiation protection/mitigation other than that directly targeting the cellular DNA repair mechanisms (Table 12.1). There are considerations other than actual alteration of radiation repair genes and radiation resistance genes that were discussed in the previous chapter.

Methods for facilitating adaptation of experimental animals to ionizing irradiation include focus on epigenetic [36, 37], as well as genetic changes. The concept of epigenetic modulation is relatively new in molecular biology, as applied to

Table 12.1 Target of genetic engineering of an organism to resist radiation damage

Pathway	Success of experiment	Problem for a complex
DNA strand break repair	Deinococcus radiodurans	Multicellular organism with multiple physiologic pathways and multiple organ systems All cells could not be expected to express the amplified genes consistently
Epigenetic gene activation	Transgenic mouse with active methylation or acetylation gene	Impractical
Epigenetic gene inactivation	Transgenic animal with deleting methylation gene	Impractical
Inflammatory response to radiation	TGF-B−/− mice, IL-1−/− mice	Pleotropic effects of this approach prevent "normal" response to other conditions

experimental animal system and also eventually in humans [36]. Targeting epigenetic mechanisms of gene regulation to increase irradiation resistance is an attractive and testable mechanism. Targets for radiation mitigation/protection would first consider the epigenetic mechanisms of methylation and/or demethylation of genes that would likely be altered by each form of ionizing irradiation [36]. Acetylation on genes is another biochemical strategy for gene regulation [36]. Epigenetic regulation is based on the knowledge that genes are transcribed into RNA and then translated into proteins at specific times in the cell cycle. A target for epigenetic change of the DNA for a particular gene that is exposed (made available) to the enzymes, would then facilitate transcription.

The "S" phase on the cell cycle is where DNA is exposed, where RNA polymerases bind to the promoters of these genes, and where the transcription occurs. The "S" phase is also the place, where cell doubling is initiated, so there is a dynamic of the reproduction copying of each gene expression. Epigenetic modulation to facilitate radiation protection/mitigation would involve using the methylation of a specific gene promoter to either prevent RNA polymerase for an inhibitory gene from binding and thus prevent transcription or preventing methylation of that gene to increase its transcription. This epigenetic modulation could also remove the methylation for specific gene promoters to allow undisturbed RNA polymerase binding and the transcription of that gene. The strategy of epigenetic modulation assumes that the new transcripts or blocked transcripts will be either translated into proteins in adequate amounts to "make a difference" with respect to neutralizing or blocking radiation damage to those cells or blocking the translation of inhibitory proteins. Thus, there are two ways to use epigenetics to provide such resistance to cell damage by irradiation induce more resistance genes or block the expression genes that initiate cell death pathways. At present, this approach is theoretical due to the promiscuous pathways of methylation and acetylation. The gene of interest would not be a specific target.

The previous chapter described the genetic engineering techniques and targets for directly modifying the mammalian cellular genome to provide a better response of cells, tissues, organs, and organ systems to fix the DNA damage caused by ionizing irradiation. The previous chapter also focused on the direct effects of radiation on cells including DNA double-strand breaks and induction of the genes that are involved in cell death pathways. There are other indirect ways by which to use genetic engineering to provide radiation resistance. The concept of "indirect" genetic engineering would also be a way to increase survival of irradiated animals, but to do so by focus on modifying the damage response to radiation-induced DNA damage (Fig. 12.1). This approach would target genetic pathways separate from direct DNA strand breaks and their repairs.

There are three potential systematic ways to use genetic engineering to achieve indirect protection/mitigation of radiation damage: (1) modification of the inflammatory response to ionizing irradiation; (2) preventing new induced irradiation-induced epigenetic changes; and (3) targeting "master regulator genes" including genes for specific tyrosine kinase signaling molecule that then induce a cascade of effects that activate a continuous damage response to irradiation, which is deleterious to the organism [31, 32]. The third category of targets would be analogous to an activated fire alarm that could not be switched off and which kept a siren blaring day and night with no respite. The challenge of identifying a master regulator gene for the radiation response is great. Even greater is determining how to silence this pathway to facilitate radiation resistance. Finally, the third challenge is to determine the safety of such a target. Would shutting of the fire alarm also shut off all electricity and prevent temperature control.

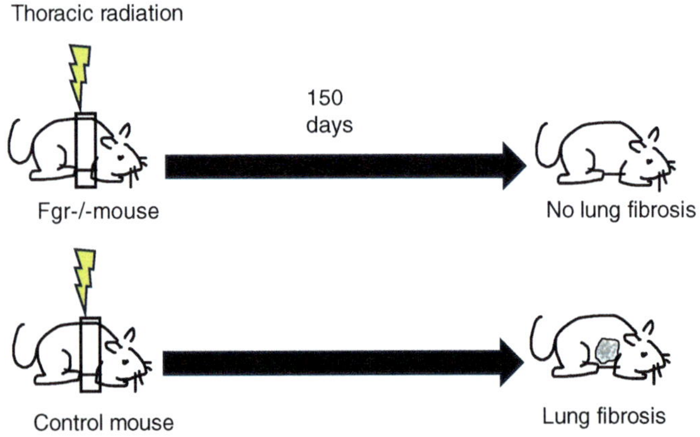

Fig. 12.1 Genetic alteration that produces radiation resistance. An example of genetic alteration, which profoundly influences radiation resistance is that of the deletion of the tyrosine kinase, Fgr. As shown in the top panel, thoracic irradiation of mice that are deleted by homologous recombination deletion (knockout) for Fgr and who receive thoracic irradiation (note the block placed over the radiation device, which prevents radiation to the lower body), develop a markedly reduced or absence of late effects at 150 days later. These animals have no lung fibrosis. In contrast, in the bottom panel, wild type mice that are controls receiving the same irradiation will develop lung fibrosis at around 150 days. The mechanism of this lack of fibrosis by Fgr deletion is the subject of intense investigation [31, 32]

Genetic Engineering to Modify the Inflammatory Response

It is well known that the response to an injury, in some cases, can be worse than the injury itself. One example is the inflammatory response that follows the infection by the virus that causes rabies [30]. The inflammatory response to the virus is associated with severe neurological responses that can cause death [30]. The virus enters the victim's nervous system usually from a bite wound. The saliva of an infected animal contains the virus, and after a bite, the virus targets the sensory nerves (afferent nerves). By tracking through these afferent nerves of the peripheral nervous system, the virus reaches the central nervous system (spinal cord and brain), where a severe inflammatory reaction to the virus is generated. The inflammation involves both humoral (cytokine levels elevation) and cellular (lymphocytes, monocytes, neutrophils) expansion, and their secondary release of more cytokines. The cytokines induce brain swelling, vascular permeability, and associated symptoms of seizures and sensory/motor effects. The afferent nerves (sensory nerves coming from the point of the virus entry to the central nervous system) start the process, which can take days to reach the brain and then produce infection of the motor nerves (efferent nerves) with other neurological effects (from the central nervous system out to the periphery). The efferent nerve produces the muscle spasms that cause difficulty swallowing and produce the term "hydrophobia" or an aversion to water or anything that might be swallowed [30].

In severe cases of rabies, and under situations where the inflammatory response to the virus cannot be lessened in time by starting vaccination with rabies antiserum in a series of injections to neutralize the virus proliferation, some patients have presented with uncontrollable and thus unmanageable seizures. Some of these patients have been placed into a medical coma by administering drugs that produce deep anesthesia. The seizure activity is quieted and allows the body's cellular and humoral immune response to neutralize the virus without the serious effects of the cytokine storm that caused the seizures. The coma condition prevents the neurological complications of seizures and other muscle spasms rather than eliminating the virus itself. Thus, inflammation is the cause of death not the virus. With ionizing irradiation, particularly, partial body irradiation, the bone marrow-derived inflammatory cells migrate via the circulation into the irradiated area to cause swelling and release of cytokines that can further damage tissues. That is why corticosteroids are used to decrease radiation pneumonitis (inflammation of the lung) [28].

There are other situations in which the response of the virus or infectious agent can be worse than the infection itself, as was seen in the first COVID-19 patients, who required respirator care for their lung swelling [28].

A similar indirect inflammatory response occurs with exposure to ionizing irradiation. At the cellular level in experimental systems with cells in culture, the radiation-induced nuclear DNA double-strand breaks occur, but are repaired within minutes after the irradiation beam is turned off [5]. However, signals from the cell nucleus, where the DNA double-strand breaks occurred, are transmitted to the mitochondria in the cellular cytoplasm. There may be hundreds or thousands of mitochondria in any single cell [7]. Mitochondria are the engines for oxidative metabolism and are found in all oxygen consuming cells.

In the mitochondria, which sit in the cytoplasm, the signals from the nucleus, where the DNA double-strand breaks occurred, may have already been repaired, reach the mitochondria, and activate a cascade of effects starting in the outer mitochondrial membrane and lead to changes in the inner mitochondrial membrane, and in the membrane bound molecules call complexes of the electron transport chain to oxidize the lipids in the membrane and cause membrane permeability [6, 7]. These oxidized lipids allow the release into the cytoplasm of enzymes such as cytochrome C, which then activate other components of a cascade of events in pathways, such as apoptosis, that induce cell death [6, 7]. The actual irradiation-induced original injury in the nucleus, which is rapidly repaired by the DNA repair enzymes starts a death process that is outside the nucleus. The cytoplasmic events in mitochondria have been termed the result of the "horse is out of the barn" and cannot be recalled [7]. Once the signaling from nuclear DNA damage has been communicated to the mitochondria, any effort to block cell death should be directed to mitochondria, not the nucleus. Therefore, recent approaches toward preventing irradiation-induced cell death have appropriately targeted the mitochondria [8]. One strategy for genetic engineering of mitochondrial targets is based upon data with mitochondrial-targeted drugs.

Delivering antioxidant molecules to mitochondrial membrane to stop the membrane lipid oxidation. One strategy for targeting an antioxidant drug to the mitochondrial membrane was realized by using the molecular structure of triphenylphosphonium, attached to the antioxidant tempol [8]. In another strategy, the tempol was attached to a component of the hemigramicidin antibiotic, which also targets the mitochondrial membrane [18, 19]. This mitochondrial targeting approach concentrated antioxidant drugs to the mitochondrial membrane by up to 600-fold [6]. This strategy was also an approach to limit irradiation-induced secondary effects from transport of signals from nucleus to the mitochondria at the single-cell level. To change a gene or genes to achieve this goal without the use of drugs, one must identify a critical gene that induces cell death that follows oxidative stress. Theoretically, the mitochondrial genome (32 genes) could be genetically engineered to control antioxidant levels in the mitochondria and prevent oxidation of the mitochondrial membrane [7].

With respect to irradiation that is specific such as head and neck irradiation, genetic engineering might produce protection and/or mitigation of radiation injury. Irradiation, which can produce severe oral cavity and oropharyngeal inflammation mucositis, can be mitigated by the delivery of antioxidant and mitochondrial stabilizing drugs into the oral cavity [11, 18, 19]. An organ-specific way to prevent secondary radiation effects could be expanded to the whole body. Mitochondrial targeting also prevents death of mucosal stem cells and allows the organ to repair [11, 18, 19]. At the systemic level, the inflammatory response is broader and can be a significant cause of multiple systems morbidity and death. The MnSOD transgenic mice are an example of how this could work [2].

Total body irradiation is associated with not only DNA double-strand breaks in many cells, tissues, and organs, but also the induction of the release of cytokines from the irradiated tissues including cells that are repairing radiation damage and will not die. These cells release cytokines including interleukin 1, tumor necrosis factor-alpha, tumor growth factor-beta, and many others [18–20]. Within minutes of irradiation, the transcription of genes for inflammatory cytokines is elevated and within hours plasma levels of inflammatory cytokines are increased. Inflammatory cytokines are also chemokines and recruit inflammatory cells. In the case of targeted irradiation or subtotal body irradiation, inflammatory cells leave the bone marrow in unshielded/unirradiated areas and migrate through the plasma/circulation to sites of irradiation. With total body irradiation exposure, there is no "sacrosanct" (unirradiated) area from which to recruit bone marrow cells and thus the entire system is in a crisis mode with inflammatory cytokines mobilizing cells from the marrow, lymph nodes, spleen, and integrating migration to sites of injury.

With total body irradiation, all bone marrow cell containing areas are injured and the trafficking of inflammatory cells is not focused on a specific area. The storm of cytokines that follows irradiation and the associated recruitment of the migration of inflammatory cells that release secondary cytokines and cause further injury is occurring everywhere after total body irradiation (TBI) (Table 12.1).

Irradiation inflammation exacerbates the initial radiation damage response. There are time-based syndromes of the response of animals and humans to TBI. One phenomenon leading to rapid organ system failure occurs in the intestine and is called the gastrointestinal (GI) syndrome [22]. Another, more delayed failure after TBI occurs with the blood-forming organs, which involves the bone marrow and is termed the hematopoietic syndrome [22]. The mechanism of both the acute GI syndrome and the acute hematopoietic syndrome and gastrointestinal syndrome involves death of stem cells for each organ system. The released inflammatory cytokines from each organ will induce damage in the other. Both the severity of each syndrome are worsened by the total volume of radiation exposure and the radiation dose. The quality of irradiation (gamma rays, protons, GCR, neutrons, or mixed beam) and the dose rate of exposure are also directly related to the severity of each syndrome.

How can one use genetic engineering to limit a response to total body irradiation? Animals that lack the gene for a specific inflammatory cytokine or a master regulator to turn on cytokine genes have been shown to tolerate larger doses of total body irradiation [31, 32]. The tolerance is related to the absence of an inflammatory cytokine can be confirmed by giving utilizing antibodies to specific cytokines. Genetically engineering animals to produce a specific cytokine have been carried out in model systems, and these animals are also radiation-resistant (Fig. 12.1). Is this approach any more practical than the one described in the previous chapter in which DNA repair genes are amplified or restored?

Genetic engineering of inflammatory cytokines, either shutting off their response to irradiation, or limiting production of gene products has the potential complication of secondary induction of other compensatory mechanisms. For example, experimental animal is genetically engineered to produce TGF-β, other inflammatory cytokines may be upregulated, and the overall inflammatory response can be the same or even more severe [33].

Genetic engineering that can be used to alter the immune response is a strategy, but a more feasible approach would be to neutralize the products of the inflammatory response genes themselves (Fig. 12.1). The basis for anti-inflammatory drugs to dampen the effects of the induced gene product responses was first established with the use of corticosteroids [28]. Delivering steroids after total body irradiation or hemi-body irradiation in the case of thoracic or lung irradiation was shown to blunt the inflammatory response [29]. In addition to causing lysis of inflammatory T lymphocytes and B lymphocytes and reducing levels of inflammatory cell migration, steroids have been shown to lessen radiation-induced permeability of blood vessels, decrease tissue swelling, and limit cell death [22]. However, a problem with steroid administration has been a phenomenon of "rebound" also seen in steroid responses in other diseases [29].

Whole-brain irradiation in clinical radiotherapy is associated with normal tissue swelling. Patients, who are likely to develop seizures from the tissue swelling can be treated with steroids, but when the level of steroids is tapered, the patients develop a rebound phenomenon in which the original tissue swelling comes back [29]. This rebound has also been observed with radiation pneumonitis or lung inflammation that can be decreased by the administration of steroids, but the rebound effect is also detectable. Would this apply to the various forms of irradiation obtained during space travel? Limited experience with large volume proton irradiation in clinical radiotherapy has also been shown to produce inflammatory responses similar to that with gamma rays/X-rays. Thus, the same genetic engineering approaches or drug neutralization approach to limit the inflammatory response would likely be applicable to proton irradiation from SPEs. There is little information on the effect of genetically engineering the inflammatory response or using anti-inflammatory drugs with respect to high LET-charged particle irradiation, typical of GCR [24]. Limited information is also available on neutron-induced cell damage, leading to an inflammatory response.

Radiation causes direct cell death, but injured and potentially recovering cells release inflammatory cytokines including chemokines that recruit inflammatory cells to the site of irradiation, and these inflammatory cells release cytokines that produce further damage. Thus, all forms of irradiation would be expected to induce an inflammatory response that could be lessened by genetically engineering a decrease in production of inflammatory cytokines, or by giving neutralizing antibodies. How these principles would apply to continuous low-dose irradiation, mixed-beam irradiation from multiple sources of irradiation, and the accumulated dose of irradiation from a 180-day cruise exposure from a trip to Mars, 500 days on the Martian surface, and another 180 days for return is unknown [24].

Preventing by Genetic Engineering Other Irradiation-Induced Epigenetic Deleterious Methylation and Demethylation of Other Genes and Pathways

Basic biology textbooks refer to the lack of evidence for the inheritance of acquired characteristics. The inheritance of acquired characteristics was proposed in the century by the biologist Lamarck. Lamarckian biology, which was described centuries ago, has been dispelled as wrong, the theory suggested that characteristics acquired during one generation could be transferred by inheritance to subsequent generations. The Lamarckian biology was discarded. A classic example was circumcision of male infants by some cultures for millennia, which never leads to the absence of the foreskin on newborn male infants of subsequent generations [38].

However, now generations later, the phenomenon of epigenetic alterations leading to transfer of altered characteristics to the progeny of animals with epigenetic alteration has been documented to occur [38] in cancer-prone mouse strains showing then progeny of epigenetic-altered animals have the inherited characteristic of proneness to that same cancer [39]. The experimental result brings back a consideration of this phenomenon of inheritance of acquired characteristics. Is this the creation of a mouse with and epigenetic change, so is this an inherited acquired characteristic?

Genes are regulated binding of promotors to sequences in the gene, in specific chromosomal locations, leading to transcription of mRNA. RNA sequences in a single site can lead to production of a small protein by translation. Splicing of RNA from different sites on different chromosomes was demonstrated in the 1970s [40, 41] and sections of DNA transcribed from different sites on different chromosomes can be assembled and attached together to produce a mRNA that leads to translation of a protein. An initial step on promoter binding to the initiation sites of transcription of a gene is the basis for gene activation. Promoter binding to a particular gene activates transcription and then RNA goes onto translation and production of the gene product.

The phenomenon of epigenetic regulation of gene activation is a recently described phenomenon that relates to potential for genetic engineering of the pushing or silencing of gene transcription [36]. Epigenetic modulation of gene transcription follows a principle of availability of the DNA to RNA polymerases that initiate transcription. Methylation of DNA shows the structure of the DNA so that the polymerases cannot bind and initiate the transcription. There are examples of both hypermethylation and hypomethylation that can alter DNA transcription. The methylase or enzymes that methylate DNA provide a target for regulation of gene activation and essentially a second method by which to genetically engineer response to a physical agent or infectious agent including ionizing irradiation. The unfolding of DNA during the S-phase of the cell cycle makes areas of the DNA in the chromosome available for promoter binding and thus initiation of transcription. If these unfolded and exposed and available sections of DNA are methylated in areas, where the promoter would bind to initiate transcription, then that particular gene will not produce RNA and will not produce protein. Recent evidence that an epigenetic change can be induced in one generation of mice and essentially inherited in a second generation was a groundbreaking discovery [39]. Inheritance of targeted methylation or demethylation could be genetically engineered to produce alteration of specific genes, but can it be targeted to select genes? The CRISPR/CAS-9 method may facilitate this [4]. Thus, it is possible to genetically engineer a mouse strain to be sensitive to irradiation by blocking transcription of genes for antioxidants or DNA repair enzymes. It is also possible to use epigenetic modification to accelerate production of anti-inflammatory mediators that would counteract the induction of inflammatory mediators. Experiments in this area are being carried out and provide a secondary approach to using genetic engineering to modify the radiation response.

Targeting by Genetic Engineering a Master Gene Regulator of the Radiation Response

Is there a master regulator of radiation damage such that its modification would lead to radiation protection/mitigation at all levels? The identification of such a master regulator gene would provide a target for solving all the problems of radiation exposure. There are candidate genes that are being studied. One such gene is that for the tyrosine kinase Fgr (Table 12.1) [31, 32]. A tyrosine kinase is an enzyme that adds a phosphate group to the amino acid tyrosine on specific proteins. The Fgr kinase is specific and separate from many other protein kinases. Recent data presented suggest that Fgr could be a master regulator of irradiation damage [32]. Furthermore, Fgr may be a regulator of both acute and chronic/delayed radiation injury. With respect to acute injury, mice lacking Fgr are radiation resistant [31, 32]. These same mice do not develop late radiation-induced lung fibrosis [31, 32]. The late injury may also be inflammatory and the mechanism of this master regulator Fgr may be also based upon its anti-inflammatory actions (Fig. 12.1; Table 12.1).

A master regulator must work through modulation of the known pathways of the effect being regulated. The proven effect of an abundance of antioxidants or DNA repair enzymes, to confer radioresistance on cells in animals, demonstrates that overabundance of specific gene products can be helpful in neutralizing the effects of ionizing irradiation. These experiments relate to the genetically altered mouse strains that can overproduce the antioxidant manganese superoxide dismutase (MnSOD), copper/zinc superoxide dismutase (Cu/ZnSOD), catalase, or peroxidase [5]. Animals that overproduce these antioxidant enzymes are resistant to ionizing irradiation. Is this a form of genetic engineering? These inbred mouse strains pass on the overproduction of the radioprotective enzymes from one generation to another.

Compensatory downregulation of other radiation resistance-inducing gene products can occur, and thus, animals might show no detectable radioresistance. How to modulate this form of overproduction of radioprotective genes without inducing a compensation mechanism is a challenge.

At present, we are far from being able to duplicate an experimental animal for the selection of a radioresistant animal, such as Deinococcus radiodurans [35]. In the example of natural selection, which occurred in continuous irradiation of meat products and the generation of a Deinococcus variant that had amplification of multiple copies of DNA repair and antioxidant genes, the natural selection process took many generations, and the replication of bacteria with a 4-h cycle provided opportunity to select such a variant. With more complex animal models, such a program of natural selection to produce radioresistant organisms would be impractical. However, there is evidence of a first step *C. elegans* flatworms can become radioresistant if grown in any antibiotic culture [21]. The antioxidant facilitates radioresistance. Discovery of which genes were modified and how to target that with epigenetics could now follow.

Thus, the strategy of genetic engineering to essentially reproduce an artificial "end-game of natural selection" has been one theoretical strategy to produce radioresistance by introducing a new gene or neutralizing an overactive inflammatory response gene. These techniques are theoretical and research in this area continues [39–41].

References

1. Dahlstrom E, Pozza MA. New risks of future lunar landings. In: Pozza MA, Dennerley JA, editors. Risk management in outer space activities. Springer Nature; 2022. p. 221–39.
2. Mazzucato M, Robinson DKR. Co-creating and directing innovation ecosystems? NASA's changing approach to public-private partnerships in low-earth orbit. Technol Forecast Soc Chang. 2018;136:166–77.
3. Witze A. NASA's Artemis moon mission is set to launch: here's the science on board. Nature. 2022; https://doi.org/10.1038/d41586-022-02293-8.
4. Asmamaw M, Zawdie B. Mechanism and applications of CRISPR/Cas-9-mediated genome editing. Biologics. 2021;15:353–61. https://doi.org/10.2147/BTT.S326422.
5. Epperly MW, Bray JA, Kraeger S, et al. Prevention of late effects of irradiation lung damage by manganese superoxide dismutase gene therapy. Gene Ther. 1998;5(2):196–208. https://doi.org/10.1038/sj.gt.3300580.
6. Kagan VE, Wipf P, Stoyanovsky D, et al. Mitochondrial targeting of electron scavenging antioxidants: regulation of selective oxidation vs random chain reactions. Adv Drug Deliv Rev. 2009;61(14):1375–85. https://doi.org/10.1016/j.addr.2009.06.008.
7. Kagan VE, Bayir HA, Belikova NA, et al. Cytochrome c/cardiolipin relations in mitochondria: a kiss of death. Free Radic Biol Med. 2009;46(11):1439–53. https://doi.org/10.1016/j.freeradbiomed.2009.03.004.
8. Stoyanovsky DA, Huang Z, Jiang J, et al. A manganese-porphyrin complex decomposes H(2)O(2), inhibits apoptosis, and acts as a radiation mitigator in vivo. ACS Med Chem Lett. 2011;2(11):814–7. https://doi.org/10.1021/ml200142x.
9. Epperly MW, Gretton JE, Bernarding M, et al. Mitochondrial localization of copper/zinc superoxide dismutase (Cu/ZnSOD) confers radioprotective functions in vitro and in vivo. Radiat Res. 2003;160:568–78.

10. Epperly MW, Sikora C, Defilippi S, et al. Manganese superoxide dismutase (SOD2) inhibits radiation-induced apoptosis by stabilization of the mitochondrial membrane. Radiat Res. 2002;157(5):568–77. https://doi.org/10.1667/0033-7587(2002)157[0568:msdsir]2.0.co;2.
11. Willis J, Epperly MW, Fisher R, et al. Amelioration of head and neck irradiation-induced mucositis and distant marrow suppression in Fanca−/− and Fancg−/− mice by intraoral administration of GS-nitroxide (JP4-039). Radiat Res. 2018;189(6):560–78. https://doi.org/10.1667/RR14878.1.
12. Epperly MW, Travis EL, Whitsett JA, et al. Overexpression of manganese superoxide dismutase (MnSOD) in whole lung or alveolar type II (AT-II) cells of MnSOD transgenic mice does not provide intrinsic lung irradiation protection. Int J Cancer. 2001;96(1):11–21. https://doi.org/10.1002/1097-0215(20010220)96:1<11::aid-ijc2>3.0.co;2-r.
13. Rhieu GH, Shinde A, Epperly MW, et al. Organ-specific responses of total body irradiated doxycycline-inducible manganese superoxide dismutase Tet/Tet mice. In Vivo. 2014;28(6):1033–43.
14. Stoyanovsky DA, Vlasova II, Belikova NA, et al. Targeting and activation of NO donors in mitochondria. Peroxidase metabolism of (2-hydroxyamino-vinyl)-triphenyl-phosphonium by cytochrome c releases NO and protects cells from apoptosis. FEBJ Lett. 2009;583:2000–5.
15. Epperly MW, Sacher JR, Krainz T, et al. Effectiveness of analogues of the GS-nitroxide, JP4-039, as total body radiation mitigators. In Vivo. 2017;31(1):39–43. https://doi.org/10.21873/invivo.11022.
16. Tyurina YY, Tyurin VA, Epperly MW, et al. Oxidative lipidomics of γ-irradiation induced intestinal injury. Free Radic Biol Med. 2008;44:299–314.
17. Tao M, You C-P, Zhao R-R, et al. Animal mitochondria: evolution, function, and disease. Curr Mol Med. 2014;14(1):115–24. https://doi.org/10.2174/15665240113136660081.
18. Berhane H, Shinde A, Kalash R, et al. Amelioration of irradiation induced oral cavity mucositis and distant bone marrow suppression in Fancd2—(FVB/N) mice by intraoral JP4-039/F15. Radiat Res. 2014;182(1):35–49. https://doi.org/10.1667/RR13633.1.
19. Shinde A, Berhane H, Rhieu BH, et al. Intraoral mitochondrial-targeted GS-nitroxide, JP4-039, radioprotects normal tissue in tumor-bearing radiosensitive Fancd2−/− (C57BL/6) mice. Radiat Res. 2016;185(2):134–50. https://doi.org/10.1667/RR14035.1.
20. Rajagopalan MS, Gupta K, Epperly MW, et al. The mitochondria-targeted nitroxide JP4-039 augments potentially lethal irradiation damage repair. In Vivo. 2009;23(5):717–26.
21. Melov S, Ravenscroft J, Malik S, et al. Extension of life-span with superoxide dismutase/catalase mimetics. Science. 2000;289(5484):1567–9. https://doi.org/10.1126/science.289.5484.1567.
22. Prasad KN. Chapter 19. Acute radiation syndromes. In: Pizzarello D, editor. Radiation biology. 1st ed. Boca Raton, FL: CRC Press; 2020.
23. Epperly MW, Sikora CA, Defilippi S, et al. Bone marrow origin of myofibroblasts in irradiation pulmonary fibrosis. Am J Respir Cell Mol Biol. 2003;29(2):213–24. https://doi.org/10.1165/rcmb.2002-0069OC.
24. Durante M, Cucinotta FA. Heavy ion carcinogenesis and human space exploration. Nat Rev Cancer. 2008;8(6):465–72. https://doi.org/10.1038/nrc2391.
25. Cohen S, Janicki-Deverts D, Doyle WJ, et al. Chronic stress, glucocorticoid receptor resistance, inflammation, and disease risk. Proc Natl Acad Sci USA. 2012;109(16):5995–9. https://doi.org/10.1073/pnas.1118355109.
26. Badhwar GD, O'Neill PM. Galactic cosmic radiation model and its applications. Adv Space Res. 1996;17(2):7–17. https://doi.org/10.1016/0273-1177(95)00507-b.
27. Friedel RH, Wurst W, Wefers B, et al. Generating conditional knockout mice. Methods Mol Biol. 2011;693:205–31. https://doi.org/10.1007/978-1-60761-974-1_12.
28. Imai R, Ro S, Tomishima Y, et al. Steroid resistance and rebound phenomena in patients with COVID-19. Respir Investig. 2021;59(5):608–13. https://doi.org/10.1016/j.resinv.2021.05.007.
29. Long V, Yew YW, Chandran NS, et al. Psoriasis flares and rebound phenomenon following exposure and withdrawal of systemic steroids: a systematic review and meta-analysis. J Am Acad Dermatol. 2022;87(3):660–1. https://doi.org/10.1016/j.jaad.2022.01.006.

30. Bastos V, Pacheco V, Rodrigues EDL, et al. Neuroimmunology of rabies: new insights into an ancient disease. J Med Virol. 2023;95(10):e29042. https://doi.org/10.1002/jmv.29042.
31. Mukherjee A, Epperly M, Shields D, et al. Ionizing irradiation induced Fgr in senescent cells mediates fibrosis. Cell Death Discov. 2021;7(1):349. https://doi.org/10.1038/s41420-021-00741-4.
32. Mukherjee A, Epperly MW, Fisher R, et al. Inhibition of tyrosine kinase Fgr prevents radiation-induced pulmonary fibrosis (RIPF). Cell Death Discov. 2023;9(1):252. https://doi.org/10.1038/s41420-023-01538-3.
33. Galbreath E. Overexpression of TGF-β1 in the central nervous system of transgenic mice results in hydrocephalus. J Neuropatholo Exp Neurol. 1995;54(3):339–49.
34. Mukherjee A, Epperly MW, Fisher R, et al. Silica induced lung fibrosis is associated with senescence, Fgr, and recruitment of bone marrow monocyte/macrophages. In Vivo. 2021;35(6):3053–66. https://doi.org/10.21873/invivo.12601.
35. Cox MM, Battista JR. Deinococcus radiodurans—the consummate survivor. Nat Rev Microbiol. 2005;3(11):882–92. https://doi.org/10.1038/nrmicro1264.
36. Kane AE, Sinclair DA. Epigenetic changes during aging and their reprogramming potential. Crit Rev Biochem Mol Biol. 2019;54(1):61–83. https://doi.org/10.1080/10409238.2019.1570075.
37. Issa J-P. Age-related epigenetic changes and the immune system. Clin Immunol. 2003;109(1):103–8. https://doi.org/10.1016/s1521-6616(03)00203-1.
38. Martin C, Zhang Y. Mechanisms of epigenetic inheritance. Curr Opin Cell Biol. 2007;19(3):266–72.
39. Lind MI, Spagopoulou F. Evolutionary consequences of epigenetic inheritance. Heredity (Edinb). 2018;121(3):205–9. https://doi.org/10.1038/s41437-018-0113-y.
40. Sharp PA. Split genes and RNA splicing. Cell. 1994;77(6):805–15. https://doi.org/10.1016/0092-8674(94)90130-9.
41. Ghai M, Kader F. A review on epigenetic inheritance of experiences in humans. Biochem Genet. 2022;60(4):1107–40. https://doi.org/10.1007/s10528-021-10155-7.

Chapter 13
Cryopreservation for Long-Term Space Flight

The moon is a relatively close target for space travel. As of January 2024, there have been 5 moon landings from 5 countries (USA, USSR, China, India, and Japan) for space vehicles delivered equipment. The last U.S. mission was completed in 1972 (Apollo, 1972). The India mission was India (Chandra year-3); Japan (SLIM lander). However, there are other failed missions: USSR (Luna 5) crashed, Israel: Con Space II, 2019 failed; NASA/Astrobotic—Peregrine lander (failed). The recent Peregrine crash was the first NASA/Private company attempted collaboration. The India mission was directed to the South Pole of the Moon in search of a source of water/ice. The private company with NASA plans collaborative missions Houston-Based Intuitive Machines. These are all attempts at contracted moon landings.

Now, fast forward to the future. How can we plan for astronaut travel to locations that are light years away. Given the life span of humans, it is not possible for the same humans, who departed from Earth to arrive at a location 100 light years away or even to a location 100 years away. We do not have Star-Trek type "warp" space drive nor do we have the ability to travel the distance that light travels in 1 year = 5.87863×10^{12} miles or 9.46073×10^{12} km, let alone 100 light years away.

For space travel trips of this magnitude of light years distance and longer duration, the current astronauts must either be genetically engineered to have greatly increased lifespan or be cryopreserved to allow them to have viability once the journey is complete. This later strategy would account for human limited lifespan. Yet another strategy is to plan to have generations of humans, bred, and educated on route to the target.

An incremented approach to deal with a huge challenge is clearly prudent. First for travel to Mars, travel time 180 days, then to the Moon of Jupiter, Europa [1–3], travel time Galileo October 18, 1989, to December 23, 1995, satellite data. Six-eight 1/2 years travel time for the mission: 6 years travel to Jupiter, and two-and-a-half years to orbit Europa [3]. This time frame is possible for astronauts, who leave Earth when in their 20 s or 30 s.

J. Greenberger, *Radiation Oncology and Radiation Biology*,
https://doi.org/10.1007/978-3-031-66300-0_13

A discussion of space flight for the anticipated trip to Mars (over one-year duration) and the trip to Europa (12+ years) is possible without discussing cryopreservation of astronauts. However, subsequent trips outside the solar system (many more years or decades duration) must take into account the fact of human aging and human lifespan.

Cryopreservation has already been established for single cells [4–23], but not for tissues or organs. Simple organisms have been cryopreserved [24, 25]. The current knowledge is that the galactic cosmic irradiation, which reaches our lunar surface and which reaches the Martian surface at any given instant, represents energy and particles arriving at that moment from supernovae, which occurred hundreds of years previously [26]. This radiation of space travel will affect frozen cells and organisms [27]. The GCR radiation at the time that it reaches a lunar or Martian habitat, or the space vehicle that is transporting the astronauts to these sites represents a supernovas event, which is long gone. The light from that event traveling at the speed of light arrives later. This concept is one with which astrophysicists and astronomers may be comfortable, but may be a concept, which for many biologists is unfathomable. Travel beyond light speed is also theoretical at present, but may soon be possible [28, 29]. If travel speeds are increased, then cryopreservation of astronauts may not be necessary; however, it is a valuable discussion at present.

The supernova represents the death of a star, which was similar to our sun, but for a distant solar system that death of that star occurred in an instant, but led to transmission of charged high molecular weight (high LET) atoms across vast expanses of space. Traveling at the speed of light for years (light years), these solar particles include the high LET (linear energy transfer) ions composing galactic cosmic irradiation (GCR). Cryopreserved astronauts will be irradiated and will have biologic effects as do frozen single cells [27].

The number of supernovae has been estimated to be thousands per year [26] and the number whose GCR products reach the astronauts at any one time may represent the particle records of events that occurred hundreds of light years away. The particles that hit the spacecraft or habitat are those relevant to the time of arrival at any one time.

The Curiosity Rover experiments [25] recorded radiation events that were experienced by the spacecraft delivering the Martian rover to the Martian surface. Those events occurring on the Martian's surface provided the data by which a calculation was made as to the cumulative radiation exposure that would be experienced by astronauts during the planned Martian mission. The current calculations for the Martian mission relate to plans for approximately 180 days travel of the spacecraft to Mars and 180 days return trip (Table 13.1). The mission plan includes an estimated 500 days on the Martian surface, which would be a total of 850 days [30] (Table 13.2). That time of 850 days, while still a challenge for physicians and radiation biologists to plan for radiation shielding and for administration of medical and, perhaps, dietary radiation countermeasures is still a manageable timeframe.

The Mars Mission of 850 days is not shocking given the scope of current concepts of time for human aging. The mission appears to be feasible. However, the concept of a space mission for travel to Europa (the Moon of Jupiter) 12+ years,

Table 13.1 Challenges to radioprotection of mammalian frozen cells, tissues, organs, and organ systems

Human	Organisms
Cryopreserved sample (DMSO)	**Results of thawing**
Sperm	Success
Oocytes	Success
Fertilized zygote	Success
Hematopoietic stem cells	Success
Mobilized peritoneal blood	Success
Umbilical cord blood	Success
Skin for engraftment	Success
Other organs corneas	In progress
Experimental animal studies	
Mouse kidney	In progress
Liver	In progress
Whole embryo	In progress
Invertebrates	In progress
Radiation biology of cryopreserved cells	Effect of MnSOD overexpression

Table 13.2 Targeted locations for next NASA missions and estimated travel time given currently available vehicles and propulsion systems

Location	Distance from Earth (miles)	Travel times
Moon	238,900 miles	4 days 6 h (based on Apollo missions)
Mars	140 million miles	8–9 months (based on curiosity rover Mission)
Europa	390,400 million miles	5 ½ years (based on voyager 1 and 2, Galileo missions, and planned clipper probe)

Speed of light = 186,282 miles per second
Light year = 5 × 10e12 miles

plus time on the surface, or to a location outside our current solar system is one in which human aging may make such a mission difficult or even impossible unless the aging of the human astronauts can be somehow modulated. This conclusion assumes that travel faster than the speed of light [28, 29] will not be available before a solution to human aging is available.

To approach the modulation of aging for prolonged space travel, there are two new exciting scientific disciplines, both of which are in their infancy. One is the concept of travel beyond light speed. This speed of travel makes it possible to compress the idea of light years to a manageable distance. The other concept is that of using cryopreservation of the astronauts to stop the human biological clock until such time has passed to allow for the travel from the Earth to a target in a distant solar system. These two scientific disciplines are currently both in the realm of theoretical, but neither can we avoid the need to consider the radiation biology involved.

Regarding travel at and beyond the speed of light, there have been scientific papers published estimating the amount of energy that must be consumed to produce a condition in which the conversion of a space vehicle containing human passengers to convert the vehicle and its biological material to energy, then transport that energy to a distant location and then reconstitute that energy back to the materials of the space vehicle, and its occupants, which will be biological material [29]. Teleportation is theoretical, but is one way to potentially travel beyond light years in a time frame that would not consume the life of the astronauts. The other theoretical approach is to utilize the curvature of space, or its recently discovered wormholes and black holes to cut travel time, but all of these ideas are speculative and theoretical.

There also have been theoretical scientific papers published on the amount of energy that would be required for producing travel speed faster than the speed of light. These physical and theoretical areas are in their infancy. No one has addressed the concept of the combined injury, which would follow such an energy delivery system for any novel methodology, when combined with the components of space irradiation. Combining the effect on the human body of such a new theoretical energy for travel beyond light speed with radiation exposure is beyond the scope of even a theoretical treatise at the present time.

However, the other concept of modulation of human aging is a discussion that has already begun, and experiments are focused on safe cryopreservation [31–33]. There are still controversies about ethics of storage [34]. To freeze the aging process, one can speculate a possible pathway for research. The technique of cryopreservation as a method by which to freeze human aging is already being applied with human cells in the disciplines of fertilized ova (embryos) and bone marrow stem cell cryopreservation for marrow transplant. Cryopreservation or other freeze-dry techniques have historically preserved tissue structure, but not life [35–37]. There are successful cryopreservation new experiments in progress [38–42].

Cells, tissue, organs, and whole animals including humans can be frozen to preserve architecture and structure. The discovery of frozen whole animals from thousands of years ago (woolly mammoth [36]), and other preservation techniques have been known to preserve anatomy (mummies) [35], and, of course, formalin fixation for modern pathology, but none can preserve life.

Successful Cryopreservation of Single Cells

There are currently multiple examples of published evidence that cryopreservation of biological materials is a real phenomenon [22]. There are reports of the recovery of frozen microbes from unplanned cryopreservation events. One such example is that of the arctic and Antarctic explorers, whose cryopreserved bodies were found decades after being lost and presumed dead [37]. Recovery of materials at autopsy led to the discovery in human remains of viruses and bacteria [37]. These microbes were recovered from individuals' decades after the freezing process. The discovery of the flu virus from the 1919 epidemic is one example in which the virus was recovered, from a frozen-infected person, then genetically sequenced, and its components compared to more recent epidemic influenza viruses [37]. Even more dramatic was the discovery of cryopreserved plants and animals from Permafrost regions of the arctic [19]. Seeds and spores have been recovered. Paleontologists celebrated the recovery of an intact juvenile mammoth from the permafrost in Russia, which was cryopreserved in excellent condition [36]. The frozen animal was intact for evaluation of organs, organ systems, skin, and hair [36], and the digestive system contents revealed evidence of the dietary component that had been consumed thousands of years ago [36]. These events can be termed accidents of nature. There were no plans for thawing and rejuvenation in these specimens, but their examples provide evidence of the potential feasibility of preserving the anatomy of biological materials for study. It is a very different challenge to plan for freezing and then later thawing by a process to safely reconstitute a viable organism. Organ transplantation is a real phenomenon for fresh tissues [43–47]. Cryopreserved tissue transplant works in some tissues, such as hematopoietic cells and stromal cells [4, 10, 41], but radiation affects on the biology of these cells and their capacity to express late effects has not been reported [27, 48–50].

The examples of successful cryopreservation in the modern era include data with sperm, oocytes, fertilized ova, and hematopoietic stem cells (Table 13.1). The first successful cryopreservation techniques were developed for cells in culture. The molecule dimethylsulfoxide (DMSO) was discovered to be a potent antifreeze [6, 7]. Its small molecular weight allowed interculation of the DMSO molecule into all major sensitive components of the biological systems in single cells, namely, DNA, RNA, and lipids comprising the organelles nuclear, and cell membranes. Prior to the use of DMSO (dimethylsulfoxide) as a cryoprotectant, attempts to freeze cells and thaw them for use in tissue culture revealed the problem was crystallization of water during the freezing of cells. The crystallization of water molecules within cells was destructive, such that the thawing procedure led to toxicity of these crystals for the critical molecular events that are required for cell survival and cell replication.

The use of DMSO was as an antifreeze to prevent crystallization of water [27]. The thawing process for single cells presented the secondary problem that was solved by DMSO. Removing frozen cells from liquid nitrogen, or a −80 ° storage freezer had to be carried out in a measured, and not precipitous fashion. Slow thawing with periodic addition of culture medium was required to allow the DMSO to diffuse out of the cells as they warmed and culture medium entered with nutrients. The molecular escape of DMSO from proteins, lipids, and carbohydrates, and its replacement by nutrients in culture medium was slow and allowed cellular structures to recover from freezing at the same time that new nutrients were provided in the tissue culture media to allow cell survival.

The first cryopreservation experiments were performed with cell lines [5]. The next experiments with fresh tissues were carried out with freezing of sperm (Table 13.1). These experiments revealed that after thawing these cells recovered active flagellar motion and were capable of fertilizing ova in culture [25]. Subsequent experiments with frozen ova that were recovered from induced ovulation in experimental animals including mice followed [38], then experiments with fertilization of ova in vitro and cryopreservation of inducible stem cells or embryos fertilized ova [10] led to pioneering experiments in which patients could cryopreserve their fertilized ova for later implantation into the uterus [12].

Planned cryopreservation of sperm and ova was helpful under conditions in which patients (both men and women) were scheduled to undergo either pelvic radiotherapy, chemotherapy, or combination therapies for cancer. There was not only the concern about potential for the radiation and/or chemotherapy toxicity to cause death of the germ cells (spermatogonium, oogonium), but also that low-dose non-lethal levels of these toxic anti-cancer modalities would induce mutations in germ line cells that could lead to a teratogenic effect in a subsequent pregnancy. The successful germ cell and embryo cryopreservation techniques have facilitated reimplantation of thawed fertilized ova (embryos) from in vitro fertilization and subsequent successful live healthy births [9]. The first successful birth of a healthy child from the implantation of a cryopreserved fertilized ovum (embryo) was an epic event and its publication led to a now-established method to facilitate planned pregnancies [32].

As a research tool, cryopreservation is routinely used in laboratories in which permanent cell lines for future experimental use are cryopreserved and stored [22]. Cryopreservation not only facilitates recovery of resources from experiments that are sometimes decades old, but also is cost effective as it obviates the need to continue to passage cell lines in vitro. Most importantly, continuous passage of cell lines was impractical, because of the constant threat of contamination of cell lines in culture, possibility of incubator and tissue culture accidents, and the cost ineffectiveness of keeping so many cell lines in live culture [22]. Central repositories for frozen cell lines, experimental animal sperm, and embryos are maintained and distributed to laboratories worldwide for research use. One such resource is the ATCC (American Type Tissue Culture), which has a catalog of available cryopreserved cell and animal specimens available for distribution [22]. Cryopreservation is also now used routinely to store seeds, records of plant species that have either become extinct, or are no longer viable candidates for survival in a changing environment. Storage facilities as a "record" of agriculture and animal husbandry has become a basic element of current science (a repository of seeds at the North Pole) [39].

Another major success of cryopreservation, which is relevant to modern medicine, is the cryopreservation of bone marrow stem cells [23]. This was first carried out in experimental animals including mice and dogs, hematopoietic stem cell sorting, concentration, and cryopreservation led to the successful thawing of such cells and intravenous injection into total body irradiated recipients.

The success with cryopreserved marrow stem cells has also been valuable for understanding the biology of the shielded limb experiments, where a small percentage of the bone marrow is protected from, otherwise, total body radiation proved that bone marrow stem cells migrate to distant sites through the circulation. There were also the parabiosis experiments in irradiated animal models, which also conclusively proved that hematopoietic stem cells could traffic from irradiated environments to other environments [46]. In this model, a total body irradiated mouse shared its peripheral blood circulation with a non-irradiated (control) mouse. The control mouse bone marrow migrated into the irradiated mouse and reconstituted the hematopoietic system of the irradiated mouse [46]. The concept of cryopreservation of hematopoietic stem cells and successful thawing allowed this scientific observation to be adapted for clinical use. Bone marrow stem cell transplantation is now possible in both the autologous and heterologous settings. Patients can have their own bone marrow stem cells harvested, sorted, and cryopreserved for later infusion (autologous marrow transplant) after they have received hematopoietic-lethal doses of total body irradiation and/or chemotherapy to treat their cancer [33]. The patient's marrow can be harvested from their marrow or stem cells, be mobilized by administering the cytokine G-CSF (granulocyte colony-stimulating factor) to enter the peripheral blood, and the cells are sieved out of the blood by a machine as they are traveling in the blood. This process of leukapheresis allows collection of the person's own hematopoietic stem cells from his blood without the need for a marrow biopsy [45] (Table 13.1).

Hematopoietic stem cells can be delivered by intravenous injection from prior cryopreserved samples and have been shown to successfully reconstitute hematopoiesis in individuals. An even more dramatic use of autologous stem cells came from the work with umbilical cord blood stem cells [33]. After delivery, the obstetrics patient's own umbilical cord blood cells were found to contain totipotential stem cells of fetal origin that were already trafficking during gestation [35]. The cells could be recovered from the placenta and umbilical cord and cryopreserved for later use if that baby decades later as an adult ever needed an autologous source of bone marrow stem cells at some time in life. The frozen cells from cord blood are stable for decades. A company (Biocyte, Corp.) provides this storage service [33]. There is also a possibility of sharing of stem cells, but the genotyping for histocompatibility may not be perfect as it is with autologous stem cell transplant. Heterologous cell populations in the concept of allogeneic marrow transplantation have also been highly successful. The treatment of graft-vs.-host disease has advanced to the stage where allografts of hematopoietic stem cells are now possible [37]. Entire new research fields of transplant immunology and development of measures to prevent transplant rejection were advanced by the availability of cryopreservation of hematopoietic stem cells. The bone marrow stromal cells of the hematopoietic microenvironment (mesenchymal stem cells) [41], adipose stem cells [48], and endothelial cells [34] have also been cryopreserved and then thawed and transplanted.

Cryopreservation of Organs

Experiments were carried out with cryopreservation of kidneys from experimental mouse models. Kidney transplantation was the first successful solid organ transplantation [43] and bone marrow [44]. The kidney for the first human renal transplant came from an identical twin donor and was freshly removed with no need for temperature manipulation. In contrast, for experimental animal studies with cryopreserved organs in rodents, the kidneys that were used in these first experiments were cryopreserved in DMSO. Supportive evidence came from the observation that DMSO could permeate multiple cell phenotypes within the kidney and suggested that the thawing process could be facilitated just as easily as it was with single cells in the sperm/ova/embryo/bone marrow stem cell experiments. The kidney cryopreservation experiments focused on microsurgical techniques required for anastomosis of renal artery and vein, and urethral urine collection systems [43]. The microsurgery was successfully completed, and reperfusion of blood from the recipient into the donor kidney was successful. However, the complexity of the physiology of the glomerular filtration apparatus, the countercurrent physiology of the renal collecting tubules, and interaction of the different cell phenotypes including endothelial cells, renal epithelial cells, and the effect of circulatory leukocytes from the recipient, now infiltrating the donor organ posed a problem that could not be solved by simple cryopreservation and thawing techniques.

Other organs have also been used as experimental targets for cryopreservation, and the results with these organs have also been inconclusive. An intermediate step of cryopreservation of these cellular organisms has been successful, and this has been carried out with arthropods (Freeze-drying as a method of preservation) [24], C. elegans [49], Drosophila [50], and other more complex cellular systems [25].

The lack of current success in organ transplantation from mammals is an evolving science and will lead to better results in the future. However, at the present time, organ cryopreservation is not a viable option. Low temperature preservation is used routinely to facilitate donor organ harvest for kidney transplant, cardiac pulmonary transplant, intestinal transplantation, and other complex human transplantation experiments. Cryopreservation is not a reality, but low temperature/hypothermia is a reality for increasing the duration of organ survival during planned medical organ transplantation.

The Effects of Ionizing Irradiation on Cryopreserved Cells

Questions that can be answered with available versions of cryopreservation. The effects of ionizing irradiation on cryopreserved cells have been reported in some available studies [27] (Fig. 13.1). Cryopreservation of cell lines including "normal tissue" developed cell lines has been a routine practice for basic science laboratories for decades. Since the availability of DMSO, cell lines and subclonal lines have provided a basis for current radiobiology and general biology experiments in laboratories throughout the world.

One cell line, which has been of great interest in both genetic engineering and understanding the role of oncogenes in malignant transformation is that of the progenitor hematopoietic cell line, 32D cl 3 [51] (which was derived from a mouse long-term bone marrow culture) (Figs. 13.2 and 13.3; Tables 13.3 and 13.4). The 32D cell line and subclonal lines that have over expressed transfected oncogenes, growth factor receptors, and murine or human transgenes, have provided many

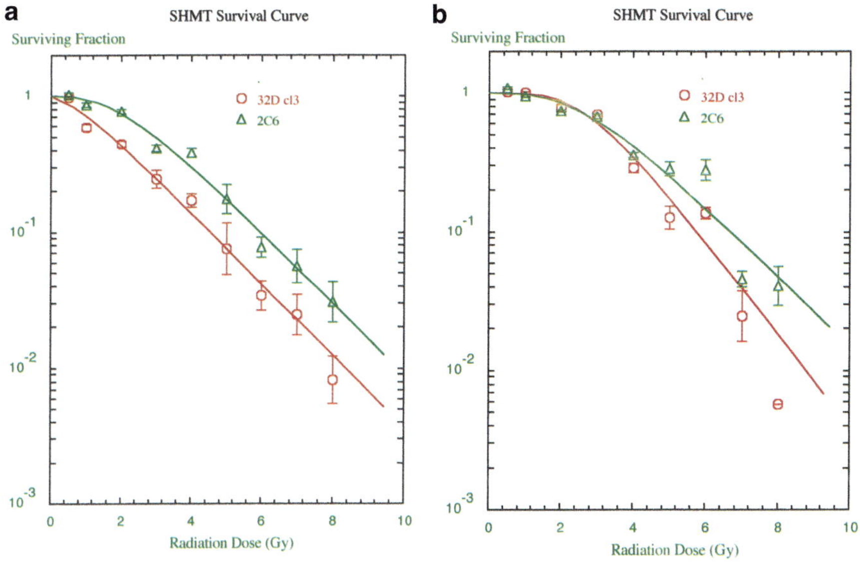

Fig. 13.1 Radiation survival curves for 32D cl 3 (○) and 2C6 (Δ) cells irradiated in culture at 24 °C (**panel a**) or −80 °C (**panel b**). Data from three experiments were fitted using the linear-quadratic model

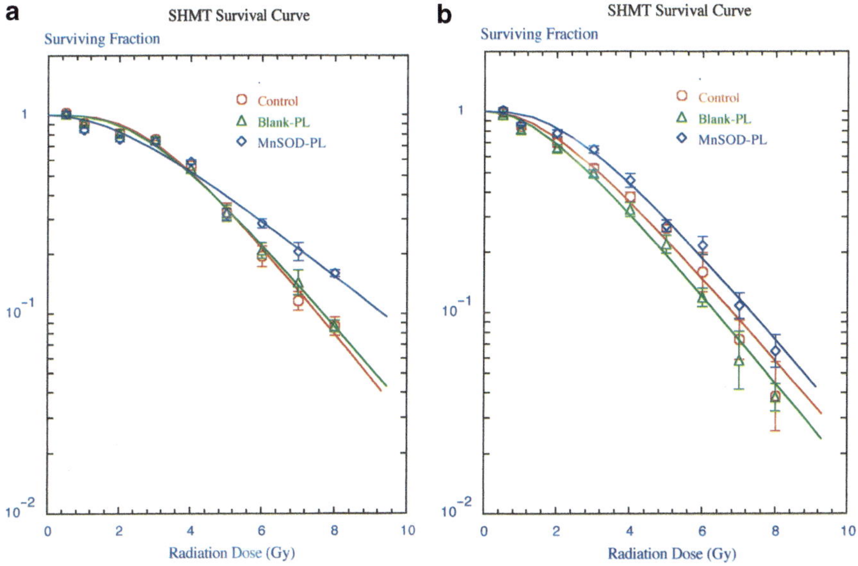

Fig. 13.2 Radiation survival curves for mouse bone murine marrow that was transfected in vitro with MnSOD-PL to produce 2C6 (◇) or blank plasmid PL (Δ) (see Materials and Methods [27]), or was not transfected (○). Data from three experiments were analyzed using a linear-quadratic model

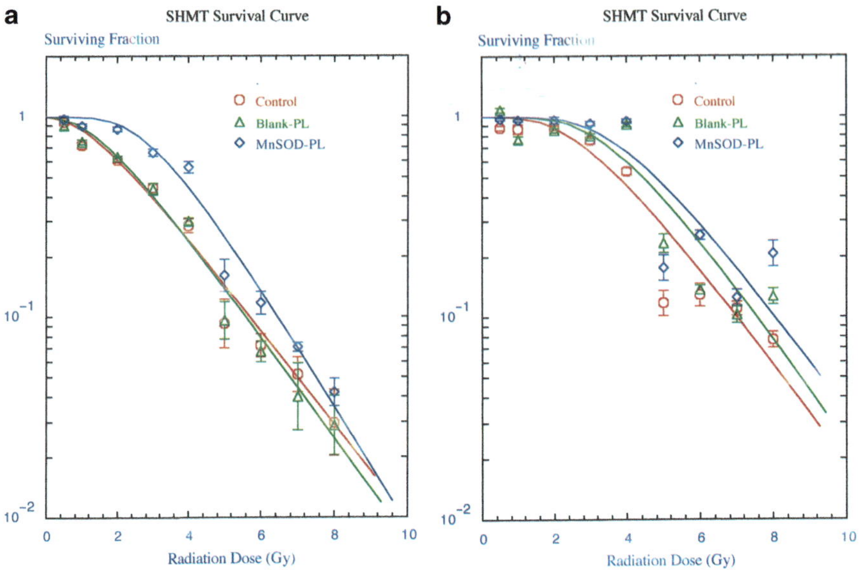

Fig. 13.3 Radiation survival curves for mouse bone marrow that was transfected in vivo 24 h prior to explant with MnSOD-PL (◇) or blank plasmid PL (Δ)or was not transfected (○). Bone marrow was harvested 24 h after injection of MnSOD-PL and either immediately irradiated (**panel a**) or frozen and irradiated while frozen (**panel b**). Data from three experiments were analyzed using a linear-quadratic model

laboratories with the basis for studies of the molecular biology of gene activation

Table 13.3 Analyses of survival data for 32D cl 3 and 2C6 cells irradiated at 24 °C compared to −80 °C

	Irradiated at 24 °C		Irradiated at −80 °C	
Cells, experiment no.	D_0	$\tilde{n}$	D_0	$\tilde{n}$
32D cl 3				
1	1.15	1.70	1.26	14.11
2	1.25	2.14	1.65	10.991
3	1.42	1.11	1.46	12.00
Average	1.27 ± 0.08	1.65 ± 0.30	1.46 ± 0.11	12.55 ± 0.90
2C6				
1	1.97	5.25	1.81	4.31
2	2.11	4.90	2.26	6.81
3	2.30	4.95	2.04	6.00
Average	2.13 ± 0.09 (p = 0.0024)	5.03 ± 0.11 (p = 0.0004)	2.04 ± 0.130 (p = 0.0276)	5.56 ± 1.25 (p = 0.0038)

and interaction with cellular processes [51]. 32D cells are cryopreserved in DMSO and thawed with a high rate of success with minimal alteration of biological function.

Table 13.4 Effect of transfection in vitro or in vivo with either MnSOD-PL or Blank-PL on survival of mouse bone marrow irradiated at 24 °C or −80 °C

Transfection in vivo, experiment no.	Irradiated at 24 °C		Irradiated at −80 °C		Transfection in vitro, experiment no.	Irradiated at 24 °C		Irradiated at −80 °C	
	D_0 (Gy)	$\tilde{n}$	D_0 (Gy)	$\tilde{n}$		D_0 (Gy)	$\tilde{n}$	D_0 (Gy)	$\tilde{n}$
Control					Control				
1	1.45	6.03	1.54	6.21	1	1.80	6.36	2.60	1.09
2	1.45	1.37	1.77	7.52	2	1.84	3.08	2.44	1.15
3	1.58	3.62	1.66	6.50	3	1.81	6.00	2.54	1.00
Average	1.56 ± 0.06	3.67 ± 1.35	1.66 ± 0.64	6.75 ± 0.40	Average	1.81 ± 0.01	5.15 ± 1.04	2.53 ± 0.05	1.08 ± 0.04
Blank-PL					Blank-PL				
1	1.45	3.19	2.17	3.50	1	1.98	5.04	2.92	1.00
2	2.03	1.11	2.46	2.70	2	1.84	2.99	2.16	1.28
3	2.34	3.17	2.04	5.77	3	1.96	5.15	2.33	1.86
Average	1.94 ± 0.26	2.49 ± 0.69	2.22 ± 0.12	3.99 ± 0.92	Average	1.93 ± 0.04	4.39 ± 0.70	2.47 ± 0.23	1.38 ± 0.25
MnSOD-PL					MnSOD-PL				
1	2.09	2.36	2.13	4.38	1	2.48	3.28	3.19	1.09
2	2.60	1.00	1.96	4.21	2	2.13	2.71	3.17	1.00
3	1.88	4.12	2.21	3.11	3	2.43	3.32	3.47	1.00
Average	2.19 ± 0.21 ($p = 0.047$)	2.49 ± 0.90	2.10 ± 0.07 ($p = 0.017$)	3.90 ± 0.40 ($p = 0.024$)	Average	2.35 ± 0.11 ($p = 0.0087$)	3.08 ± 0.19	3.42 ± 0.13 ($p = 0.0026$)	1.03 ± 0.03

Notes: Data were analyzed using a single-hit, multitarget model to obtain D_0 and $\tilde{n}$. Pooled data are shown in Figs. 13.2 and 13.3. Significance of difference from control was assessed using Student's *t*-test

Epperly MW, Epperly LD, Niu YY, Wang H, Zhang X, Franicola D, Greenberger JS. Overexpression of the MnSOD transgene product protects cryopreserved bone marrow hematopoietic progenitor cells form ionizing radiation. Radiat Res. 2007;168: 560–566

In one radiobiology study, 32D cells and subclone 2C6 overexpressing the gene for MnSOD were cryopreserved, and then at liquid nitrogen storage temperatures close to absolute zero, the vials of frozen cells were irradiated while frozen and a dose response curve of radiation was performed [27]. Thawed cells then were assayed for viability, recovery of viable cells, clonogenicity, and stability of the irradiated compared to non-irradiated frozen cryopreserved cells. The results were very interesting in two regards. The cryopreservation process itself was toxic. Thawing cells after cryopreservation in DMSO led to a reproducible loss of cells during the thawing process [27]. Different rates of addition of culture media and removal of DMSO led to improved survival, but the toxicity of thawing itself was detectable and was quantifiable.

Irradiation of cryopreserved cells proved to be an additive toxicity to that of the thawing process. Irradiated cells did suffer DNA double-strand breaks and the repair of double-strand breaks did occur either during the cryopreserved state or during the thawing state such that there was a measurable effect of oxidative stress of irradiation above and beyond that demonstrated by the DMSO/thawing toxicity. In these experiments, a subclonal line of 32D, 2C6 which was overexpressing the antioxidant gene MnSOD [27], was shown to be protected from the process of cryopreservation and thawing better than the control 32D parent cell line [27]. The antioxidant effect of MnSOD could have been expressed during the frozen state or at the time of thawing. The experimental techniques available at the time of this publication could not differentiate between the timing of the DNA repair process relative to the frozen or thawing state.

Other publications measuring the effects of irradiation on cells in a cryopreserved state have supported this original publication [35]. Further studies will be required to determine whether irradiation of cryopreserved organs and organ systems will also facilitate radiation resistance. The effect of transgene integration into cryopreserved cells can also be measured in these types of experiments. Future studies should uncover many valuable principles of the role of cryopreservation in radiation protection and radiation resistance.

Whether cryopreserved animals and humans can withstand galactic cosmic irradiation that would be experienced during years or decades of cryopreservation is a question that cannot be currently answered. However, if cryopreservation is proven efficient and safe, it could be designed to limit aging and essentially "freeze" the aging process allowing astronauts to travel vast distances over vast periods of time, [52, 53] then be thawed and not age, must require decades of research in understanding the radiobiology of aging. At the present time, it is known that irradiation accelerates aging [54, 55], and this has been described in previous chapters and is a mainstay of the understanding of late effects of irradiation in clinical radiotherapy, as well as that would be applied to space irradiation [56, 57]. Much work is yet to be done.

References

1. Bland MT, Weller LA, Archinal BA, et al. Improving the usability of Galileo and Voyager images of Jupiter's moon Europa. Earth Space Sci. 2021;8(12):e2021EA001935. https://doi.org/10.1029/2021EA001935.
2. Chyba CF, Phillips CB. Europa as an abode of life. Orig Life Evol Biosph. 2002;32(1):47–68. https://doi.org/10.1023/a:1013958519734.
3. Kloster KW, Petropoulos AE, Longuski JM. Europa orbiter tour design with Io gravity assists. Acta Astronaut. 2011;68(7–8):931–46.
4. Guillaumet-Adkins A, Rodriguez-Esteban G, Mereu E, et al. Single-cell transcriptome conservation in cryopreserved cells and tissues. Genome Biol. 2017;18(1):45. https://doi.org/10.1186/s13059-017-1171-9.
5. Wu SZ, Roden DL, Al-Eryani G, et al. Cryopreservation of human cancers conserves tumour heterogeneity for single-cell multi-omics analysis. Genome Med. 2021;13(1):81. https://doi.org/10.1186/s13073-021-00885-z.
6. Satpathy S, Thomas BE, Pilcher WJ, et al. The simple preservation of single cElls method for cryopreservation enables the generation of single-cell immune profiles from whole blood. Front Immunol. 2023;14:1271800. https://doi.org/10.3389/fimmu.2023.1271800.
7. Wohnhaas CT, Leparc GG, Fernandez-Albert F, et al. DMSO cryopreservation is the method of choice to preserve cells for droplet-based single-cell RNA sequencing. Sci Rep. 2019;9(1):10699. https://doi.org/10.1038/s41598-019-46932-z.
8. Lee JS, Yi K, Ju YS, et al. Effects of cryopreservation and thawing on single-cell transcriptomes of human T cells. Immune Netw. 2020;20(4):e34. https://doi.org/10.4110/in.2020.20.e34.
9. Taylor MJ, Weegman BP, Baicu SC, et al. New approaches to cryopreservation of cells, tissues, and organs. Transfus Med Hemother. 2019;46(3):197–215. https://doi.org/10.1159/000499453.
10. Li R, Yu G, Azarin SM, et al. Freezing responses in DMSO-based cryopreservation of human iPS cells: aggregates versus single cell. Tissue Eng Part C Methods. 2018;24(5):289–99. https://doi.org/10.1089/ten.TEC.2017.0531.
11. Yango P, Altman E, Smith JF, et al. Optimizing cryopreservation of human spermatogonial stem cells: comparing the effectiveness of testicular tissue and single cell suspension cryopreservation. Fertil Steril. 2014;102(5):1491–8. https://doi.org/10.1016/j.fertnstert.2014.07.1250.
12. Wilton LJ, Shaw JM, Trounson AO. Successful single-cell biopsy and cryopreservation of preimplantation mouse embryos. Fertil Steril. 1989;51(3):513–7. https://doi.org/10.1016/s0015-0282(16)60564-2.
13. Meryman HT. Cryopreservation of living cells: principles and practice. Transfusion. 2007;47(5):935–45. https://doi.org/10.1111/j.1537-2995.2007.01212.x.
14. McRae A, Ricardo-Silgado ML, Liu Y, et al. A protocol for the cryopreservation of human intestinal mucosal biopsies compatible with single-cell transcriptomics and ex vivo studies. Front Physiol. 2022;13:878389. https://doi.org/10.3389/fphys.2022.878389.
15. Deutsch M, Afrimzon E, Namer Y, et al. The individual-cell-based cryo-chip for the cryopreservation, manipulation. And observation of spatially identifiable cells. I: methodology. BMC Cell Biol. 2010;11:54. https://doi.org/10.1186/1471-2121-11-54.
16. Jang TH, Park SC, Yang JH, et al. Cryopreservation and its clinical applications. Integr Med Res. 2017;6(1):12–8. https://doi.org/10.1016/j.imr.2016.12.001.
17. Bhattacharya S. A review on cryoprotectant and its modern implication in cryonics. Asian J Pharmac. 2016;10(3):154.
18. Shannon JE, Macy ML. Chapter 8—Freezing, storage, and recovery of cell stocks. In: Kruse PF, Patterson MK, editors. Tissue culture: methods and applications. Patterson, Academic Press; 1973.
19. Engelmann F. Plant cryopreservation: progress and prospects. In Vitro Cell Dev Biol Plant. 2004;40:427–33.
20. Anger JT, Gilbert BR, Goldstein M. Cryopreservation of sperm: indications, methods, and results. J Urol. 2003;170(4 Pt 1):1079–84. https://doi.org/10.1097/01.ju.0000084820.98430.b8.

21. Lavappa KS, Macy ML, Shannon JE. Examination of ATCC stocks for HeLa marker chromosomes in human cell lines. Nature. 1976;259(5540):211–3. https://doi.org/10.1038/259211a0.
22. Arav A, Rubinsky B, Seren E, et al. The role of thermal hysteresis proteins during cryopreservation of oocytes and embryos. Theriogenology. 1994;41(1):107–12.
23. Berz D, McCormack EM, Winer ES, et al. Cryopreservation of hematopoietic stem cells. Am J Hematol. 2007;82(6):463–72. https://doi.org/10.1002/ajh.20707.
24. Sahgal G, Sundrasekar J, Subramaniam S. Brine shrimp cytotoxicity activity for different parts of Hymenocallis Littoralis. Rapports De Pharmacie. 2017;3(4):423–8.
25. Kuzmic M, Galas S, Lecomte-Pradines C, et al. Interplay between ionizing radiation effects and aging in C. elegans. Free Radic Biol Med. 2019;134:657–65. https://doi.org/10.1016/j.freeradbiomed.2019.02.002.
26. Holwerde BW, Knabel S, Steele RC, et al. The observable supernova rate in galaxy-galaxy lensing systems with the TESS satellite. Mon Not R Astron Soc. 2021;505(1):1316–23.
27. Epperly MW, Epperly LD, Niu YY, et al. Overexpression of the MnSOD transgene product protects cryopreserved bone marrow hematopoietic progenitor cells from ionizing radiation. Radiat Res. 2007;168(5):560–6. https://doi.org/10.1667/RR1071R.1.
28. Faulkner DR. Astronomical distance determination methods and the light travel time problem. Answers Res J. 2013;6:211–29.
29. Hill JM, Cox BJ. Einstein's special relativity beyond the speed of light. Proceedings of the Royal Society A Mathematical, Physical, and Engineering Sciences, October 3, 2012.
30. Vasavada AR. Mission overview and scientific contributions from the Mars science laboratory curiosity rover after eight years of surface operations. Space Sci Rev. 2022;218(3):14. https://doi.org/10.1007/s11214-022-00882-7.
31. Yang D, Brown SE, Nguyen K, et al. Live birth after the transfer of human embryos developed from cryopreserved oocytes harvested before cancer treatment. Fertil Steril. 2007;87(6):1469.e1–4. https://doi.org/10.1016/j.fertnstert.2006.07.1546.
32. Smithi LK, Roots EH, Dorsett MJO. Live birth of a normal healthy baby after a frozen embryo transfer with blastocysts that were frozen and thawed twice. Fertil Steril. 2005;83(1):198–200. https://doi.org/10.1016/j.fertnstert.2004.07.953.
33. Ballen KK, Gluckman E, Broxmeyer HE. Umbilical cord blood transplantation: the first 25 years and beyond. Blood. 2013;122(4):491–8. https://doi.org/10.1182/blood-2013-02-453175.
34. Mitchell P. European researchers condemn US firm's cord-blood-storage patent. Lancet. 1997;349(9060):1232. https://doi.org/10.1016/S0140-6736(05)62436-1.
35. Bomhard AV, Elsasser A, Ritschi LM, et al. Cryopreservation of endothelial cells in various cryoprotective agents and media—vitrification versus slow freezing methods. PLoS One. 2016;11(2):e0149660. https://doi.org/10.1371/journal.pone.0149660.
36. Kato H, Anzai M, Mitani T, et al. Recovery of cell nuclei from 15,000 years old mammoth tissues and its injection into mouse enucleated matured oocytes. Proc Jpn Acad Ser B Phys Biol Sci. 2009;85(7):240–7. https://doi.org/10.2183/pjab.85.240.
37. Worobey M, Han G-Z, Rambaut A. Genesis and pathogenesis of the 1918 pandemic H1N1 influenza A virus. Proc Natl Acad Sci USA. 2014;111(22):8107–12. https://doi.org/10.1073/pnas.1324197111.
38. Gerritse R, Beerendonk CCM, Tijink MSL, et al. Optimal perfusion of an intact ovary as a prerequisite for successful ovarian cryopreservation. Hum Reprod. 2008;23(2):329–35. https://doi.org/10.1093/humrep/dem384.
39. Lynnerup N. Mummies. Am J Phys Anthropol Suppl. 2007;45:162–90. https://doi.org/10.1002/ajpa.20728.
40. Zittoun RA, Mandelli F, Willemze R, et al. Autologous or allogeneic bone marrow transplantation compared with intensive chemotherapy in acute myelogenous leukemia. N Engl J Med. 1995;332(4):217–23. https://doi.org/10.1056/NEJM199501263320403.
41. Anklesaria P, Kase KR, Glowacki J, et al. Engraftment of a clonal bone marrow stromal cell line in vivo stimulates hematopoietic recovery from total body irradiation. Proc Natl Acad Sci USA. 1987;84(21):7681–5. https://doi.org/10.1073/pnas.84.21.7681.

42. Burdette EC, Wiggins S, Brown R, et al. Microwave thawing of frozen kidneys: a theoretically based experimentally-effective design. Cryobiology. 1980;17(4):393–402. https://doi.org/10.1016/0011-2240(80)90046-2.
43. Merrill JP, Murray JE, Harrison H, et al. Successful homotransplantation of the human kidney between identical twins. JAMA J Am Med Assoc. 1956;160(4):277–82. https://doi.org/10.1001/jama.1956.02960390027008.
44. Thomas ED, Lochte HL Jr, Lu WC, et al. Intravenous infusion of bone marrow in patients receiving radiation and chemotherapy. N Engl J Med. 1957;257(11):491–6. https://doi.org/10.1056/NEJM195709122571102.
45. Bendall LJ, Bradstock KF. G-CSF: from granulopoietic stimulant to bone marrow stem cell mobilizing agent. Cytokine Growth Factor Rev. 2014;25(4):355–67. https://doi.org/10.1016/j.cytogfr.2014.07.011.
46. Kamran P, Sereti K-I, Zhao P, et al. Parabiosis in mice: a detailed protocol. J Vis Exp. 2013;6(80):50556. https://doi.org/10.3791/50556.
47. Harris AC, Ferrara JLM, Levine JE. Advances in predicting acute GVHD. Br J Haematol. 2013;160(3):288–302. https://doi.org/10.1111/bjh.12142.
48. Ejaz A, Greenberger JS, Rubin PJ. Understanding the mechanism of radiation induced fibrosis and therapy options. Pharmacol Ther. 2019;204:107399. https://doi.org/10.1016/j.pharmthera.2019.107399.
49. Glenister PH, Whittingham DG, Lyon MF. Further studies on the effect of radiation during the storage of frozen 8-cell mouse embryos at −196°C. J Reprod Fertil. 1984;70(1):229–34. https://doi.org/10.1530/jrf.0.0700229.
50. Moskalev A, Zhikrivetskaya S, Krasnov G, et al. A comparison of the transcriptome of Drosophila melanogaster in response to entomopathogenic fungus, ionizing radiation, starvation, and cold shock. BMC Genomics. 2015;16 Suppl 13(Suppl 13):S8. https://doi.org/10.1186/1471-2164-16-S13-S8.
51. Greenberger JS, Sakakeeny MA, Humphries KC, et al. Demonstration of permanent factor-dependent multipotential (erythroid/neutrophil/basophil) hematopoietic progenitor cell lines. Proc Natl Acad Sci USA. 1983;80(10):2931–5. https://doi.org/10.1073/pnas.80.10.2931.
52. Ihle J, Keller J, Greenberger JS, et al. Phenotypic characteristics of cell lines requiring IL-3 for growth. J Immunol. 1982;129(4):1377–83.
53. Epperly MW, Bray JA, Esocobar P, et al. Overexpression of the human MnSOD transgene in subclones of murine hematopoietic progenitor cell line 32D cl 3 decreases irradiation-induced apoptosis, but does not alter G_2/M or G_1/S phase cell cycle arrest. Radiat Oncol Investig. 1999;7(6):331–42. https://doi.org/10.1002/(SICI)1520-6823(1999)7:6<331::AID-RO13>3.0.CO;2-M.
54. Epperly MW, Sikora CA, DeFilippi SJ, et al. Pulmonary irradiation-induced expression of VCAM-1 and ICAM-1 is decreased by MnSOD-PL gene therapy. Biol Blood Marrow Transplant. 2002;8(4):175–87. https://doi.org/10.1053/bbmt.2002.v8.pm12014807.
55. Seed TM, Carnes BA, Tolle DV, Fritz TE. Blood responses under chronic low daily dose gamma irradiation: I. Differential preclinical responses of irradiated male dogs in progression to either aplastic anemia or myeloproliferative disease. Leuk Res. 1989;13(12):1069–84. https://doi.org/10.1016/0145-2126(89)90152-5.
56. Lee H. Ex situ conservation efforts for plant diversity protection with a focus on seeds. Open Agric J. 2023;17:230822.
57. Horne WH, Volpe RP, Korza G, et al. Effects of desiccation and freezing on microbial ionizing radiation survivability: considerations for Mars sample return. Astrobiology. 2022;22(11):1337–50. https://doi.org/10.1089/ast.2022.0065.

Chapter 14
Identification and Management of Radiation Late Effects in Humans

Over 120 years of experience with ionizing irradiation exposure of humans during the advent and development of diagnostic radiology, nuclear medicine, and radiation oncology have provided physicians and scientists with a great deal of information regarding the hazards of radiation and, most prominently, the pathophysiology of the late effects [1–4]. This clinical patient information will be of great value in the coming decades and will help the development of countermeasures for ionizing irradiation associated with nuclear war, radiation counter-terrorism, and space radiation. The history of understanding late effects of ionizing irradiation primarily comes from therapeutic radiology, in recent decades, renamed radiation medicine or radiation oncology [1–4]. The majority of patients, who have been treated with ionizing irradiation, have been those with cancer. As radiation doses for treating cancer increased over the decades from the 1960s to the decade of 2010 subsequently have decreased with the knowledge that there is a threshold beyond which additional radiation doses do not provide greater local control or cure.

The specialty of diagnostic radiology has also focused on reducing radiation exposure to patients for diagnostic purposes. Shielding devices, radiation beam intensifiers, and other techniques have been used to minimize the dose of radiation required to provide adequate imaging for computerized actual tomography (CAT scans) and all forms of radiation-requiring imaging. The same strategy has been applied to decreasing the amount of tracer that is required for diagnostic positron emission tomography (PET) scanning.

Information from patients, who received clinical radiotherapy (therapeutic radiology) during the decades from 1900 to 2010, is the basis for our understanding of organ-specific radiation late effects [5–19]. The clinical outcomes information has been exceedingly important for basic radiation biology, but also to provide the background information for development of radiation countermeasures (our best response to the threat of nuclear war or nuclear reactor accidents) and prepare to safely treat astronauts for space travel.

J. Greenberger, *Radiation Oncology and Radiation Biology*, https://doi.org/10.1007/978-3-031-66300-0_14

The history of radiation oncology is one that is both unique to that specialty and also consistent with all other specialties in clinical medicine [19]. The observation that a new technique or new treatment works to achieve the goals of that therapeutic intervention is always followed by clinical trials focused on determining the minimum dose of a therapeutic agent that is required and the toxicity of a maximum dose. The same principles hold true for use of radiation oncology (therapeutic radiology) to treat cancer [19].

Understanding radiation late effects based on all the data accumulated in the last 120 years from the use of radiotherapy to treat cancer must credit those pioneers of the specialty in their attempts to cure cancer also provide valuable information on late effects.

In the early part of the twentieth century, radiation oncologists in the United Kingdom and France provided valuable information on radiation late effects because radiation was used more frequently than today and was used to treat benign noncancer diseases (Table 14.1).

Table 14.1 Clinical uses of ionizing irradiation: historical perspective

Type of radiation	Use	Approximate years
1. Roentgen ray	Cancer	1900
2. Radium	Cancer	1900
3. Radiation elixir	Rejuvenation	1920s
4. Orthovoltage X-ray	Fluoroscopy Arthritis, tonsillitis, cancer, shoe size measure	1920s–1960s
5. Cobalt^{60} teletherapy	Cancer	1966
6. Radioiodine	Thyroid cancer	1960
7. Linear accelerator	Cancer	1970
8. Electron beam	Cancer	1970
9. High-energy X-ray >10 MV	Cancer	1974
10. Gamma knife radiosurgery	Cancer, vascular malformation	1982
11. Collimation of beam	Cancer	1990
12. Moving gantry and micro-leaf collimator	Cancer	1990
13. High dose rate brachytherapy, fractionated iridium implants	Cancer	1995
14. Linear accelerator adaptation for SRS, SRT, SABR	Cancer	1995
15. Proton beam	"	1980
16. Neutron beam	"	1980
17. PI-Meon beam	"	1976
18. Carbon ion beam	"	2000
19. FLASH irradiation	"	2005
20. Radioisotope therapy injector	"	2000

To develop appropriate treatment for head and neck cancers, Honore Baclesse, determined the size of the radiation field delivered to the head and neck region, was associated with greater toxicity of the same radiation dose [1–4]. Decreasing the field size and volume of tissue treated "the shrinking field technique," which was reported by Baclesse provided the most valuable information on how to safely control cancer. The earliest patients, who had local control and long-term survival, who were followed, and whose case presentations were reported in the 1930s, first uncovered the phenomenon of radiation late effects. Pathologists analyzed the tissue in irradiated patients and determined that there was fibrosis consisting of dense collagen [11–18]. The replacement of flexible tissues with fibroblasts and structural abnormalities in the tissues was associated with loss of flexibility and the scar formation [12]. The radiation-induced scars that present late radiation effects in skin, muscle, and other soft tissues were similar in many ways to those that were reported by pathologists looking at healing of areas of thermal burn, chemical burn, and healing large surgical wounds. In the use of radiotherapy, both external beam and brachytherapy (implantation of radiation-emitting sources, initially radium, and then cesium), gynecologic oncologists also reported late radiation effects and the histopathology was also consistent with fibrosis, the tissue looking very much the same as that in the head and neck regions of "cured" patients [9, 10].

The clinical observations and multiple publications by Gilbert Fletcher, primarily during his years at the M.D. Anderson Hospital in Houston, Texas, led to secondary understanding of radiation late effects, namely organ dysfunction [1]. Fibrosis alone, while prominent, was not the most debilitating late side effect of therapeutic radiation. Organ dysfunction was observed in both head and neck cancer patients and gynecologic oncology patients. These two populations were intensively studied by Gilbert Fletcher and his multiple surgeon colleague. Gilbert Fletcher also pioneered the concept of multimodality therapy due to his intense collaboration with surgeons [1–4]. Head and neck surgeons carried out excision of primary squamous cell carcinomas of the head and neck regions and also did extensive neck dissections. Neck dissections facilitated precise understanding of the regional lymph nodes, nodal stations, and the progression of head and neck cancers. The work of Fletcher and Jesse [1] including their epic textbook provided information about nearly every anatomic site of head and neck cancers, and the likely areas, where lymph node metastasis would be detected. For example, in this textbook and multiple publications, Fletcher and Jesse defined the nodal stations, which were likely to be positive in patients with primary tumors of the sphenoid sinus, compared to those with cancer originating in the base of the tongue, floor of the mouth, or retromolar trigone. These diagrams provided generations of radiation oncologists and surgeons with the information necessary to determine what nodal station should be sampled (if a full dissection was not to be planned) or, in the case of radiation oncologists, what area should be included in the radiation fields to attempt to control microscopic disease, since those particular nodal stations were likely to be the first echelon of spread of the cancer. Head and neck cancer patients were some of the first to be "cured" and who survived 10–20 years after surgery and radiotherapy [11, 12]. Chemotherapy was not added to regimens for treating head and neck cancers for decades after surgery and radiotherapy had become the standard of care for head and neck cancer. Also, the experiments in which Fletcher and colleagues would eliminate brachytherapy implantation of sources in head and neck region in an attempt to cure the cancers with external beam alone led to the observations that the integration of external beam and brachytherapy was the optimum way to deliver high doses to tumor volumes and minimize late effects. Gilbert Fletcher led to the training of generations of specialists with expertise in treating head and neck cancer [9, 19].

Rodney Million, at the University of Florida in Gainesville, C.C. Wang at the Massachusetts General Hospital associated with Harvard Medical School and others, expanded the body of data to optimize radiation dose, treatment planning, and integration of brachytherapy with external beam cured thousands of patients. Their work added to a significant body of data on radiation late effects. Fibrosis was the primary discovery, but organ dysfunction rapidly became a category of late effects, which needed observation. For head and neck cancer, pharyngeal constrictor muscles and muscles involved in the larynx and speech were those that led to the first clinical observations of organ dysfunction. Difficulty swallowing due to pharyngeal muscle fibrosis and change in voice including fatigue in speaking and change in quality and pitch of voice presented as early onsets of symptoms from late effects, even before soft tissue fibrosis was detected [12]. For those patients treated to oral cavity tumors and salivary gland tumors, it was observed that xerostomia (dry mouth) was an early sign of late effects on the salivary glands and led to the modified use of blocking or sparing contralateral parotid glands or portions of the glands to maintain saliva production.

Surgeons and radiation oncologists dealing with the management of head and neck cancer patients began to understand the relative risk for side effects in surgical compared to radiotherapy approaches. Combined modality approaches led to cooperation between these specialists, in some cases minimizing the volume of tissue removed for treatment of primary head and neck cancers and replacement with external beam radiotherapy or brachytherapy implants in some cases. In other cases, it was determined that the radiation dose required to control a tumor might produce more side effects than an intensive composite resection. The cooperation between otolaryngologists/head and neck cancer surgeons and radiation oncologists became the standard for the development of the specialty of radiation oncology and training residents during the twentieth century.

Gynecologic oncologists and their interaction with radiation oncologists presented the second large group of collaborators to provide valuable information on radiation late effects [20]. The same principles applied to understanding the optimal way to treat cervix cancer, endometrial cancer, and vulvovaginal cancer and also led to an understanding of the best management of patients with bladder cancer and anal/rectal cancers since the normal tissues in the pelvic region responded to radiation independent of where the primary tumor was diagnosed. The most valuable information on late effects came from those patients with cervix cancer. Gilbert Fletcher and colleagues, as well as, the other radiation oncologists mentioned above dealing with head and neck cancer patients, provided the most important information on dose-response curves and the role of volume in managing the late effects of treatment of cervix cancer. Gilbert Fletcher reported that brachytherapy [1] was a critical component of the management of cervix cancer. Delivering the dose to the cervix, parametria was a critical part of the management and attempts to substitute external beam alone were not as effective as controlling disease and produced more late effects. The combination of brachytherapy with external beam radiotherapy became standard theraputic irradiation. The development of brachytherapy applicators to concentrate therapeutic isotope doses to the cervix or endometrium was critical to facilitate delivery of radiation doses to those critical structures and minimize dose to areas outside the tumor volume.

The use of low dose rate brachytherapy with isotope insertion was periods of 50 h and required patients to stay in the hospital for sometimes 2 days. There were associated medical problems with prolonged bed rest including thrombosis and risk of thrombo-embolism, but also the radiation safety considerations having patients in the hospital with brachytherapy sources in place in the pelvis and requirement for training and understanding the risks of radiation dose that would be unintentionally delivered to patients family members, who visited, but also to nursing staff and hospital employees at all levels; therefore, high dose rates after loading brachytherapy was substituted for the low dose rate isotopes, but the principle was the same, namely that the delivery of radiation by brachytherapy to local structures was much more likely to control the tumor and reduce the side effects of external beam radiotherapy [21, 22]. The kinetics of radiation were described in experimental animals [23–25] and were similar to those observed in head and neck cancer patients. Late radiation fibrosis also has been observed in the heart [26–28], the kidney [29], and intestine [30, 31].

At the completion of a course of radiotherapy for cervix cancer, for example, patients would recover from any acute effects of irradiation, enter into a "eclipse" or stationary phase, and then during follow-up over the next 2 years begin to experience radiation late effects. Fibrosis in the tissues was histopathologically very similar to that found in head and neck cancer patients. Organ dysfunction was associated with radiation damage to the organs in the field. Depending on the treatment planning and the technique of delivering external beam radiation to the cervix, there were complications of results from late effects on the anus and rectum and also interiorly in the bladder. Fibrosis of the bladder leads to reduced bladder volume, frequency and urgency, or incontinence. Fibrosis in the rectum led to presentation of patients with late effects including painful bowel movements and rectal bleeding. Depending on the positioning of radiation beams, particularly, prior to the availability of intensity-modulated radiotherapy (IMRT), patients presented with hip dysplasia and fracture from lateral beams. Obese patients often suffer from skin lesions, ulceration, and tissue breakdown from anterior radiation fields.

While patients with head and neck cancer and those with gynecologic cancers provided the largest groups of patients with respect to volume of data reported and precise identification of optimal dose-response curves to achieve local control/cure with minimal side effects [12], there was also a great availability of data with respect to bladder cancer and rectal cancer (Tables 14.2 and 14.3).

Table 14.2 Reported late effects of radiation exposure organ-specific or total body irradiation (TBI)

Late effect	Reported
1. Skin fibrosis and ulceration	1920
2. Lymphoma/leukemia	1920s
3. Anemia/marrow failure	1920s
4. Tissue fibrosis (skin)	1930s
5. Organ failure: Kidney, liver, intestine, bone marrow	1940s
6. Lung fibrosis	1940s
7. Infertility	1940s
8. Cancer	1940s
9. Neurocognitive loss:	1970s
Pediatric	1970s
Adult	1971
10. Osteoporosis	1970s
11. Wound healing failure, cardiac fibrosis, erythema in nonhuman primates	1980s
Diabetes, stroke-vessel damage, brain necrosis	1990s
12. Leukoencephalopathy	1990s
13. Brain necrosis	2000

Table 14.3 Evidence linking radiation acute effects to late effects

Clinical evidence	Proposed mechanism
1. Observations of lung cancer survivors	Slow proliferating cell populations
2. Delayed immune response	Tissue injury
3. Molecular biomarkers of late effects in C3H/H- vs. C57BL/6 mice	TGF-β, IL-1, TNF-α
4. Master regulator genes induced by ionizing irradiation	Fgr

For these two anatomic sites: (1) head and neck and (2) cervix and endometrium, surgeons and radiation oncologists collaborated on studies to determine whether preoperative radiation was superior to postoperative radiation, and in these categories, controversies in these strategies led to randomized perspective trials and valuable information about advantages and disadvantages of giving the radiotherapy prior to surgical excision [1–3]. For both rectal/anal cancers and bladder cancers, preoperative radiation shrunk the tumor volume and facilitated surgical excision that required less normal tissue resection. However, there was a problem recognized that often microscopic disease was not detected at the time of surgery, and there were positive resection margins. In contrast, allowing surgery to precede radiotherapy, larger volumes of tissue were resected and there were in many publications reports of fewer patients with positive resection margins, and, accordingly, less postoperative radiation dose required. Many publications reported advantages and disadvantages of each approach. There were also studies to determine the time after surgical resection when postoperative radiotherapy could be started. Some reports indicated 2–4 weeks after surgical excision was required for adequate wound healing, and there was concern that postoperative radiation would result in delayed wound healing. The controversy still persists. The one observation which was generally agreed upon was that surgery and radiation led to a form of combined injury and that late effects were likely to be associated with greater radiation dose. The advent of chemotherapy in the latter part of the twentieth century led to introduction of the third modality of cancer care to all patients with pelvic malignancies including gynecologic neoplasms, bladder, and anal and rectal cancer. Using chemotherapy as a third modality allowed protocols to include reduced radiation doses. This led to decreased side effects. Organ dysfunction remained a major category of side effects and was the main focus of follow-up of patients with cancer of the pelvic regions including all those listed above [20].

This chapter will serve as a bridge between the three scientific disciplines that are involved in this book: (1) clinical radiation oncology; (2) the development of medical countermeasures against radiation terrorism or nuclear power station accidents; and (3) space radiation.

Radiation late effects are defined by the radiobiologists and radiation oncologists, as those, which appear months to years after the completion of clinical radiotherapy or some other form of radiation exposure [5–7]. The concept of late effects assumes that the irradiated animal or human has recovered from any acute radiation effects and has then entered what is commonly called the "latent period" in which no specific symptoms or signs of radiation exposure are detectable. One of the critical and as yet unanswered questions in radiation biology is the mechanism of release from the latent period and initiation of the late effects [1]. Much of the information that is currently available on radiation late effects comes from the medical specialty of clinical radiotherapy, also called radiation medicine or radiation oncology.

The first reports of radiation late effects came from the discoveries of radium by the scientists, Marie and Pierre Curie during the first years of the 1900s [32]. Around that same time, Conrad Roentgen carried out the first experiments using the cathode-ray tube (X-ray machine) to image organs in the human body [1]. These pioneers of the field of radiation biology and clinical radiology in their first work with their scientific investigations focused little attention on the biology of ionizing irradiation. The potential medical uses of radium and X-irradiation led to their first use in humans and the inevitable discovery of late effects from their own exposure to this new form of irradiation [3].

The First Publications of Radiation Late Effects

The use of radium to treat cancers came from the first observations of the induced skin erythema and later ulceration when radium sources were kept near the human body [6]. It was observed that radium caused normal tissue damage. The first implantation of radium sources into human cancer was published in the early 1900s

[1, 32]. Therefore, it was thought that radiation damage to normal tissue could be controlled and utilized to localize that damage to a cancer in a patient with a gynecologic cancer, patient with cervical cancer [33], and then later in another patient with head and neck cancer [1].

The first use of the cathode-ray tube used the X-irradiation emitted from the cathode-ray tube to treat an enlarged spleen in a patient in Chicago, Illinois [1–4]. This application to a cancer patient also followed the observations of the toxicity of the X-ray tube for normal skin. The clinical adaptation of an X-ray machine was also the result of the observation that prolonged exposure to X-rays by the technical person who turned on the machine and displayed skin erythema (redness) as an effect of exposure to the X-ray beam. There were visible skin changes and in damage the thought was very similar to that with radium exposure, namely that such a toxic effect could be localized to treat cancer [1–4]. One of the first patients, who was treated with the Roentgen ray was a female, with what appears to have been a case of whether chronic myelogenous leukemia, or myeloid metaplasia, either of which could have produced the splenomegaly, which caused painful enlargement of the spleen [34]. The technique is still being used [34] with modern linear accelerators. These first clinical adaptations of the use of radium and X-rays were initially successful and led to the widespread further uses of these modalities to treat cancer patients.

In addition, in the early days of use of radiation to treat cancer, other uses emerged. The pharmaceutical use of radiation-emitting isotopes was in an advertised and sold concoction called: "radithor"—[35–37].

The publication on radithor [35] recalled that in the 1920s and 1930s, there was much charlatanism and hucksterism in clinical medicine. Other examples include the use of the tesla coil to generate static electricity, which was applied to treat arthritic joints and painful areas. In the era before antibiotics, clinicians reached for any new approach to treat fatal diseases including infections and other effects of aging [37]. Radithor was sold in bottles and can still be found in antique stores, the same bottles from that era. An old bottle of radithor (empty) found in an antique store still had traces of radium and was detectable by a Geiger counter, which was reported in his publication [35, 36]. The radium was considered to be magic such that its consumption would lead to rejuvenation and youthfulness [35, 36] (Table 14.1).

The use of both radium and the cathode-ray tube by physicians was primarily palliative and most patients did not survive long enough to allow observation of late effects, which would have been observed in "cured" cancer patients. These modalities produced serious side effects both acute and late [38–41]. The collection of large amounts of data on radiation late effects was delayed for decades until the widespread use of orthovoltage X-ray machines became available [40]. The initial use of X-ray machines was for diagnostic purposes, not for the treatment of cancer (Table 14.1). Radiation induction of cancer was a prominent late effect [40–43]. Other late effects included cataracts [44–46]. Radiation delivered to children was particularly devastating as it caused cognitive dysfunction and growth abnormalities [20, 47–50]. Modifications in brain irradiation followed [50], as well as, concern for the effects of space radiation cognitive function [51]. However, those first uses in diagnostic radiology did lead to prolonged exposure of people using the machines. Fluoroscopy was used by most physicians in the early twentieth century and now is known to have been quite dangerous. The fluoroscope leaves the X-ray beam on for minutes and allows the radiologist or technician to observe organ motion real time. Imaging many patients per day led to hours of exposure to the fluoroscopist and serious side effects. The first reports of drops in peripheral blood counts from the radiation killing of lymphocytes were only detected as fatigue and loss of energy. Assay for peripheral blood counts were not routinely available, and only skin changes in the fluoroscopist were a detectable indication of toxicity. These early fluoroscopists suffered radiation-induced acute effects (Table 14.2), and the survivors did have late effects, as well. Decades later with the advent of cobalt-60 teletherapy machines (Table 14.1), the use of ionizing irradiation to treat cancer then allowed a retrospective analysis of the toxicity of those early uses of diagnostic orthovoltage X-ray machines (Table 14.1).

Late Effects on Atomic Bomb Survivors

Much information on radiation late effects has been obtained from the meticulous follow-up of survivors of the Hiroshima and Nagasaki atomic bombings and also from the survivors of the Marshallese Islander fusion/thermonuclear bomb testing, primarily on the island of Rongelap. The valuable information that has been obtained from these follow-up protocols must be credited in a large part to the work of William C. Moloney, M.D. (Fig. 14.1), the past Professor of Emeritus of Medicine at Harvard Medical School and the Brigham and Women's Hospital, and past Director of the Division of Hematology at Brigham and Women's Hospital.

Dr. Moloney was one of the first physicians, who had arrived at the Atomic Bomb Casualty Center in Hiroshima, Japan (Fig. 14.1a–e). He worked with Japanese physicians to meticulously catalog the types and magnitudes of radiation-induced injuries in the Japanese survivors. His work was seminal, because his past experience in the United States Army during World War II led him to become an expert in clinical hematology, and this was perfect for the task of evaluating peripheral blood samples and bone marrow samples from the atomic bomb survivors. His many achievements, his paper published in Science, 1955, cataloged the types of leukemia that were observed in the Japanese survivors. This work led him to document that the chronic myelogenous leukemia, which was detected in a significant number of Japanese patients, was not a radiation-induced leukemia, but was part of the genetic background of the Japanese population at that time. There were publications in the literature at that time documenting irradiation-induced leukemia in animal models, principally mice (RF strain at Oakridge Laboratories, Jim Otten), and the work on retrovirus (C-type virus)-induced leukemias in mouse models (Ruscher Moloney, Friend, Kaplan, reference book on viruses). Dr. Moloney's work led to the conclusion that ionizing irradiation was a very poor leukemogen for humans and that the

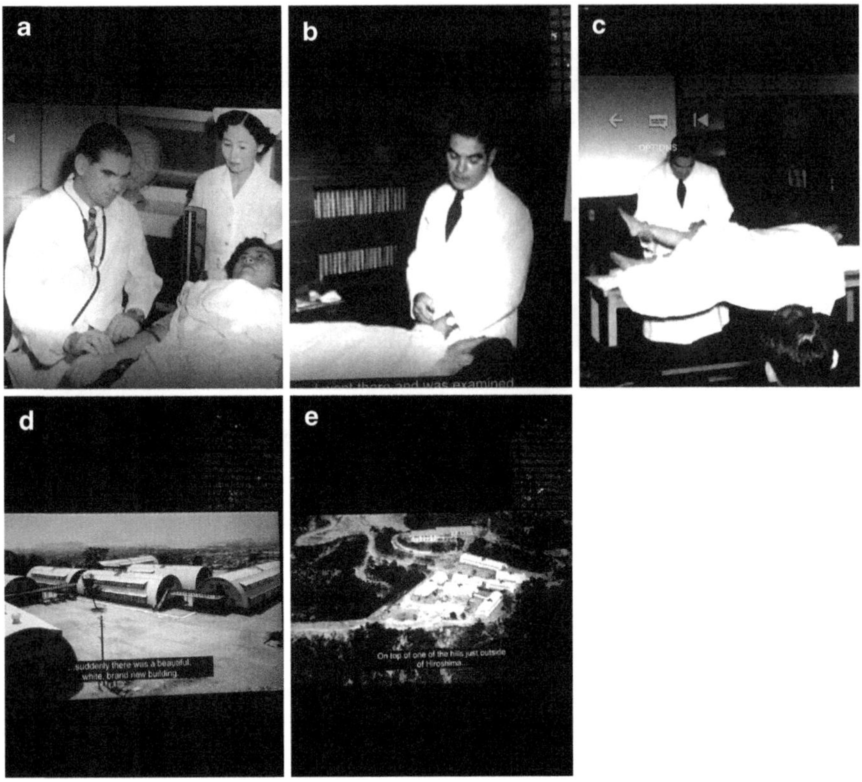

Fig. 14.1 Hiroshima Atomic Bomb Casualty Commission first physician on site: Dr. William C. Moloney (Panels **a**–**e**)

work in animal models could not be related to the Atomic Bomb Casualty Center survivors. His work on irradiation-induced acute effects was primarily that related to epilation, thermal burns, and concussions (Fig. 14.1).

The identification of irradiation-induced cancers in the Japanese survivors was to be the work of the next decades. Studies on the children and grandchildren of the atomic bomb survivors have been published, and there is a mass of literature on possible radiation late effects. These data have become a primary source for establishing protocols and methodology for following total body irradiated cancer patients, who were prepared for bone marrow transplantation and suffered the same acute and late effects of total body irradiation in the clinical setting. There continues to be a wealth of information generated by the follow-up of the now three generations of the Hiroshima and Nagasaki survivors.

Additional information on radiation late effects came from the close follow-up of Marshallese survivors of the fusion/thermonuclear bomb testing, primarily, on the island of Rongelap. Sites for testing of thermonuclear weapons in the late 1950s led military experts to target the Marshallese islands. The prevailing winds were projected to carry the radioactive fallout out to sea, but on the day of one of the largest tests, the wind had changed and fallout was directed to the island of Rongelap. Dr. Moloney and a team of physicians visited the Marshallese islanders on Rongelap and found that many people were living underneath huts. They already sustained radiation burns from the fallout, primarily, of radioiodine and cesium. The documentation of skin burns from fallout radiation created a significant body of literature, which is important for understanding acute radiation burns, skin ulceration, and secondary infections, the development of acute countermeasures for radiation burns, and the observation of the timing of the development of radiation skin and subcutaneous fibrosis. The data led to publications, which have been important for modern radiation oncologists, who treat patients with electron beam (beta-radiation), which simulates the skin reaction seen in the beta-irradiation radioactive fallout, and also the early publications demonstrating that the new technique of intensity-modulated radiotherapy (IMRT).

IMRT is based on three-dimensional treatment planning to deliver a highly collimated photon (X-ray) irradiation resulting in the same skin reactions. Development of treatments for beta-radiation (electron beam)-induced skin burn came largely from the data collected on radioactive fallout from the Marshallese islanders. There was an additional complication with the Marshallese islanders in that many of the survivors ingested and inhaled radioisotopes, as well. Argonne National Laboratories developed a whole-body irradiation (whole-body burden) scanning technique and algorithms for estimating the total dose of radioisotopes that had been inhaled/ingested. The patients at an in-patient facility at Brookhaven National Laboratories were assessed for whole-body burden of isotopes and followed for development of acute and late effects. These patients were primarily those from radiation accidents in the United States during the decades of the "Cold War." Techniques for managing whole-body burden of inhaled or ingested isotopes were also valuable for the development of chelators by scientists at the Lawrence Livermore Laboratories in the 1980s and 1990s.

Much of the information on the diagnosis and management of radiation late effects came from military operations. The survivors of the Hiroshima and Nagasaki atomic bombings, the survivors of the Rongelap/Marshallese Islander exposure to radioactive fallout from the fusion bomb testing, and other military incidents comprised much available information on radiation late effects. These data have been of great value in clinical medicine, preparing generations of radiation oncology residents to manage the side effects of therapeutic radiation.

In addition, to having served as the Director of the Division of Hematology in the Department of Medicine at Brigham and Women's Hospital (BWH) of Harvard Medical School, and prior to that in the Thorndike Laboratories in Boston City Hospital, Dr. Moloney contributed numerous seminal medical publications to the medical literature. His research team at BWH contributed the first multiagent chemotherapy regimen for management of leukemia (the VMP regimen), which preceded the more commonly cited MOPP regimen for Hodgkin's disease that was developed by Vincent Di Vita, George Canellos, and colleagues at the National Cancer Institute. Chemotherapy drugs for the treatment of leukemia and lymphoma have become the mainstay of therapy and persist to this day.

The advent of targeted therapies, immunotherapy, and other systemic administered non-cytotoxic drugs will eventually replace chemotherapy agents that produce systemic toxicity to normal tissues. However, the history of chemotherapy started with the work of Sidney Farber, at Harvard Medical School, with the first development of anti-folate drugs. Aminopterin and methotrexate are drugs designed to produce DNA damage by mimicking folate, which was required for normal hematopoiesis, but also for the proliferation of leukemia cells. Pediatric patients at the "Jimmy Fund" of Children's Hospital of Harvard Medical School, Dr. Farber, and his hematology colleague, William C. Moloney.

William C. Moloney pioneered the use of sequential single-agent chemotherapy in children with Leukemia and other pediatric cancers. Many of these children also received radiotherapy of bulky mass disease, primarily, in lymphoma and pediatric Hodgkin's disease during the 1960s and 1970s. However, the first chemotherapy protocols were sequential single-agent delivery systems. Patients received methotrexate and had a predictable fall in white blood cell counts as this drug killed leukemia cells, but there was rapid recurrence. They then received 6-mercapoturine (6-MP), which was another antimetabolite that focused on the purine component of DNA replication. Children, who failed this second regimen were placed on, then-new drug, Vincristine. Other drugs were tested at the Jimmy Fund, including L-Asparaginase, all as single agents. Combination chemotherapy followed was designed to target the nadir of white blood cell counts, which occurred at different times, and interdigitate the delivery of multiple agents based on their normal tissue toxicity. For example, one drug, which produced a drop in blood counts could be given, and then at the nadir blood counts, a second drug could be administered, which did not have a toxicity, primarily, on the bone marrow. While this work was being carried out in pediatric leukemia patients at the Jimmy Fund, Dr. Moloney developed the combination chemotherapy approach of outpatients at the Brigham and Women's Hospital, Division of Hematology, resulting in the VAMP regimen of (vincristine, aminopterin, methotrexate, and prednisone).

In addition to training generations of hematology fellows and general medicine residents, Dr. Moloney cataloged his own work on the translation of the valuable lessons he learned at the Hiroshima Atomic Bomb Casualty Center (Fig. 14.1) to his practice of medicine in the modern era. His book "Pioneering Hematology" provides a useful reference for the new generation of physician-scientists. While caring for pediatric and adult leukemia patients, Dr. Moloney developed a model system for testing drugs in the rat. While RNA virus-induced leukemias in rats was not detected with the frequency and diversity, as it was in mouse models, he discovered ways to use the rat model as a way to develop treatments for central nervous system recurrence of leukemia. During these same decades, genetic inbred strains of mice and rats were being developed by investigators including Jacob Furth. His work provided the genetically inbred mouse strains and rat strains that are now used to develop new targeted therapies with less normal tissue toxicity.

Understanding the late effects of irradiation is a topic of great interest in the years after the atomic bombing of Hiroshima and Nagasaki. Beginning with Cold War and with the advent of thermonuclear weapons with greater destructive power and greater scope of production of fallout, there were medical-legal consequences of the atmospheric atomic bomb testing in the late 1940s and 1950s.

At the atomic bomb test center in Nevada, soldiers were tasked with carrying out maneuvers at some distance from the detonation of nuclear weapons. These studies with the military personnel followed work using animal model systems including: pigs, cattle, and other animals that were placed close to the blast zone and in the setting of susceptibility to fallout. Much of these data have recently been declassified, and the atomic bomb test museum in Las Vegas, Nevada, has both physical evidence and video documentary presentations that are available to the general public to describe this era in the US development of nuclear weapons. While atmospheric testing of nuclear weapons ceased in the decade after the 1960s, there is evidence that the atomic bomb detonations during that era produced radioactive fallout, some of which was carried as far east as states on the Atlantic seaboard. Studies were done to demonstrate that inhalation of radioisotopes from the fission reactions in Nevada could be detected in the bone marrow cells of individuals, who were breathing air during the late 1950s. In addition, facilities that produced fissionable materials for the plutonium pits, fission core of nuclear weapons, in the 1950s and 1960s were the subject of litigation regarding leakage of radioisotopes from these facilities and potential exposure of individuals in the communities adjacent to the facilities. In both the situation of the soldiers in proximity to atmospheric testing of the atomic bombs in the 1950s, and in individuals and communities adjacent to facilities that were producing fissionable material for nuclear weapons, policies were targeted at the government or private sector of individuals, who were responsible for these test sites/facilities.

In the course of preparation of data for litigation, background levels of radioisotopes from fission bombs were detected in humans in multiple locations. With the sensitivity of detection of extremely small quantities of radioisotopes including both short-lived and long-lived isotopes (long-lived isotopes being uranium 235 and plutonium 239), the sensitivity of detecting small numbers of molecules has been reported. The, then significant fear of radiation in the United States in the 1950s and 1960s, following the Atomic bombings in Japan, and the fusion bomb testing in the Marshallese islands, and the then "Cold War" concern for military use of nuclear weapons by the United States and/or then Soviet Union, there was a continuing concern for late effects of radiation, primarily the induction of cancer. Environmental contaminants in addition to irradiation and radioisotopes have been implicated in the induction of cancer (asbestos, talc containing asbestos, and other environmental contaminants), all of which have been the subjects of discussion for litigation. A primary concern for late effects of any form of irradiation is that of the induction of cancer [40–43].

The topic of radiation carcinogenesis relates to the late effects of therapeutic radiation, radiation nuclear weapons, and radiation terrorism, as well as concern about the effects of space radiation. One unifying concept in this book is the fact that radiation is a carcinogen and presents a risk factor for humans in any situation, whether clinical application of radiation, or as a consequence of environmental exposure (both accidental and willful), and remains a major concern for the preparation of astronauts for missions in which significant long-term exposure to radiation will be a reality.

Late effects of irradiation include but are not limited to carcinogenesis and leukemogenesis. The collection of data with respect to human exposure and late effects began with the discovery of radioisotopes (Marie and Pierre Curie and Bacquerel [32]) and with the discovery of the Roentgen ray. There were individual case reports during this era, but the major collection of data began after the Hiroshima/Nagasaki bombings in World War II, and the massive development of nuclear weapons, which followed. The use of radiation in clinical management of cancer patients led to further acquisition of data. The available evidence now is copious.

The best approach to understanding radiation-induced cancer is to look at each tissue, organ, and organ system, but also with respect to the age of the individual, comorbid disease, genetic factors in the background, and medical history. Several major conclusions can be drawn from this plethora of data. Radiation exposure to radioactive iodine does lead to thyroid cancer [41]. Total body irradiation exposure does lead to both aplastic anemia and leukemia. Therapeutic radiation to specific sites leads to the generation of radiation-induced sarcomas that are directly dependent upon radiation dose, volume of tissue treated, and fraction size [42]. Some of these data do relate to experiments in animal models, but not all. In cancer patients, who received radiotherapy in addition to combination chemotherapy, attempts have been made to determine, which of the components of multimodality agents could be considered the most significant in the induction of a subsequent second cancer.

The role of radiation in treating Hodgkin's disease was important, but did lead to secondary cancers including large B-cell lymphomas [52]. This work followed similar studies in pediatric patients, who received combination chemoradiotherapy [40].

Documentation of Radiation Late Effects in Cancer Patients Who Were Treated in the Early Twentieth Century

The diagnostic X-ray machines that were used in the first decades of the twentieth century produced orthovoltage X-rays (Table 14.1). These machines produced a spectrum of X-ray energies all below 1 megavoltage energies. These X-rays could be tuned to eliminate certain low energies by filtering the beam with aluminum or copper leaflets that absorbed the low energies (1–4). This filtration was important since the low-energy X-rays delivered dose deposition primarily to the skin surface of patients. The energies of X-rays with energy below 1 MEV were usually in the range of 100–250 KVP (Kilovoltage). The orthovoltage X-rays had a depth dose distribution, which produced significant deposition of the radiation on the skin surface or at several millimeters depth. The low-voltage X-rays also had a large component of backscatter [1]. Backscatter is caused by X-ray protons hitting and ejecting electrons from atoms in tissue and some rebounded backwards like the rebound of a basketball from the rim or backboard of the goal. The orthovoltage X-rays that hit tissues under the skin produced electrons that backscattered to the skin creating even more significant erythema during the acute phase of radiation delivery and also led to the first observations of clinical late effects in these patients, who were treated for either benign conditions/diseases or were treated for localized tumors, which may have recurred after surgery or had been controlled for months to years and then recurred at a time when the patient was no longer a candidate for surgical re-excision.

These patients were treated with a diagnostic X-ray machine that was primarily used for diagnostic X-rays, but now was directed to kill cancer cells by leaving the beam on for longer. Diagnostic radiologists delivered the first radiotherapy. There was, at this time, no separate specialty of therapeutic radiology (now called radiotherapy) [19]. There were no separate departments of radiation oncology in hospitals. There was no separate board certification for therapeutic use of radiation. In fact, during the transition years before the creation of a separate specialty of radiation oncology, physicians were "double-boarded" in both diagnostic and therapeutic radiology.

The first reported appearance of radiation acute and late effects were by diagnostic radiologists, who were the only physicians that were board certified to use X-ray machines for both diagnostic and then late treatment of cancer. By the 1940s, there began decades of experience by radiologists documenting the appearance of scar tissue in previously irradiated skin tissue [9]. These observations led to the condition now known as radiation fibrosis, which resulted from changes in the skin that were reminiscent of thermal burns, chemical burns (including those from mustard gas exposure during World War I), and traumatic abrasions. The early reports provided the first clinical patient evidence of late tissue fibrosis, which was analyzed by pathologists, who were the ones reporting changes at autopsy [10]. The physicians, who followed their patients, treated the fibrosis much as they would with patients, who presented with fibrosis from other causes including applying moisturizers and skin creams and also delivering physical therapy or massage to attempt to improve skin elasticity. The pathologists found in microscopic examination of the areas of scarring that there was a large component of proliferation of fibroblasts in the radiation-induced scar tissues at the sites of prior radiation.

In the modern era, cases of radiation fibrosis are limited to patients, who were cured of head and neck cancers or lung cancers, and presented decades later with radiation fibrosis [11]. Rare severe cases are currently being treated with plastic surgery that removes the fibrotic areas and may perform reconstruction with vascularized skin flaps that are transferred from adjacent unirradiated tissues [12]. Even more recent research programs are now focused on the elucidation of the mechanism of the effectiveness of injecting into the radiation fibrotic area, the patient's own adipocyte stem cells that are harvested from fat tissue from the abdominal wall. Another approach has been to use allograft fat tissue that is harvested from donors [14–18].

One such source of allograft adipocyte stem cells is from donors, who are undergoing resection of adipose tissue from their abdominal wall as part of a program of weight reduction, cosmetic surgery, or as part of a program of bariatric surgery. This donor adipocyte tissue is transplanted/injected into the fibrotic areas of radiation fibrosis [14–18]. The fibrosis remodeling effect of adipocyte injection is remarkably well tolerated, and there is no significant graft rejection phenomenon. New therapeutic approaches also include recent research into the effectiveness of injection into the fibrotic area of extracellular matrix from the adipocyte stem cells that are grown in vitro [17, 18].

Thus, the first publications of radiation fibrosis that were induced by the then-new Roentgen ray modality in the early decades of the twentieth century described fibrous tissue very similar to scar tissue from thermal burns or chemical injury [5–7]. Decades later, the molecular mechanisms that are involved in radiation fibrosis were shown to be also evolving and causing much more significant late effects, causing much more deleterious effects in multiple organs other than the skin [17, 18].

Furthermore, the other observations from the early twentieth-century use of orthovoltage radiation was that of the cumulative effects of low dose radiation exposure by people including physicians, who were constantly working in proximity to the radiation sources. These people include not only the physicians using such sources for medical treatments, but also in the case of X-ray machines, those people, who were carrying out fluoroscopy and not using appropriate lead shielding, such as lead aprons to protect themselves from radiation. One serious late effect, namely infertility, was due to the non-appreciated radiosensitivity of spermatogonia and oogonia. In the case of the physicians, physicists, or technicians, who were performing fluoroscopy, this was a serious late effect.

Diagnostic X-rays have been used for over 100 years routinely for medical management, and there is a plethora of publications from such radiation exposure during the early twentieth century. These publications document the ability of X-rays to detect abnormalities in bone including bone tumors and fractures. The data led to widespread use of radiation machines for diagnosis or many patient presentations and by not medical personnel. In fact, before X-ray machines were limited to availability in healthcare facilities, shoe salesmen often used fluoroscopy to measure the foot size for determining the appropriate shoe size (Table 14.1). There were other multiple examples of the use of X-radiation machines to treat disease states other than cancer, and these uses resulted in the exposed people living for decades, such that long-term follow-up of irradiated people led to the detection of many radiation late effects.

In the early twentieth century, wristwatch dials were marketed as having numbers that glowed in the dark. This strategy was used to advertise the sale of watches that were fluorescent at night. Radium was initially applied in a liquid that was painted onto the numbers and the hands of the watches. Radium was used to paint the numbers on the watch dials, because the capacity of radium225 in its degeneration led to emission of photons in the visible fluorescent light range [42]. In fact, the name radium was given to that purified element by its discover, Marie Curie. She and her husband, Pierre, purified radium from pitch blend, and it was she, who first noticed that the purified element was radiant [32]. The early watch-dial painters would often lick the brushes that were used to put the liquid radium on the watch dials. Decades later, it was observed that radium had accumulated in the oral cavity tissues in the mouth and was deposited in the bones of the head and neck region producing oral cavity cancers, primarily those in the jaw. While Marie and Pierre, themselves, suffered late effects of carcinogenesis for radium exposure [32], these data from many watch-dial painters were one of the first examples of a serious and life-threatening "late effect" of irradiation, namely carcinogenesis [38–40].

In the early and mid-twentieth century, X-ray machines were used to treat many benign diseases, because of the capacity of X-rays to reduce/decrease the volume of tissues whether they contained cancer or not, physicians through the X-rays could provide a safe and effective nonsurgical approach to reducing the volume of enlarged lymphoid tissues, such as tonsils (Table 14.1). The use of orthovoltage radiation to treat the spine in patients with painful ankylosing spondylosis (curvature of the spine causing deformities including kyphosis) led to clinical application in which multiple small-volume sites (several vertebral bodies) in the thoracic and lumbar spine were treated with orthovoltage irradiation [40]. Other studies documented the widespread use of orthovoltage X-rays to treat this not benign condition (but not cancer) of the spine with X-ray treatments. Physicians documented the induction of leukemia in these patients, who had multiple courses of X-ray treatments with orthovoltage X-rays over decades [40]. Most recently, in the 1940s, orthovoltage X-rays were used to treat children with enlarged tonsils and who presented with repeated tonsillitis and associated infections (Table 14.1). The thinking at the time was that irradiation could reduce the size of these large lymph nodes (tonsils and adenoids) and prevent infection without the need for surgery, which was then tonsillectomy and adenoidectomy. The follow-up of many of these individuals showed that many suffered the induction of lymphoma and other cancers in the irradiated volumes (Table 14.1). The observation extended to the induction of noncancerous hematologic conditions including the histiocytosis [40]. Another example of irradiation-induced cancer as a late effect of orthovoltage radiation of the head and neck region was after its use to treat acne and other benign skin diseases [40]. Children, who were treated with orthovoltage radiation for acne, often developed skin fibrosis and in some developed skin or thyroid cancer. The collimation of early X-ray machines was imperfect, and many of these patients had scatter irradiation to the thyroid, which may have led to the developed of thyroid cancer.

This setting-up of orthovoltage radiation fields in the early and middle twentieth century was not precise and did not always limit the deposition of radiation from the external beam of orthovoltage X-rays to the target only. The irradiation often produced significant dose distribution to the thyroid [41].

There was a second and entirely different mechanism of thyroid carcinogenesis from radiation exposure. This carcinogenesis came from the ingestion of radioiodine (I-125 or I-131), which accumulated in the thyroid. Unintentional administration of radioiodine is different from the use of therapeutic radioiodine to treat thyroid cancer [43]. In fact, this conundrum is representative of the overall inherent contradiction of radiotherapy. Stated simply, high doses of targeted radiation kill cancer, while lower doses or repeated smaller doses cause cancer. The deposition of iodine radioisotopes in the organ is caused by the biology of the thyroid itself, namely the need for iodine in the synthesis of thyroid hormones including thyroxine.

The human diet requires iodine uptake by the thyroid. The absence of iodine in the diet causes the thyroid to enlarge and causes goiters. Radioiodine can be targeted to its uptake by the thyroid tissues and once accumulated kills the thyroid cells (Table 14.1). For some forms of thyroid cancer that have intact iodine uptake, this radioiodine therapy will work. Undifferentiated thyroid cancers that will not concentrate iodine cannot be treated this way. A test of uptake of thyroid scan using nontherapeutic iodine precedes the use of ablative radioiodine, to be sure that the patient's tumor will accumulate the therapeutic radioiodine that will be administered later. Higher doses of irradiation such as used to treat lung cancer were reported to induce sarcomas [42].

Thyroid accumulation of a carcinogenic radioisotope iodine occurs from radioactive fallout that has appeared at both fission and fusion bomb test sites [41]. In the cases of the Japanese Hiroshima and Nagasaki atomic bombings, the data collection revealed fallout containing radioiodine. Radioiodine accumulation also was a concern after radiation nuclear reactor accidents, with both the Chernobyl and the Fukeishime Dai Ichi [43] nuclear reactor accidents. All of these data demonstrated that the thyroid was a target for carcinogenesis by X-ray exposure from accumulation of nontherapeutic levels of radioiodine. Therefore, two major late effects of ionizing irradiation in humans have been well documented from several data sets and include the "benign" tissue effect of radiation fibrosis, primarily, in skin, and the malignant side effect of induction of malignancy.

By the 1950s, any delivery of therapeutic radiation, whether by radioisotope administration or external beam irradiation required both: (1) mandatory monitoring of radiation dose and volume treated and (2) an informed consent process to explain to patients in detail the risks of the acute, as well as the late effects of irradiation. Patients were then and must now be informed about fibrosis and carcinogenesis/leukemogenesis [12, 21, 22].

How Does the Data Obtained from Medical Identification of Radiation Late Effects Apply to Development of Countermeasures for Radiation Terrorism and Help Prepare for Managing the Irradiation During Space Flight?

Nearly, 100 years of data acquired from treating patients with radiotherapy for cancer has produced a vast storehouse of information on radiation late effects. These data now can be applied to understand the effects of ionizing irradiation for total body, partial body irradiation, and organ-specific radiation [1, 4]. As a medical specialty, radiation oncology has developed protocols for treating nearly every form and presentation of cancer. Furthermore, the radiation therapy beams for patient irradiation have continually evolved and changed over the last 100 years to the point now where orthovoltage radiation machines have been replaced by extremely sophisticated delivery systems. In the 1960s, the introduction of the use of cobalt-60 teletherapy machines became the state of the art. Teletherapy units, which delivered gamma radiation at 1.0 MeV, were touted as "skin-sparing" radiation. The major advantage of cobalt 60 was in its ability to target the radiation dose deeper into the patient and repeatedly spare the skin (Table 14.1). The concept of electron "build up" to reach a Dmax (depth in tissue from the skin surface to the 100% dose from a single beam) greatly reduced the dose that had to be delivered to reach the tumor within the patient. The cobalt unit delivered a 100% prescribed dose to a 1.0 cm. depth not to the skin surface. Thus, the skin did not receive a dose greater than that which was prescribed for the tumor and skin burns (erythema, ulcers, and moist desquamation-weeping lesions did not occur as rapidly as had been the case with orthovoltage irradiation). The depth dose characteristics of cobalt-60 also reduced backscatter and eliminated much of the acute skin damage that was associated with orthovoltage irradiation.

The orthovoltage irradiation that preceded the use of cobalt-60 when compared provided much of the information on radiation late effects on skin, to the underlying muscle, and to soft tissues, primarily in the head and neck region for treatment of oral and oropharyngeal cancer, but also with the treatment of breast cancer, and pelvic cancers including cancers of the cervix, endometrium, vulvovaginal region, and colorectal cancers [22]. These patients all had in common the ability of irradiation to provide long-term local control or in many cases cure of their cancer with less skin fibrosis. The cobalt-60 machines allowed patients to survive years and decades. They did, however, develop late effects in other organs and many such late effects could be explained in part by the same process of radiation fibrosis. The clinical radiotherapy of the 1920s through 1950s did provide the basic data for dose-response curves, dose volume relationships, radiation fractionation, and the different types of radiation beams that could deliver radiation dose to specific sites and tissue.

The first radiation oncologists (who were, in fact, diagnostic radiologists using the Roentgen ray to treat cancer) [1–3] made the initial observations that are the foundation of modern radiotherapy. These individuals include Drs. Baclesse, Papillion, Gilbert Fletcher, and Piercain. These individuals made the key observations that the magnitude of the damage to normal tissue caused by irradiation was dependent on three critical factors: (1) volume of tissue treated; (2) the dose delivered per fraction in fractionated irradiation; and (3) the total number of fractions (total dose) delivered.

The fractionation protocols, which continue in modern-day radiotherapy, have their basis in the work of these pioneers in large part, because the radiobiology has not changed.

While 100 years may seem like a long time, a lesson comes from the history of aviation. If one looks at the biplane flown by the Wright Brothers in 1909 sitting on a runway next to a modern F15 Strike Eagle, one must conclude that the basic principle of flight has not changed. Lift must be achieved by the same combination of thrust and wing curvature. Similarly, over the same 100 years comparing the first Roentgen ray tube treatment machine with our modern stereotactic linear accelerator, the basic radiobiology of cells, tissues, organs, and volume treated has not changed. The clinical radiation oncologists of the 1930s and 1940s proved that normal tissues could better tolerate radiation if there was a time between the delivery of lower doses per day rather than giving a larger dose in a single day. Fractionation schemes devised decades ago have led to our now standard fractionation protocols, which have persisted in clinical radiotherapy through the early 2000s.

By the year 2000, nearly all orthovoltage radiation machines and all but a few cobalt-60 units had been replaced by linear accelerators to deliver radiation at energies that were tunable to the depth dose curves that were desired by the clinician. Four MeV linear accelerators were the mainstay of radiotherapy in the 1970s. These machines were replaced by higher energy machines delivering X-rays up to 23 MeV and higher (Table 14.1). Also, these linear accelerators could deliver electron beam irradiation by bypassing the tungsten targets that were hit by electrons in the waveguide to produce X-rays. Thus, the linear accelerators could deliver X-rays (photons) and negatively charged electrons, both with tunable energies. This flexibility of radiation beam construction provided the clinician with the ability to target the depth to underlying tumor volumes in large patients, sometimes, 20–30 cm. deep by using the high-energy photon beams. The availability of electron beam delivery by the same machines allowed targeting of superficial tumor volumes, since the electrons stopped in tissues at more superficial depths (Table 14.1). The potentially most effective use of proton beam irradiation, is due to its delivery of the dose deep in tissue and has the advantage of stopping at depth-based upon the the rapid fall of the dose at the Bragg-peak. The physics of proton travel in tissue is dramatic. This allows deposition of the major energy deep in tissue. The Bragg peak of energy deposition is due to the slowing down or stopping point of the heavier particle-weight of protons producing an even more precise depth dose curve to deliver the dose precisely and far from the skin [4]. The ability to use these linear accelerators or proton machines each with programmable and tunable energy led to a better outcome for patients, but also provided more critical information on radiation late effects.

Combinations of electron beam energies (generated by removing the tungsten target from the electrons traveling down the waveguide in the linear accelerator) allowed the electrons to directly hit the patient-provided depth dose curves that could enhance radiation dose to volumes several centimeters deep rather than the very deep targeting by high-energy X-rays.

Electron beam irradiation was also used extensively in the 1970s and 1980s and even today to treat breast cancer patients, who had recurrence on the chest wall and also head and neck cancer patients, who had tumor recurrence in lymph nodes. Long-term cancer survivors of the use of these modalities developed significantly less late fibrosis in the skin in the treated area. Management of radation treatment plans is focused on reduction of the tissue volumes treated, and optimal use of fractionation protocols including hyperfractionation to further improve treatment outcomes. Hyperfractionation is a scheme in which two or more doses of radiation are given per day, separated by 4–6 h. The time allows for normal tissue repair and also allows radiation oncologists to manage the concepts of volume, total dose, and fraction size to get the optimal cancer control results and to minimize the acute and late toxicities of radiotherapy. All of these studies, which have accumulated over decades of clinical research have led to a clear understanding of the pathophysiology of radiation acute effects, but also have provided a window to understand late effects in many normal tissues within the transit volume of the X-ray/electron/proton beams.

What has been to date, an underestimated and not a focus of concern by radiation oncologists and radiation physicists, has been the production of neutrons by X-ray machines that deliver radiation in excess of 10 MeV [53–56]. Neutrons are generated by the X-rays hitting the components of the shielding in the collimator, which is composed of depleted uranium or other heavy metals [54]. Neutrons are detected and assayed/quantitated at the time of acceptance testing of newly installed linear accelerators. There is currently no mandate for routinely measuring the levels of neutron that are generated and contribute to patient irradiation during radiotherapy protocols. At the present time, it is accepted that patients are receiving some dose of whole-body neutrons [54]. This topic will be more relevant to understanding the role of neutrons, as a component of space irradiation, particularly after the structural components of the space vehicle have been decided upon. The study of the radiobiological late effects of neutron irradiation is now being studied by a few research groups that have neutron generating machines available. There are some reports from experimental animal studies (Colorado State University, Columbia, Brookhaven, Europe, and China) [55].

The concept of late effects, as with acute radiation effects, focused on the three major components of clinical radiotherapy with respect to normal tissue tolerance: (1) volume treated; (2) dose per fraction; and (3) total dose. This being the case, there is a plethora of data regarding late effects for each of the multiple organs that were irradiated during the treatment of patients for cancer. Data concerning radiation late effects led to several conclusions regarding common biological processes like fibrosis, but also individual organ-specific effects that are relevant to that organ and its adjacent anatomic structures.

A discussion of clinical radiation oncology late effects in each of several normal organs and organ systems may be helpful to understand the late effects of space irradiation. Clinical radiotherapy-induced late effects led radiobiologists to develop radiation countermeasures. Thus, clinical radiotherapy provides a basis for the use of organ-specific information for multiple applications of newly discovered medical radiation countermeasures.

Late Effects of Brain Irradiation

One of the major reports of analysis of data in the 1970s came from multiple studies of children with leukemia, who received whole-brain irradiation to be prophylactic to nests cells of leukemia cells that were lodged in the brain and could not be reached by the then-available chemotherapy agents [47]. Whole-brain radiation was delivered to children at usually around 20 Gy in 10 fractions of 2 Gy delivered over 14 days [47]. Hundreds of children received cranial radiotherapy (whole-brain irradiation) and were followed for years and multiple reports documented cognitive deficits, which appeared years after irradiation, while it was assumed during the 1970s that this radiation would be "safe" and that the risks of any damage would be greatly outweighed by the prevention of recurrence of leukemia provided one of the first dramatic reports of an unanticipated late effect, which changed therapeutic programs. Whole-brain irradiation has been now essentially eliminated from the treatment of leukemia except for rare T-cell variants and other variants that have a propensity for local recurrence in the brain. Another exception to the elimination of whole-brain radiation from clinical protocols is the rare cancers that place the entire craniospinal volume at risk for tumor spread such as medulloblastoma [48]. New chemotherapy drugs, which penetrate the blood/brain barrier and reach the cerebral spinal fluid, are being modified to replace radiation delivery to this large volume. Another exception, which may require whole-brain irradiation, is in some adult patients with small-cell lung cancer, which is known to recur in the brain [49]. Randomized perspective clinical trials are still in progress to either deliver prophylactic whole-brain radiation after local control of the initial cancer has been documented and after an appropriate interval has passed after the completion of chest radiation and chemotherapy is completed. This modality is then applied compared to no delivery of radiation at all. Other than these limited examples, the use of whole-brain radiation for prophylaxis against the suspected risk of local recurrence of the tumor in the brain has been minimized or eliminated due to both the availability of stereotactic radiosurgery beams (Table 14.1), but also due to the toxicity and late effects.

In more recent years, clinical studies have reported the use of a whole-brain radiation technique, which could spare the hippocampus region [50]. When whole-brain radiation is used now in protocols for the exceptions including T-cell leukemia and protocols for small-cell lung cancer, the addition of specific shielding of the hippocampus is now routinely carried out. In protocols for treating pediatric and adult patients with primary brain tumors or in some cases metastasis, hippocampal sparing is routinely carried out. It has been demonstrated in animal models and in patients that sparing the hippocampus and the neural network that goes through the hippocampus greatly reduces the cognitive deficit that was seen in the early experiments for childhood whole-brain radiation for prophylaxis against recurrence in the brain in the 1970s [49, 50]. The general concept now is to reduce the use of brain irradiation, to any volume, and certainly to minimize and use of whole-brain irradiation, if possible. The only exceptions to the routine use of whole-brain irradiation now appear to be in cases of palliation of significant symptoms of cancer recurrence including seizures activity and pain or in situations in which the chemotherapy available cannot effectively control disease that has metastasized to the brain.

Protocols for the use of immunomodulatory therapies including point inhibitors and CAR-T-cell therapies are now in clinical trials with a major goal of improving the rate of cure, decreasing morbidity, and also eliminating the need for radiation. The overall conclusion from this assessment of historical data must be that ionizing radiation to the brain is deleterious. As regarding the effects of radiation on the brain in both radiation counter-terrorism and space irradiation, there is a recent report of significant cognitive deficits that are induced in experimental animals that are exposed to components of galactic cosmic radiation (GCR) [51]. There is also a program of research that is promulgated by NASA to develop medical countermeasures for space radiation induction of cancer and neurocognitive deficits [51].

Radiation Effects on the Eye

The late effect of cataract formation in the eyes is a documented event. Cataracts have been observed in patients receiving irradiation, where the lens is in the field. There is also clearly documented evidence of increase in cataract size and earlier onset in the astronauts going back to the first space program missions [44–46]. Many of these astronauts are developing cataracts. There are data to support the increased risk for cataracts in individuals exposed to high LET particle irradiation, protons, and neutrons [53–56]. The molecular mechanism of cataracts is associated with increased deposition of crystalline components of the lens. These molecular mechanism and biochemistry are very similar to that occurring in other cells and cell types after radiation exposure and will be discussed in the context of both the inflammatory response that follows the onset of late effects of radiation in multiple organs and the damage in both epithelial and endothelial cells, which occurs in accumulating fashion and may be part of the mechanism by which late effects are initiated after the latent period [24, 25].

In brain irradiation protocols including radiotherapy of orbital lymphoma or lymphoma recurrence in the posterior orbit of the eye, the lens is shielded, if possible [46]. Individuals being treated for leukemia or lymphoma recurrance and with presentation of cancer cells in the retro-orbital space or other patients with cancer of the ethmoid sinuses or frontal sinus, challenged dosimetrists to design plans that shield the lens of the eyes. Shielding the lens prevents cataract formation. Similarly, treating choroid melanoma or other tumors of the retina, using microbeam irradiation can protect the lens. The microbeam is a recent technology that has provided targeting of very small (millimeter diameter volumes), so that the lens is shielded. Anticipated cure of many forms of cancer near the eye always takes into account the known risk factor of cataract formation [46].

Head and Neck Region Tissues

A major dataset has accumulated on the hundreds of survivors of head and neck cancer, who have had radiation. A recent research program [15] focuses on the trajectory of onset of radiation fibrosis in multiple tissues within the target volume of patients treated for head and neck cancer. Prominent is the initiation of fibrosis in the pharyngeal constrictor muscles resulting in delayed, severe dysphagia, difficulty swallowing, and the alterations in voice resulting from fibrosis of the muscles in the larynx. This collection of patients in the survivorship clinics of many medical centers provides a focus for studying both ways to prevent late effects and manage the early onset and the use of new drugs as radiation countermeasures to treat fibrosis. Depending on the radiation dose delivered, interaction with combination chemotherapy, and site of the initial head and neck cancer, cured patients may be at risk for radiation induction of soft tissue sarcomas. This is in the category of radiation carcinogenesis, very similar to what was described above in the early radiation population.

Thyroid

Thyroid cancer caused by external beam radiation and radioisotopes is a real problem, and the thyroid should be shielded. Tissues that are positive for radioiodine uptake have been calculated [41]. The use of radioiodine to ablate the thyroid for thyroid cancer results in placing that organ at risk for thyroid carcinogenesis. Thyroid ablation to treat hyperthyroidism is still a clinical modality and risks must be explained to patients (Table 14.1). How these areas of the head and neck region including soft tissues, thyroid, the eye, and the brain are very relevant to the discussions of space radiation and radiation counter-terrorism.

Thoracic Irradiation

The thoracic irradiated volume, total dose delivered, and dose fractionation scheme are critical in placing the lung at risk for radiation-induced pulmonary fibrosis (RIPF) [23–25]. The mechanism of lung fibrosis is currently being studied intensively. The role for the Fgr kinase [24] has been important. For kinase is a gatekeeper for genes involved in regulating profibrotic genes including those controling the deposition of collagen, increasing TGF-β production, and is also involved in producing inflammatory cytokines that recruit monocytes from the bone marrow into tissues including the lung, where they produce profibrotic factors. Preventing fibrosis has been focused with lung, because of the increasing number of patients, who are at risk for this late radiation side effect. Up until the 1970s, thoracic irradiation was common for patients with Hodgkin's disease [52]. Because of the side effects of damage to lung and heart, radiotherapy has now been eliminated or restricted to very small numbers of Hodgkin's disease patients. Combination chemotherapy, which is effective has been used nearly exclusively. Radiation fibrosis of the lung has many factors in common with that of environmental lung disease including silicosis and post-viral causes, including that which is now being reported among COVID-19 survivors [57]. In conclusion, RIPF has in common a potential gatekeeper (Fgr kinase), which may be involved in many forms of lung fibrosis, which may be a target for the development of an effective radiation countermeasure.

Cardiac Late Effects

Until the 1970s, it was assumed that heart irradiation to doses up to 40 Gy would be safe, and thus, Hodgkin's disease was routinely treated by either the mantle or the thunderbird treatment volume. Henry Kaplan et al. [52] defined in their textbook the techniques for delivery chest irradiation while blocking normal lung as best possible, but including all the lymph nodes and lymph node chains in Hodgkin's disease [52]. Cardiac irradiation was minimized by putting a block over the left ventricle as the mantle blocks were designed. Patients were treated with an anterior and posterior field every day to this volume. Some patients also received irradiation to para-aortic lymph nodes or pelvic lymph nodes. In rare protocols, patients received liver irradiation, as well. Many patients had splenectomy to remove sites of Hodgkin's disease recurrence. With the advent of better chemotherapy, radiotherapy has been greatly reduced to the lung and heart [26–28]. The radiation damage to the heart has since been shown to be similar to that in other organs and includes fibrosis, which can compromise cardiac function of cardiomyocytes, but also damage the cardiac conduction system reducing arrhythmias [26–28]. The phenomenon appears to be radiation dose, volume, and fraction size dependent, but with children recent reports indicate that any cardiac irradiation as part of the treatment of Hodgkin's disease or other lymphomas is deleterious and produces late cardiac damage. Placing patients at higher risk for myocardial infarction in subsequent decades has all but eliminated the use of thoracic irradiation for lymphoma renal damage from irradiation [26–28]. Dose-response curves clearly indicated the dose to the kidney, which produced kidney failure [29]. The mechanism is that of fibrosis, endothelial damage, and physiological damage.

Kidney Damage

The kidneys are routinely identified and imaged by CAT scan, previously by intravenous pyelogram, and are blocked or left out of the field. Patients with a pelvic kidney are at great risk for pelvic radiotherapy to treat malignancies in the pelvis and during CAT scan imaging, a pelvic kidney usually means that radiotherapy should not be used. Radiation oncology residents are taught that 12 Gy to the whole kidney produces a risk of renal damage. Three-dimensional and intensity-modulated radiation therapy (IMRT) isodose planning can limit renal damage [29].

Liver Damage Late Effects

The liver is very sensitive to ionizing irradiation, and thus, whole liver irradiation was virtually eliminated in the 1970s [52]. Radiation hepatitis is lethal, and attempts to treat hepatocellular carcinomas or other liver tumors or patients with multiple liver metastases were eliminated, and other modalities chosen include injection of drug-containing microspheres, ablative surgical techniques, or surgical excision. Small-volume treatment of liver metastasis is now common using stereotactic radiosurgery in which very small volumes can be treated with high-dose radiation in very few fractions. The majority of the liver is out of the radiation field, and thus, the radiation hepatitis is minimized.

Abdominal Organs Late Effects

Radiotherapy of the pancreas as part of abdominal irradiation for Hodgkin's disease led to pancreas carcinogenesis. Radiation carcinogenesis is another reason that abdominal radiotherapy was eliminated as the para-aortic field to treat para-aortic lymph nodes and was eliminated because of the dose to the pancreas [52].

The stomach, small intestine, and colon demonstrate significant radiosensitivity, again, dependent upon volume, total dose, and fraction size. Intestinal stem cells in the ilium are killed in a dose-response fashion but recover. Late effects in the intestine include significant component of combined injury. Those patients, who had prior surgery, developed fibrotic lesions and adhesions between different loops of bowel. The reduced bowel motility leads to rapid onset of fibrosis. Fistula formation which is a communication of a bowel loop with another loop occurs through a channel that is caused by fibrosis, Sinus formation: intestine [58–60] communicates with the skin is usually due to adhesions that result from prior surgery, and is exacerbated by irradiation. Other side effects of abdominal irradiation limit its use. Abdominal wall irradiation can be used for palliation or for controlling tumor recurrence postoperatively, but the volume is minimized. Intensity modulated radiotherapy (IMRT) treatment planning greatly enhances the ability of irradiation to avoid the intestine [58–60].

Patients receiving pelvic radiotherapy for gynecologic neoplasms, which can be cured by radiotherapy, the intestine is moved as best possible to an area cephalad to the pelvis. This can be achieved by positioning the patient, so that the intestine falls out of the field. In some cases, intestinal loops can be moved surgically to keep them out of an irradiated field. Whole abdomen irradiation was used to treat ovarian cancer in past decades. This complication has been eliminated, because of the sensitivity of the intestine to the acute effects of irradiation. With the availability now of research tools to protect intestinal stem cells including *Lactobacillus reuteri*, which has been genetically engineered to produce either IL-22 or interferon-β [58–60], the intestine can be protected from whole abdomen irradiation, and patients with ovarian cancer can receive whole abdomen irradiation as a component of their therapy. This genetically engineered probiotic may not come into use as a theraputic for some time due to the availability of better chemotherapy drugs and immunotherapy drugs including checkpoint inhibitors that can target ovarian cancer and eliminate the need for radiation [58–60].

Late Effects of Irradiation on Pelvic Reproductive Organs

Germ line cells, like lymphocytes, are easily destroyed by ionizing irradiation. The molecular mechanism of the radiosensitivity of these cell phenotypes is a subject of intense research. Any planned therapeutic irradiation must include a discussion with the patient and family of the expected and anticipated risk of subsequent infertility for both males and females. Sperm banking for males and oocyte cryopreservation for females must be discussed, and for married couples, a discussion of in vitro fertilization and embryo cryopreservation should be included [20]. In the treatment planning, radiotherapy for prostate cancer is an established modality. Depending on dose, volume, and fraction size, bladder fibrosis is a significant complication. Rectal stricture caused by fibrosis of that organ is another significant damage of prostate radiotherapy. The use of implantation of the prostate with radioiodine or gadolinium seeds can limit radiation dose to that organ and decrease the dose to normal tissues (Table 14.1). The use of IMRT and stereotactic radiosurgery techniques and high-dose small-fraction treatments can reduce the risks for rectal and bladder fibrosis.

These are two major side effects of pelvic radiotherapy. In patients with bladder cancer, who receive partial bladder or whole bladder irradiation, the same side effects apply to the rectum. With regard to side effects of pelvic radiotherapy, the best examples come from gynecologic neoplasms. As with head and neck cancer that is cured by irradiation in conjunction with chemotherapy, there are hundreds and thousands of patients, who are long-term survivors and have provided major clinical information on radiation late effects. The same holds true for patients with gynecologic neoplasms including cervix cancer, cancer of the uterus, vulvovaginal cancer, all of whom have received curative doses of radiation delivered by combinations of radioisotope implantation using intercavitary devices or cesium needles, plus external beam radiation. The use of IMRT in minimizing radiation dose to intestine, rectum, and bladder has facilitated a lower incidence of effects on these organs. There are thousands of long-term survivors of pelvic radiotherapy, who are at risk for radiation fibrosis. Both the head and neck cancer population and pelvic radiotherapy population provide many patients for testing new antifibrotic drugs [23–25].

Late Effect of Radiation Carcinogenesis

There is much information that indicates that there is a genetic component of sensitivity to this late effect. Mouse models show certain strains that are induced to develop leukemia or solid tumors by whole-body irradiation, while others are not. The genetics of this phenomenon is still in its infancy. With cancer patients, it is clear that a risk of carcinogenesis must be described for every patient receiving radiotherapy. Two examples of great concern for radiation carcinogenesis: High-dose radiation that is usually delivered to head and neck region or lung cancer in the range of 60–70 Gy is known to induce soft tissue sarcomas [30]. Patients cured of their lung cancer with surgery followed by chemoradiotherapy, who have received high doses of radiation, are at risk for development of sarcomas. For example, as in the curative radiotherapy of patients with benign diseases such as giant cell tumor of bone, these patients are at risk for radiation-induced secondary bone cancer or sarcoma, which can appear decades later. In conclusion, the basic concepts of volume, radiation dose, and fraction size do relate to the risk of carcinogenesis, as well as to the other late effects of ionizing irradiation. However, with radiation carcinogenesis and leukemogenesis, there is a recognized additional significant genetics component to assessing risk and actual outcomes.

References

1. Fletcher GH. Regaud lecture perspectives on the history of radiotherapy. Radiother Oncol. 1988;12(4):iii–v, 253–71.
2. Connell PP, Hellman S. Advances in radiotherapy and implications for the next century: a historical perspective. Cancer Res. 2009;69(2):383–92. https://doi.org/10.1158/0008-5472.CAN-07-6871.
3. Kogelnik HD. The history and evolution of radiotherapy and radiation oncology in Austria. Int J Radiat Oncol Biol Phys. 1996;35(2):219–26. https://doi.org/10.1016/0360-3016(96)00024-7.
4. Thariat J, Hannoun-Levi J-M, Myint AS, et al. Past, present, and future of radiotherapy for the benefit of patients. Nat Rev Clin Oncol. 2013;10(1):52–60. https://doi.org/10.1038/nrclinonc.2012.203.
5. Coia LR, Myerson RJ, Tepper JE. Late effects of radiation therapy on the gastrointestinal tract. Int J Radiat Oncol Biol Phys. 1995;31(5):1213–36. https://doi.org/10.1016/0360-3016(94)00419-L.
6. Cooper JS, Fu K, Marks J, et al. Late effects of radiation therapy in the head and neck region. Int J Radiat Oncol Biol Phys. 1995;31(5):1141–64. https://doi.org/10.1016/0360-3016(94)00421-G.
7. Coderre JA, Morris GM, Micca PL, et al. Late effects of radiation on the central nervous system: role of vascular endothelial damage and glial stem cell survival. Radiat Res. 2006;166(3):495–503. https://doi.org/10.1667/RR3597.1.

8. Yarnold J, Brotons M-CV. Pathogenetic mechanisms in radiation fibrosis. Radiother Oncol. 2010;97(1):149–61. https://doi.org/10.1016/j.radonc.2010.09.002.
9. Westbury CB, Yarnold JR. Radiation fibrosis—current clinical and therapeutic perspectives. Clin Oncol (R Coll Radiol). 2012;24(10):657–72. https://doi.org/10.1016/j.clon.2012.04.001.
10. Straub JM, New J, Hamilton CD, et al. Radiation-induced fibrosis: mechanisms and implications for therapy. J Cancer Res Clin Oncol. 2015;141(11):1985–94. https://doi.org/10.1007/s00432-015-1974-6.
11. Mady LJ, Lyu L, Owoc MS, et al. Understanding financial toxicity in head and neck cancer survivors. Oral Oncol. 2019;95:187–93. https://doi.org/10.1016/j.oraloncology.2019.06.023.
12. Nilsen ML, Mady LJ, Hodges J, et al. Burden of treatment: reported outcomes in a head and neck cancer survivorship clinic. Laryngoscope. 2019;129(12):E437–44. https://doi.org/10.1002/lary.27801.
13. Kurul S, Dincer M, Kizir A, et al. Plastic surgery in irradiated areas: analysis of 200 consecutive cases. Eur J Surg Oncol. 1997;23(1):48–53. https://doi.org/10.1016/s0748-7983(97)80142-4.
14. Ejaz S, Epperly MW, Greenberger JS, et al. Adipose-derived stem cell ameliorates ionizing irradiation fibrosis (RIF) via hepatocyte growth factor mediated TGF-β down regulation and recruitment of bone marrow cells. Stem Cells. 2019;37(6):791–802. https://doi.org/10.1002/stem.3000.
15. Chinnapaka S, Yang KS, Samadi Y, et al. Allogeneic adipose-derived stem cells mitigate acute radiation syndrome by the rescue of damaged bone marrow cells from apoptosis. Stem Cells Transl Med. 2021;10(7):1095–114. https://doi.org/10.1002/sctm.20-0455.
16. Ejaz A, Chinnapaka S, Yang K, et al. Human adipose tissue-derived extracellular matrix (Ad-ECM) mitigates radiation-induced skin fibrosis (RISF) by promoting endothelial cells mediated M2 macrophages polarization. Acta Biomater. 2024. In press.
17. Ejaz A, Greenberger JS, Rubin P. Understanding the mechanism involved in radiation-induced fibrosis development and the therapy options. Pharmacol Ther. 2019;204:107399. https://doi.org/10.1016/j.pharmthera.2019.107399.
18. Ejaz A, Egro FM, Kenny EM, et al. Current evidence for fat grating in radiation-induced soft tissue injury part II: mechanisms and animal models. 2024. In revision.
19. Wallner PE, Kachnic LA, Alektiar KM, et al. The American Board of Radiology initial certification in radiation oncology: moving forward through collaboration. Int J Radiat Oncol Biol Phys. 2019;104(1):21–3. https://doi.org/10.1016/j.ijrobp.2019.01.090.
20. Stilman R, Schiff T, Jaffe N, et al. Ovarian failure following cancer therapy in the prepubertal female. Am J Obstet Gynecol. 1981;139:62–6.
21. Montgomery C, Lydon A, Lloyd K. Psychological distress among cancer patients and informed consent. J Psychosom Res. 1988;46(3):241–5. https://doi.org/10.1016/s0022-3999(98)00089-0.
22. Shakespeare TP, Dwyer M, Mukherjee R, et al. Estimating risks of radiotherapy complications as part of informed consent: the high degree of variability between radiation oncologists may be related to experience. Int J Radiat Oncol Biol Phys. 2002;54(3):647–53. https://doi.org/10.1016/s0360-3016(02)02996-6.
23. Mukherjee A, Epperly M, Shields D, et al. Ionizing irradiation-induced Fgr in senescent cells mediates fibrosis. Cell Death Discov. 2021;7(1):349. https://doi.org/10.1038/s41420-021-00741-4.
24. Mukherjee A, Epperly MW, Fisher R, et al. Silica induced lung fibrosis is associated with senescence, Fgr, and recruitment of bone marrow monocyte/macrophages. In Vivo. 2021;35(6):3053–66. https://doi.org/10.21873/invivo.12601.
25. Mukherjee A, Epperly MW, Fisher R, et al. Inhibition of tyrosine kinase Fgr prevents radiation-induced pulmonary fibrosis (RIPF). Cell Death Discov. 2023;9(1):252. https://doi.org/10.1038/s41420-023-01538-3.
26. Wang H, Wei J, Zheng Q, et al. Radiation-induced heart disease: a review of classification, mechanism, and prevention. Int J Biol Sci. 2019;15(10):2128–38. https://doi.org/10.7150/ijbs.35460.

27. Beizile-Dugas E, Eisenberg MJ. Radiation-induced cardiovascular disease: review of an underrecognized pathology. J Am Heart Assoc. 2021;10(18):e021686. https://doi.org/10.1161/JAHA.121.021686.
28. Jaworski C, Mariani JA, Wheeler G, et al. Cardiac complications of thoracic irradiation. J Am Coll Cardiol. 2013;61(23):2319–28. https://doi.org/10.1016/j.jacc.2013.01.090.
29. Greenberger JS, Weichselbaum RR, Cassady JR. Radiation nephropathy: prevention, diagnosis, management. In: Rieseilbach RE, Garnick MR, editors. Cancer and the kidney. Philadelphia: Lee and Febiger; 1982. p. 814–23.
30. Shadad AK, Sullivan FJ, Martin JD, et al. Gastrointestinal radiation injury: symptoms, risk factors, and mechanisms. World J Gastroenterol. 2013;19(2):185–98. https://doi.org/10.3748/wjg.v19.i2.185.
31. Biete A, Valduvieoc I, Rovirosa A, et al. Whole abdominal radiotherapy in ovarian cancer. Rep Pract Oncol Radiother. 2010;15(2):27–30. https://doi.org/10.1016/j.rpor.2010.02.004.
32. Rockwell S. The life and legacy of Marie Curie. Yale J Biol Med. 2003;76(4–6):167–80.
33. Bortfeld T, Jeraj R. The physical basis and future of radiation therapy. Br J Radiol. 2011;84(1002):485–98. https://doi.org/10.1259/bjr/86221320.
34. Greenberger JS, Chaffey JT, Rosenthal DS, et al. Irradiation for control of hypersplenism and painful splenomegaly in myeloid metaplasia. Int J Radiat Oncol Biol Phys. 1977;2(11–12):1083–90. https://doi.org/10.1016/0360-3016(77)90113-4.
35. Macklis RM. Radithor and the era of mild radium therapy. JAMA. 1990;264(5):614–8.
36. Macklis RM. The great radium scandal. Sci Am. 1993;269(2):94–9. https://doi.org/10.1038/scientificamerican0893-94.
37. van Dijk B, Lemans JVC, Hoogendoorn RM, et al. Treating infections with ionizing radiation: a historical perspective and emerging techniques. Antimicrob Resist Infect Control. 2020;9(1):121. https://doi.org/10.1186/s13756-020-00775-w.
38. Martland HS. Occupational poisoning in manufacture of luminous watch dials. JAMA. 1929;92(6):466–73.
39. Abergel R, Aris J, Bolch WE, et al. The enduring legacy of Marie Curie: impacts of radium in 21st century radiological and medical sciences. Int J Radiat Biol. 2022;98(3):267–75. https://doi.org/10.1080/09553002.2022.2027542.
40. Greenberger JS, Crocker AC, Vawter G, et al. Results of treatment of 127 patients with systemic histiocytosis. Medicine (Baltimore). 1981;60(5):311–38. https://doi.org/10.1097/00005792-198109000-00001.
41. Boice JD Jr. Radiation-induced thyroid cancer-What's new? J Natl Cancer Inst. 2005;97(10):703–5. https://doi.org/10.1093/jnci/dji151.
42. Thiagarajan A, Iyer NG. Radiation-induced sarcomas of the head and neck. World J Clin Oncol. 2014;5(5):973–81. https://doi.org/10.5306/wjco.v5.i5.973.
43. Takamura N, Orita M, Saenko V, et al. Radiation and risk of thyroid cancer: Fukushima and Chernobyl. Lancet Diabetes Endocrinol. 2016;4(8):647. https://doi.org/10.1016/S2213-8587(16)30112-7.
44. Bouffler S, Ainsbury E, Gilvin P, et al. Radiation-induced cataracts: the Health Protection Agency's response to the ICRP statement on tissue reactions and recommendation on the dose limit for the eye lens. J Radiol Prot. 2012;32(4):479–88. https://doi.org/10.1088/0952-4746/32/4/479.
45. Kleiman NJ. Radiation cataract. Ann ICRP. 2012;41(3–4):80–97. https://doi.org/10.1016/j.icrp.2012.06.018.
46. Ainsbury EA, Barnard S, Bright S, et al. Ionizing radiation induced cataracts: recent biological and mechanistic developments and perspectives for future research. Mutat Res Rev Mutat Res. 2016;770(Pt B):238–61. https://doi.org/10.1016/j.mrrev.2016.07.010.
47. Fuss M, Poljanc K, Hug EB. Full scale IQ (FSIQ) changes in children treated with whole brain and partial brain irradiation. A review and analysis. Strahlenther Onkol. 2000;176(12):573–81. https://doi.org/10.1007/pl00002327.

48. Oshiro Y, Mizumoto M, Pan H, et al. Spinal changes after craniospinal irradiation in pediatric patients. Pediatr Blood Cancer. 2020;67(12):e28728. https://doi.org/10.1002/pbc.28728.
49. Slotman B, Faivre-Finn C, Kramer G, et al. Prophylactic cranial irradiation in extensive small-cell lung cancer. N Engl J Med. 2007;357:664–72.
50. Oskan F, Ganswindt U, Schwarz SB, et al. Hippocampus sparing in whole-brain radiotherapy: a review. Strahlenther Onkol. 2014;190(4):337–41. https://doi.org/10.1007/s00066-013-0518-8.
51. Parihar VK, Allen BD, Caressi C, et al. Cosmic radiation exposure and persistent cognitive dysfunction. Sci Rep. 2016;6:34774. https://doi.org/10.1038/srep34774.
52. Glatstein EJ, Coleman CN, Pistenmaa DA, et al. Research-driven radiation oncology: a narrative on the ongoing legacy of Henry S. Kaplan. Int J Radiat Oncol Biol Phys. 2021;109(1):10–4. https://doi.org/10.1016/j.ijrobp.2020.10.008.
53. Loi G, Dominietto M, Cannillo B, et al. Neutron production form a mobile linear accelerator operating in electron mode for intraoperative radiation therapy. Phys Med Biol. 2006;51(3):695–702. https://doi.org/10.1088/0031-9155/51/3/014.
54. Konefat A, Orlef A, Bieniasiewicz M. Measurements of neutron radiation and induced radioactivity for the new medical linear accelerator, the Varian TrueBeam. Radiat Meas. 2016;86:8–15.
55. Hall EJ, Novak JK, Kellerer AM, et al. RBE as a function of neutron energy: I. experimental observations. Radiat Res. 1975;64(2):245–55.
56. Stelzer KJ, Laramore GE, Griffin TW, et al. Fast neutron radiotherapy: the University of Washington experience. Acta Oncol. 1994;33(3):275–80. https://doi.org/10.3109/02841869409098417.
57. Blanco J-R, Cobos-Ceballos M-J, Navarro F, et al. Pulmonary long-term consequences of COVID-19 infections after hospital discharge. Clin Microbiol Infect. 2021;27(6):892–6. https://doi.org/10.1016/j.cmi.2021.02.019.
58. Hamade DF, Epperly MW, Fisher R, et al. Release of interferon-β (IFN-β) from probiotic *Limosilactobacillus reuteri*-IFN-β (LR-IFN-β) mitigates gastrointestinal acute radiation syndrome (GI-ARS) following whole abdominal irradiation. Cancers (Basel). 2023;15(6):1670. https://doi.org/10.3390/cancers15061670.
59. Espinal A, Epperly MW, Mukherjee A, et al. Intestinal radiation protection and mitigation by second-generation probiotic *Lactobacillus-reuteri* engineered to deliver Interleukin-22. Int J Mol Sci. 2022;23(10):5616. https://doi.org/10.3390/ijms23105616.
60. Hamade DF, Espinal A, Yu J, et al. *Lactobacillus reuteri* releasing IL-22 (LR-IL-22) facilitates intestinal radioprotection for whole-abdomen irradiation (WAI) of ovarian cancer. Radiat Res. 2022;198(1):89–105. https://doi.org/10.1667/RADE-21-00224.1.

Chapter 15
Challenges for Future Study of the Late Effects of Therapeutic Radiation in Cancer Survivors and Also Their Progeny

There are thousands of cancer survivors, who have received therapeutic radiotherapy. In the United States alone, given the proliferation of modern radiotherapy treatment facilities since the 1970s, and the widespread use of megavoltage radiotherapy, the greatest number of such cancer survivors is in the categories of: (1) patients with head and neck cancer; (2) patients with gynecologic cancer; and (3) patients, who were treated as children for pediatric cancer decades ago [1–3]. Current protocols and plans for use of radiotherapy in cancer patient management are focusing on decreasing radiation dose, volume of tissue treated, and, in some cases, eliminating radiotherapy from treatment protocols. The use of radiotherapy, in particular, for children has decreased in the past 50 years, but has created a vast database for understanding the late effects of therapeutic radiation [1]. Effects of surviving cancer have provided much information to study, not only the cancer patients but also their family members and progeny [2, 3]. To accurately focus on the outcomes of use of successful therapeutic radiotherapy, it is difficult to separate the radiation effects from those of surgery, whether for biopsy or local excision of primary cancers, and, of course, the simultaneous or subsequent use of combination chemotherapy or biological response modifiers. Nevertheless, it is instructive to look at the effects of therapeutic radiation on patients and their families, clearly, as important information as cancer treatment centers move forward to design better treatment paradigms with the goal of increasing care with decreased side effects.

Surviving cancer is increasingly common in the Western world and certainly in the United States. With improved and earlier diagnosis, and improved therapeutic options, many more patients are alive for decades after radiation therapy. There are consequences of the use of radiotherapy to treat cancer, which affect not only the patient, but his/her family, and certainly progeny.

J. Greenberger, *Radiation Oncology and Radiation Biology*,
https://doi.org/10.1007/978-3-031-66300-0_15

Head and Neck Cancer Survivors

Many cancer therapy centers have "survivorship" clinics in which patients are followed for decades after completion of therapeutic irradiation. Head and neck cancer patients, who received radiotherapy, have displayed in large numbers the late effects of radiotherapy. The most common late effect is fibrosis, which affects critical structures in the irradiated treatment volume. Most patients, who require intervention, present with difficulties in swallowing associated with fibrosis of the pharyngeal constrictor muscles and/or voice change that is associated with laryngeal muscle fibrosis. These patients also provide valuable information about how families have responded to having a cancer survivor in their life. Over the decades after successful radiotherapy, patients and their families are always "on the alert" for cancer recurrence or new cancers. Genetic testing for family members is available for informed consent before radiotherapy is given [2, 3]. How do patients adapt to cure of their cancer? After it becomes clear that there has been cure, and the number of 5 years, continues to be the number that patients and their care providers follow, the families settle into a pattern of adaptation. This adaptation is not different from that of a military veteran who has suffered injury from deployment in a battle zone, nor is it difficult from a survivor of a domestic tragedy, such as a home fire, automobile accident, or other situation, which can alter anatomy of the injured individual.

Most head and neck cancer survivors have an interrupted social interaction with their families. Assisted speech and dietary changes may be necessary after radiation late effects. The administration of therapeutics to counteract late radiation fibrosis is limited due to the unavailability of many medications. Survivorship clinics focusing on head and neck cancer have begun to study the "trajectory" of onset of symptoms and signs of late radiation effects, and biomarkers are being studied including plasma levels of microRNA, proteins associated with fibrosis, and nucleated cell diversity, which can herald the onset of inflammatory cell infiltration into irradiated areas that are associated with the onset of fibrosis. These studies are just beginning. The hope of these studies is to be able to intervene with new therapeutics to minimize fibrosis (Table 15.1). There is a challenge with many survivors of gynecologic

Table 15.1 Approaches to the management of late effects of irradiation in cancer survivors

Condition	Therapeutic approach
Fibrosis (head and neck region or pelvis)	Full thickness of skin graft—plastic reconstructive surgery
Anti-fibrotic drug	Quercetin Pentoxifylline
Senolytic drug	JP4-039
Physical therapy Drug trajectory of onset	Diagnose biomarkers of fibrosis onset and interval
Cellular therapies – Injection of adipocyte stem cells – Extracellular matrix injection	Harvest autologous Allogeneic cells or tissues Bioreactor experiments
TL02-59 target Fgr kinase	Timed delivery to prevent fibrosis

cancer, or the smaller numbers of patients, who are survivors of radiotherapy for testicular cancer, bladder cancer, colorectal cancer. There is concern about reproduction and potential dangers to children and/or grandchildren.

Survivors of Gynecologic Cancers

In contrast to the data of head and neck cancer survivors, patients, who have survived protocols of therapeutic irradiation for the treatment of cervix cancer, endometrial cancer, vulvovaginal cancer, and other pelvic malignancies, have family concerns about lifestyle and risk to children and grandchildren. The majority of long-term survivors of gynecologic cancer are those patients treated for cervix cancer. Cancer screening techniques for women have improved greatly over the last 50 years. The use of PAP smears, culdoscopy, minimally invasive biopsy techniques, therapeutic cervical cone section techniques that protect uterine integrity, and other diagnostic and therapeutic measures have increased the likelihood of cure in patients with early-stage cervix cancer. Cryopreservation of ova or fertilized embryos has been a recommendation at many cancer treatment centers for women, who are likely to receive intracavitary brachytherapy and/or pelvic irradiation for cervix cancer. Cervix cancer affects younger women compared to other categories of gynecologic cancer, and family planning issues are more prominent. Implantation of fertilized ova after a course of chemoradiotherapy and/or surgery for cervix cancer has been studied, although many women do not wish to risk potentially unsuccessful pregnancy, particularly, after brachytherapy and/or pelvic irradiation. Techniques for progesterone treatment to increase the likelihood of carrying a pregnancy to term are not a secure option for women, particularly in the setting of possible local recurrence or metastatic disease. Many women wish to avoid discussions about pregnancy after treatment for cervix cancer.

The late effects of pelvic radiation and interstitial or intracavitary brachytherapy for the patient are not only stressful during the treatment time, but also affect family life.

Sexual activity after hysterectomy, with or without bilateral salpingo-oophorectomy, is dependent upon rehabilitation, training by supportive caregivers, and the anatomy changes after surgery and/or radiation therapy. Life after successful treatment of cervix cancer is critical to optimize to restore quality of life in cured patient.

In the case of hysterectomy, the vaginal cuff anatomy is used to facilitate normal sexual activity. The use of Premarin vaginal cream or other local hormonal supplements has minimized dyspareunia. Depending on the surgical conditions of postoperative anatomy, there may be a need for significant rehabilitation processes. Local radiotherapy to the cervix, parametria, and radiation dose delivered to the bladder and rectum also may affect sexual activity. Women, who have been cured of cervix cancer, have the issues of the onset and magnitude of late effects. Fibrosis of tissues in the brachytherapy treatment volume present with the same issues as that for patients, who are survivors of head and neck cancer. The "trajectory" of onset of late effects has become a subject of investigation for gynecologic oncologists and primary care providers. The same issues of late effects and timing focus on the 2 years after completion of curative radiotherapy, but follow-up and surveillance for 2–10 years are common. Cervix cancer patients and those who have survived curative therapy for endometrial cancer, ovarian cancer, and other pelvic malignancies have been studied for genetic predisposition to develop other cancers and likelihood of transfer of increased genetic risk to children and grandchildren. Cancer survivors and their families are always concerned about the risk of cancer in children and grandchildren. Continuous surveillance and regular follow-up for family members by primary care providers are the usual policy in the modern era.

Pediatric Cancer Survivors

There is a clear trend toward decreasing the radiation dose delivered and the volume of tissue treated for pediatric cancer patients that has been prominent over the last three decades. Prior to that time and certainly in the 1970s and before, children received radiotherapy and these individuals have been followed for decades. Children treated for Wilms' tumor, rhabdomyosarcoma, Ewing's sarcoma, neuroblastoma, and other pediatric malignancies, who have been cured, displayed many late radiation effects. Families have adapted to anatomic changes, which follow surgery and chemoradiotherapy for pediatric cancers and modern radiotherapy techniques, primarily the use of intensity-modulated radiotherapy (IMRT), stereotactic radiosurgery, protons and overall reduction in radiotherapy dose that has made a concern for radiation late effects less prominent.

Those individuals treated prior to the advent of IMRT (prior to 1995) have been followed for growth abnormalities and have displayed many radiation late side effects. Asymmetric bone growth primarily in the axial skeleton is less common since the 1970s, because radiation oncologists have been trained to avoid asymmetric treatment of the developing spinal vertebrae. Radiation induced infertility and sterilization of pediatric patients and has been a subject of publications, particularly, for patients treated before the IMRT era there is a need for family planning and counseling as part of the evaluation for any patient with childhood cancer, who will receive radiotherapy.

Many uses of radiotherapy for children have been eliminated. Most prominently has been the elimination of whole-brain radiation in children with most forms of acute lymphocytic leukemia (ALL), since the cognitive deficits have been observed and published. The elimination or greatly reduced radiotherapy for pediatric Hodgkin's disease, and lymphomas is a clear trend. Those patients, who require radiotherapy for lung in Wilms' tumor, receive significantly lower doses and decreased fraction sizes, but these protocols have been relatively recent, and data from cancer survivors are currently being evaluated.

For pediatric solid tumors including medulloblastoma, ependymoma, and other rare pediatric cancers in which craniospinal irradiation for patients has been the standard of care, these children are being evaluated for the potential therapeutic benefit of using proton irradiation. The advantage of proton treatment for craniospinal irradiation is the clear decrease in radiation dose exposure to the anterior thoracic and abdominal structures compared to IMRT photon irradiation. Data are being collected with respect to the increasing numbers of cured patients now focusing on likelihood of appearance of a second cancer and radiation-induced late effects in anterior thoracic and abdominal structures. Patients and their families now pay particular attention to follow-up. There is a need to explain the risks of radiotherapy and chemotherapy for these cancers. Managing expections has been a prominent part of the treatment planning and follow-up. Most radiation oncologists agree that those disease categories, which demonstrate nearly uniform elimination of radiotherapy from the overall protocols, will be the ones for pediatric cancer patients. This principle underscores the general recognition of the late effects of radiation, and since pediatric patients are likely to have the greatest duration of follow-up (in many cases 50 or more years), the late effects issue for radiation therapy is prominent as there are many in new protocols to cure pediatric cancers.

General Considerations for Cancer Survivors and Their Families

Unlike the past decades before year 2000 in which low dose rate (LDR) brachytherapy was used for patients with head and neck cancer and gynecologic cancer, patients now receive high dose rate after loading brachytherapy. Thus, there is less concern about risks to family members, who are visiting hospitalized patients, who in the past had a therapeutic implant of radioisotope brachytherapy (radium or Cesium) for a 50-h or more brachytherapy treatment course.

These brachytherapy patients were hospitalized in the 1970s through 1990s in large numbers, before the widespread substitution of high dose rate (HDR) after loading of brachytherapy techniques. With HDR, the only source of radiation is found in the radiation oncology department. In contrast to LDR, catheters or appliances that were placed in the patient's body but and were loaded with isotopes that go back to the patient into his/her hospital room. With LDR, there was risk of exposure to people entering a patient's room. In the case of HDR brachytherapy, implants have been replaced by techniques of either loading brachytherapy sources in a remote location or the elimination of brachytherapy and use of external beam of IMRT, stereotactic radiosurgery, or other uses of external beam radiation.

Most patients and families are aware of the absence of risk to family members, particularly children by having a patient return home after external beam radiotherapy. As recently as the 1970s, patients and their families did ask radiation oncologists, whether it was safe for a patient receiving a 4–7-week external beam radiotherapy treatment course, to have a grandchild visit them. One place in which radiation emission from a radiotherapy patient is still considered relevant relates to men, who have had prostate radioisotope implantation either as permanent radioactive iridium or gadolinium seeds, or strands of seeds that are implanted. The half-life of the isotopes used for these treatments is on the level of days-weeks, so patients and their families are advised to have limited contact with other individuals for the first days of that interval. However, in the modern era, most radiotherapy patients do not have permanent implants.

The previous chapter outlined in a systematic fashion the different forms of presentation of the late effects of ionizing irradiation. Each of the organ systems was described in the chapter based on historical perspectives form the outcomes of treating cancer with radiotherapy. The types of cancer that involved each of these organ systems or tissues led to late effects of therapeutic radiation to each transit volume or target volume itself. This chapter will deal instead with associated problems of late effects in cancer survivors, who are cured and are expected to live for decades after completion of their radiotherapy. The concepts of "target volume" treated as opposed to minimum "transit volume" are a major points that must be defined. The final chapter of this book will focus on concern for the future of the medical specialty of radiation oncology. There are increasing concerns about the late effects of radiation treatment. The late effects of radiotherapy involve the noncancer tissue adjacent to the cancer or tissue that must be exposed to radiation in order to eradicate the cancer. The normal tissue exposed is of great concern for patients, who will determine the future of the medical specialty of radiation oncology.

A military analogy will emphasize the problem with therapeutic radiology and radiation oncology. A targeted attack on the enemy, particularly (in this case, the cancer), is best achieved by minimizing the killing/injury of non-combatants. This is called minimizing "collateral damage." Stereotactic radio-ablative-targeted radiotherapy [4, 5] is the current methodology to optimize the attempt to cure cancers, either at initial diagnosis or at time of recurrence. The radiation beam precisely is collimated to avoid normal tissue. The cancer is the target; but to reach it with ionizing irradiation, there must be some "collateral damage" to the cells in the noncancer tissue that must be transited by the radiation beam to reach the cancer and must have some margin to attempt to eliminate all microscopic sites of possible extension. The "transit volume" suffers the same effects of radiation, as does the cancer, although less in intensity. Treatment planning methodology to minimize collateral damage is continually improving but is still imperfect. This chapter will focus on the medical implications of late effects of ionizing irradiation on normal tissues in the "transit volume" compared to the cancer containing "target volume" itself. Once cancer cells have been eliminated, the return to precancerous tissue anatomy is desired, but may be imperfect. Individual case examples can best outline the extent to which radiation late effects can significantly alter the quality of life for cancer survivors due to late effects.

Case #1: A.C.: A 32-year-old Caucasian female, who is a primary care physician, presented with mid-thoracic back pain. After diagnostic X-ray evaluation, it was determined that there was destruction of two vertebral bodies in the region of the ninth and tenth thoracic vertebrae. A biopsy revealed giant cell tumor of bone [6]. The literature on this diagnosis is very revealing. Pathologists report that this particular histology, while not cancer, can behave in a fashion very similar to cancer. It is a tumor of so-called giant cell morphology, the cellular origin of which is probably in the macrophage-histocyte site category. The individual cells are locally aggressive and are invasive in producing enzymes that invade and destroy both bone and soft tissues. While not usually presenting with lymphatic metastasis or blood-borne hematogenous (through the blood) distant spread, this tumor is known to produce satellite lesions (tumor deposits close to primary tumor) and these have a high propensity for both local recurrence after surgical excision and regional spread. There are reports that cells that are left behind during surgical excision may produce satellite secondary lesions at the surgery site.

This patient had an extensive surgical resection with removal of the affected areas including several thoracic vertebrae and had spinal reconstruction. The reconstruction was carried out by a neurosurgeon and was necessary to stabilize her skeleton. It was carried out with insertion of metal plates fastened to the superior and inferior vertebral bodies by screws. The patient recovered well and was followed closely. Because the resection margins were negative (no evidence of tumor/disease left behind), no postoperative radiation was recommended. The risk of damage to her spinal cord in the transit volume, which could be potentially caused by the radiotherapy, was judged by the radiation oncologist to be greater than the likelihood of tumor recurrence. The patient and her husband were advised of the risks compared to the potential gain of postoperative radiotherapy at that time. The patient agreed to a plan for observation and agreed to no radiotherapy at that time. She was followed closely. She presented several months later with two isolated "satellite" lung lesions, one in each lung, that were in the anatomic proximity of the previous surgery. One lesion was surgically excised, and the histopathology was the same as the original tumor. The other lesion because of its proximity to the spinal cord and concern that surgical removal might be traumatic was treated with stereotactic body radiation therapy (SBRT) delivering a limited number of radiation fractions to the satellite lesion. The radiation dose delivered per day was a relatively high-dose radiation per fraction. The patient was immobilized, so that this stereotactic radiotherapy could be delivered to the smallest possible volume, which was around 2 cm in diameter.

There was discussion as to whether postoperative radiotherapy to the region of the original resected vertebrae and also to this recurrent lesion should be delivered. At this point, the patient was advised about the propensity of this tumor to again locally recur. After discussion with the patient, her husband, and other physicians associated with her case, it was concluded that the danger of radiation side effects to the spinal cord again outweighed its use of radiotherapy at that time.

At the time of the satellite lesions recurrence, it was 10 months since the original spine surgery. The patient had a physical foot drag, which was observed prior to radiotherapy, and was minor, but was present after the original surgery, and was considered a mild neurological deficit. While considered to be minimal and nonprogressive in nature, the risk of larger field radiation to the original surgical site exacerbating the neurological deficit was considered high. She had no sensory loss in her legs and full function. Her mobility and quality of life were excellent.

At this time, the patient had a small child and was actively involved in childcare, as well as her active primary care medical practice. She chose to have no large field radiotherapy at that time.

The patient was continually followed and presented again a year later (approximately 20 months after the original surgery) with now clear evidence of local recurrence in the areas of the originally involved vertebral bodies. While the margins of resection of the original surgery indicated no residual disease, and the discussion of using postoperative radiotherapy at that time revolved around estimating the low risk of local recurrence, the patient now did have a different presentation. This was clear local recurrence. She again desired to avoid any potential radiation toxicity to her spinal cord.

The patient sought the opinion of another neurological surgeon. She was now found to have a mass expanding anteriorly from the region of the originally removed vertebral bodies in the thoracic spine and tumor was extending anteriorly toward the thoracic aorta. At her own request, the patient was referred to another medical center, where there was a neurological surgeon with expertise in the indicated extensive reconstructive surgery that would be required to minimize another recurrence of this giant cell tumor of bone. The original spine stabilization appliance was removed, and the patient had an extensive resection of recurrent tumor in the area anterior to the original vertebral bodies. The pathology report was again consistent with giant cell tumor of bone. There were no other sites of regional or distant metastatic tumor.

A discussion between the neurosurgeon and radiation oncologist revealed several factors that led to the decision to now recommend postoperative radiotherapy. The neurosurgeon reported that the tumor recurrence was now deriving its blood supply from spinal arteries, thus vasculature arising from the spinal cord. The current wide local excision of the recurrent tumor was incomplete, and margins anteriorly were positive. The neurosurgeon reported that he was unable to dissect out (remove) more tumor from the anterior area. He was limited, because of the danger of damaging the blood supply, which was shared with the thoracic spinal cord. Although she had no further neurological deficits at presentation, the neurosurgeon reported that he was concerned that there was residual disease in the anterior location, where he could not complete a total excision without the need to risk damage to the spinal arteries and then the spinal cord itself. He indicated that should the patient have yet another local recurrence, which was likely, he would be unable to carry out further surgery without causing paraplegia. Furthermore, he reported that a need for further surgery would leave the patient with spinal cord paralysis and a severe neurological functional deficit.

The patient now agreed to receive postoperative radiotherapy. The treatment plan for intensity-modulated radiotherapy (IMRT) was to deliver 55 Gy in 5½ weeks at 1.8 Gy per daily dose to the area of suspected residual disease. The treatment plan was developed jointly by consultation between the neurosurgeon and the radiation oncologist. The patient and her husband were advised about the risks of radiotherapy, particularly now to be delivered to a twice-operated anatomic target volume near the spinal cord. They were further advised about the risks of radiation effects on the spinal arteries that were supplying the blood to both the normal spinal cord and the residual recurrent tumor. The radiation late effects on these blood vessels were described as being potentially extensive. Also, prominent was the concern that radiation would produce transverse myelitis or damage to the spinal cord resulting in sensory and motor loss and potentially paralysis despite the relatively safe planned radiation dose, fraction size, and volume to be treated. Thus, a safe fractionation scheme and safe protracted duration of the time of treatment were planned, along with use of a 1.8 Gy per day radiation fraction. There was concern that the compromised blood supply to the spinal cord in the presence of residual tumor near the spinal cord might elevate the risk of radiation damage to the spinal cord. The patient was also advised of the risk of a radiation-induced second cancer. Multiple informed consent sessions were held with the patient and her husband. Most important to these discussions was that the patient reported her desire to have a second child.

The radiation oncologist then requested a detailed analysis of the radiation dose that would be delivered to the ovaries despite their clear distance from the treatment target volume in the thoracic spine. The target volume was now in the spinal region at T9–T12. It was calculated that the 55 Gy of planned irradiation to that target volume would deliver <1% of that dose to the ovaries. Despite the calculated safe dose to the ovaries, the patient and her husband were advised to plan for a program of in vitro fertilization and cryopreservation of fertilized ova before radiotherapy was started. This procedure was carried out, and fertilized ova (embryos) were derived, cryopreserved, and maintained prior to, during radiotherapy, and for months after completion of the radiation treatment courses. The neurosurgeon advised that she could clearly carry a progeny to term given the stabilization of the spine that he had constructed.

The availability of intensity-modulated radiotherapy (IMRT) should be emphasized, as this computer-controlled delivery of targeted irradiation was now available. IMRT increased the feasibility of delivering 55 Gy to the target volume with minimal dose to lung, heart, and other associated anatomic structures in the transit volume. The patient was examined daily for any neurological side effects during the planned 5½ weeks of radiotherapy. She was examined, particularly for any worsening of the foot drag or for new or progressive neurological deficits. After surgery, but before radiotherapy, she had developed some foot drag, which suggested weakness of distal lower limb muscles possibly due to the repeated surgeries, but there was no indication of need for neurological intervention or physical therapy to strengthen the dorsal flexors of her right foot as the foot drag was mild. Her gait was clinically unaffected by this minor deficit. She was examined for sensory deficits and had no foot pain or numbness. There was no pain in any region of her legs.

During the course of radiotherapy, she displayed some observed minimal, but clear increase in the foot drag after 4 weeks of the planned 5½ week treatment course. Because of this observation, the radiotherapy was stopped earlier than the planned dose. It was stopped at 50 Gy. She was seen in follow-up for several months and was symptom-free and able to return to her medical practice.

The patient did have her embryo implantation procedure and was seen 2 years later bringing with her, her first child and a second newborn baby. Her other child was well and healthy. The in vitro fertilization and reimplantation into the uterus had clearly been successful, and she now had two children. All of these procedures were carried out with consultation with the neurosurgeon, who carried out the second operation and the spinal stabilization device, which he inserted after the second surgery. The device was designed to give her spinal support that would make a second pregnancy feasible and safe. This second spinal prosthesis reached the upper parts of the thoracic spine and into the lumbar spine since two additional vertebral bodies were now absent. Skin and musculature over the vertebral bodies of previous T9 through T12 vertebrae were thin due to the second surgery, and the IMRT radiotherapy was carefully designed to minimize radiation dose to the areas of skin overlying the surgical treatment volume.

Everything was then fine for 10 years. The patient and her husband moved to a different State, and she continued her medical practice, raising her children, and had regular follow-up with her neurosurgeon. Reports were sent to the radiation oncologist on a regular basis.

Ten years later, the patient reported new symptoms in the previously radiation treated area including pain and changes in sensory and motor function in her lower extremities. Evaluation by CAT and MRI scans revealed a mass at the site of the original tumor, at what was the T10–T12 region. This was in the irradiation treatment field. A biopsy revealed a high-grade sarcoma felt by the pathologist to be consistent with a radiation-induced sarcoma. The patient had received no prior chemotherapy and had received only postoperative radiation after the second extensive surgery. She was now treated for a high-grade sarcoma with multiagent chemotherapy. Further radiotherapy at this site was considered to be inappropriate. Despite extensive chemotherapy, the patient developed multiple distant lung metastasis and passed away 11½ years after the original diagnosis and 10 years after postoperative radiotherapy.

While there are limited reports of spontaneous malignant transformation of giant cell tumor of bone to a sarcoma, the most likely etiology of the patient's second tumor sarcoma was that it was an ionizing irradiation-induced sarcoma. The most devastating late effect of radiotherapy is induction of cancer.

Case #2: A 25-year-old Caucasian female presented with progressive lower back pain of several months duration. X-ray evaluation demonstrated lytic lesions in the region of the right sacroiliac joint and right ilium Biopsy revealed giant cell tumor of bone. This patient was diagnosed with the same histopathologic tumor as patient #1, but this patient presented 30 years prior to the patient in the previous case report. This second patient was seen prior to the availability of either 3D conformal radiotherapy or the availability of IMRT. The patient had an excisional biopsy, but not complete excision. The tumor could not be resected due to the extensiveness of the sacral and iliac bone destruction and the magnitude of tumor invasion into bone. She was seen by a medical oncologist, who recommended radiation therapy to control tumor growth, to limit further tumor invasion, and to limit further bone destruction. Chemotherapy was not recommended for this patient due to the histology, and the patient was referred for radiotherapy. The patient agreed to treatment after detailed and extensive informed consent. Cryopreservation of ova was available, but the patient did not want to initiate this program. Her tumor was clearly close to her right ovary, and there were lengthy discussions about preservation of ova.

She was planned to receive 55 Gy irradiation in 5½ weeks by parallel opposed, off-axis oblique fields that were designed to spare the contralateral left ovary. She was advised that despite this plan, the dose to the contralateral left ovary could not be guaranteed to be safe. Clearly, her ipsilateral right ovary and uterus would be irradiated, and the radiation dose could decrease the likelihood of her having a successful pregnancy. The calculated radiation dose to her contralateral ovary would deliver a dose that might prevent successful ovulation and pregnancy, but she might still become pregnant in the future, so she should not consider herself to be infertile. The treatment plan was designed to maintain hormone production by the left ovary, but she was advised that she could still be infertile.

Treatment planning revealed that the left contralateral ovary would still receive a dose in the range of 2–5% of the prescribed dose. At that time, the patient, although not married, again was advised to cryopreserve ova. She desired to forgo this procedure and did not know if she would ever desire to have children in the future. Despite consultation with family, the patient refused to carry out cryopreservation of ova.

She completed radiotherapy and was followed closely. Years later, she and her new husband moved to a distant location. The patient reported no further problems with the primary tumor or any problems with the postoperative radiotherapy. Fifteen years later, she reported to the radiation oncologist that she had a successful pregnancy and now had a 3-year-old child, who was normal in every way. She reported that she had just given birth to a second totally normal child. She carried both children to term, and both were the result of normal gestation and delivery. The radiation dose to the contralateral ovary had been calculated to be 5% of the 55 Gy delivered to the target volume and the fraction size then of 2.0 Gy per day and a treatment time of 5½ weeks apparently had not caused damage to the uterus, such that it prevented her from carrying her children to full term delivery. She is still being followed by local specialists.

This second case highlights the success of using a careful treatment plan even without IMRT or 3D planning available for a patient, who would likely be cured of this giant cell tumor of bone. Normal tissue protection was designed to allow for possible future pregnancy and child-bearing. The risk of induction of a malignant cancer by radiation was reported to her before she agreed to receive radiotherapy and that risk is still there for her as it was for the first patient. The availability of sophisticated treatment planning techniques, such as IMRT, did not prevent careful two-dimensional radiotherapy 30 years ago for this second patient. The literature on radiotherapy for giant cell tumor of bone continues to describe a definite risk of radiation-induced second tumors. These two cases indicate that the risk is real.

Case #3: F.A. was a 35-year-old female with a history of Fanconi anemia (FA) [7], who presented with a mass in her oral cavity. She was diagnosed with Fanconi anemia, as a child and received a bone marrow transplant as part of the planned therapy program to correct the anemia of this disease. As described in previous chapters in this book, FA is one of a category of diseases that make patients sensitive to ionizing irradiation. In FA, some, but not all patients, have symptoms and clinical problems caused by a defect in repair of DNA double-strand breaks. A defect in one or more of the 26 genes in the protein scaffold that surrounds a DNA strand break prevents the binding of DNA repair enzymes, so that these breaks, which naturally occur as part of normal cell divisions or exposure to an environmental toxin, remain unrepaired [7]. The anemia in patients with FA leads to loss of bone marrow hematopoietic blood stem cells causing anemia [8]. The FA genotype also makes patients at risk for mutations that can lead to cancer. FA is also known to be associated with a hypersensitivity of the bone marrow stem cells to the negative hematopoietic growth factor/regulator, TGF-β [8]. This patient was prepared for a bone marrow transplant by receiving chemotherapy drug, busulfan or fludarabine, to clean space in her marrow for transplanted cells. Bone marrow transplantation in this patient's childhood did cure her anemia. Bone marrow transplantation is now an accepted therapeutic option for patients with FA and is part of the standard of care, which is available to most patients. However, there are problems that remain in FA patients after correction of the anemia by bone marrow transplantation. The most serious problem in FA patients now is the high incidence of cancer, notably, in the oral cavity and oropharynx [9].

While most patients with FA present with anemia in childhood, but some present later in life with a history of sensitivity to DNA cross-linking agents that might have been administered for an unrelated indication [10]. This particular patient had received a successful marrow transplantation and her red blood cell count was stable, with no further indication of anemia. Even though the patient was followed closely with frequent physical examinations, there was the discovery of an oral cavity tumor on the floor of her mouth right side and lateral to her tongue. It was 2 cm. in diameter, and she had no palpable lymph nodes. A positron emission tomography (PET) scan, which was used to diagnose any regional or different metastasis was carried out. The PET scan is done by measuring the uptake of labeled sugar, which is also used in rapidly proliferating cells. In this patient, her cancer was positive for PET scan. The cancer revealed positivity only in the area of the primary tumor with no positive lymph nodes. She had a local surgical excision with clear negative margins and the diagnosis was squamous cell carcinoma.

Cancers were first reported in an increasing number of FA patients involving the oral cavity and oropharynx [9, 11]. Women with FA also presented with squamous cell cancers of the cervix or vulvovaginal region. Even more recently, FA patients have been presenting with esophageal or lung cancer [12]. The etiology of the secondary cancers is unknown but is likely related to the DNA repair defect in Fanconi anemia patients, which is occurring in cells and tissues other than those of the hematopoietic system, which has been replaced in large part by the bone marrow transplantation.

This FA patient presented with a cancer of the oral cavity, a clearly malignant lesion. The standard of care for this T2 size primary cancer with no positive nodes and no metastasis (T2N0M0) would have been to consider lymph node sampling or dissection to rule out the presence of metastasis in nodes that were too small to be detected by PET scan. An alternative treatment would be regional radiotherapy for 5–6 weeks. However, after consultation with the patient and her family, and the understanding the regional radiotherapy would likely be offered, if any positive nodes were found, she elected to be followed with further surveillance and no treatment. The radiosensitive phenotype of FA patients (some, but not all) has been a caution for offering postoperative radiotherapy for FA patients [11–13]. The patient was referred for consideration of postoperative radiotherapy at this site. During the consultation, a long discussion focused on the patient's desire to have children. She had recently married and was involved in family planning before the diagnosis of squamous cell carcinoma of the oral cavity was made.

This patient's care became focused on the informed consent process for postoperative radiotherapy and the patient's desire for family planning. Physicians, who treat Fanconi anemia, primarily pediatricians, are involved in the initial diagnosis and the plans for bone marrow transplantation. These physicians, usually pediatricians frequently are involved in the decisions regarding treatment of cancers, which appear in their patients. There can be sometimes painful discussion with FA patients regarding family planning. It was explained to this patient that whether or not she chose to have postoperative radiotherapy of the head and neck region, she would likely have no significant problem with pregnancy. However, the discussion focused on expectations for her family.

She was advised that due to the appearance of a first cancer, there would be a likelihood of eventual appearance of multiple other cancers. She might have a normal pregnancy including genetic testing of the fetus in utero to rule out whether her FA gene(s) were transmitted to her child. She was advised that due to the natural history of her FA, that she might not be alive to attend her anticipated child's high school graduation. She chose to be followed and was considering marriage and starting a family with full knowledge of the possible bad future events. This kind of discussion is necessary and is carried out with all FA patients including those that present with a cancer and those, who do not.

This patient was followed closely, and there was a second oropharyngeal cancer diagnosed within 2 years. She received surgical excision and then did receive postoperative radiotherapy. She chose to have adjuvant chemotherapy, using an investigational chemotherapy protocol, which is one of many being used in radiosensitive FA patients. Her postoperative radiotherapy treatment course was uneventful in part, because she was treated using a radiotherapy fractionation "clinical trial protocol" [13] to determine whether she was one of the FA patients, who was indeed radiosensitive.

This clinical trial protocol involved starting with a very small radiation field and low dose of 0.5 Gy per day for 7 days with daily blood count analysis and daily inspection of the normal tissues to determine whether she was a radiosensitive patient. With no blood count decreases and no erythema, a second week of treatment is continued with the same small volume receiving a clinical standard dose of 1.8 Gy per day. With no side effects of irradiation, the patient then received a third week of radiotherapy with the clinically relevant postoperative field involving all echelon lymph nodes and tissue boundaries. This third week was with 0.5 Gy per day reduced dose. The fourth week was then full dose to this clinically relevant volume delivering 1.8 Gy per day and going to the standard postoperative radiotherapy dose of 60 Gy. This patient declared herself not to be radiosensitive and completed a full course of postoperative radiation [13]. She is being followed closely for evidence of local recurrence, metastasis, or another third primary cancer.

The third case presented is unlike the first two, because of the added dilemma associated with the delivery of radiotherapy in patients with a suspected sensitivity to radiation therapy. Some candidates for postoperative treatment, like all others, require an explanation of the risks of radiotherapy including the late effects, but these patients have a special risk of receiving ionizing irradiation. FA patients with cancer, who survived a radiotherapy and/or course of chemoradiotherapy for cancer, are also quite concerned about the health of their children. They are also concerned about the potential for inheritance of cancer proneness in their children.

Cancer in the children of irradiated patients has been a concern for decades [14–16]. From the available data on the children and grandchildren of the survivors of Hiroshima and Nagasaki atomic bombs [14], and the children of individuals, who suffered radiation from fallout in the Marshallese Islands, particularly Rongelar [15], there are reports of cancer in these first-generation progeny, although there is no statistically significant increase in the incidence of cancers. Grandchildren of the survivors of the atomic bombs at Hiroshima and Nagasaki are still being evaluated for cancer incidence [16]. There is no significant data reporting increased risk. A complication of these studies has been separating the baseline genetic component of the original cancer patient or the original irradiated person in the case of nontherapy-associated radiation exposure. Animal experiments suggest that there is a mechanism of the increased cancer susceptibility [17].

The place, where genetic testing is most appropriate, is in those current cancer patients, who may have a gene of increased risk of breast, ovarian cancer, and pelvic cancer patients [2]. Those who present with BRAC1 or BRAC2 genetic alterations in their cancers have a special need for genetic counseling [3]. The BRACA1 and BRACA2 mutations are associated with a high incidence of cancer in these organs, and women are advised to consider this in family planning.

The risk of carcinogenesis in the progeny of total body irradiated individuals is also a second subject of intense investigation, particularly because of the plethora of data in experimental animal systems. Inbred mouse strains with a high incidence of spontaneous cancer have been studied for the effect of total body irradiation or other systemic agents on the incidence of cancer in first-generation and second-generation progeny [17]. There are genetic factors that increase the risk of cancers after total body irradiation, and the question of whether the progeny of these irradiated, cancer-prone mice will be at increased risk. There is conflicting data on several of these experiments, but they do suggest the importance of genetic testing in the modern era, where there are so many genes that have been identified as associated with a high incidence of spontaneous, non-irradiation-related cancer. A question for patients and care providers in the modern era is whether such patients with a genetically determined increased risk of cancer will have that risk increased in their first- and second-generation progeny. Will they still choose to receive radiotherapy as an option for treatment of their own cancer.

There is a new area of investigation in clinical medicine, and new prospective studies are underway to track the incidence of cancer after irradiation, not only in the patients themselves, but in their progeny.

References

1. Kleinerman RA. Cancer risks following diagnostic and therapeutic radiation exposure in children. Pediatr Radiol. 2006;36(Suppl 2):121–5. https://doi.org/10.1007/s00247-006-0191-S.
2. Plon SE, Cooper HP, Parks B, et al. Genetic testing and cancer risk management recommendations by physicians for at-risk relatives. Genet Med. 2011;13(2):148–54. https://doi.org/10.1097/GIM.0b013e318207f564.
3. Hall MJ, Obeid EI, Schwartz SC, et al. Genetic testing for hereditary cancer predisposition: BRCA1/2, lynch syndrome, and beyond. Gynecol Oncol. 2016;140(3):565–74. https://doi.org/10.1016/j.ygyno.2016.01.019.
4. Siva S, MacManus M, Ball D. Stereotactic radiotherapy for pulmonary oligometastases: a systematic review. J Thorac Oncol. 2010;5(7):1091–9. https://doi.org/10.1097/JTO.0b013e3181de7143.
5. Bernstein MB, Krishnan S, Hodge JW, et al. Immunotherapy and stereotactic ablative radiotherapy (ISABR): a curative approach? Nat Rev Clin Oncol. 2016;13(8):516–24. https://doi.org/10.1038/nrclinonc.2016.30.
6. Caudell JJ, Ballo MT, Zagars GK, et al. Radiotherapy in the management of giant cell tumor of bone. Int J Radiat Oncol Biol Phys. 2003;57(1):158–65. https://doi.org/10.1016/s0360-3016(03)00416-4.
7. Grompe M, D'Andrea A. Fanconi anemia and DNA repair. Hum Mol Genet. 2001;10(20):2253–9.
8. Rodriguez A, Yang C, Furutani E, et al. Inhibition of TGFβ1 and TGFβ3 promotes hematopoiesis in Fanconi anemia. Exp Hematol. 2021;93:70–84. https://doi.org/10.1016/j.exphem.2020.11.002.
9. Alter BP. Cancer in Fanconi anemia, 1927-2001. Cancer. 2003;97(2):425–40. https://doi.org/10.1002/cncr.11046.
10. Kachnic LA, Li L, Fournier L, et al. Fanconi anemia pathway heterogeneity revealed by cisplatin and oxaliplatin treatments. Cancer Lett. 2010;292(1):73–9. https://doi.org/10.1016/j.canlet.2009.11.009.
11. Lewis LM, Tang AL, Wise-Draper TM, et al. Successful use of a therapeutic trial of graduated volume and dose escalation for postoperative head and neck radiotherapy in a Fanconi anemia patient. Head Neck. 2020;42(10):E16–22. https://doi.org/10.1002/hed.26395.
12. Gardner UG Jr, Wood SG, Chen EY, et al. Use of a therapeutic trial of graduated neoadjuvant radiotherapy for locally advanced esophageal cancer in a patient with Fanconi anemia. Adv Radiat Oncol. 2021;7(1):100810. https://doi.org/10.1016/j.adro.2021.100810.
13. Greenberger JS, Epperly MW. Radiotherapy for the patient with Fanconi anemia: a challenge for the radiation oncologist. Chapter 7. In: Watanabe HS, editor. Horizons in cancer research, vol. 60. New York: Nova Science Publishers; 2016. p. 63–76.
14. Preston DL, Cullings H, Suyama A, et al. Solid cancer incidence in atomic bomb survivors exposed in utero or as young children. J Natl Cancer Inst. 2008;100(6):428–36. https://doi.org/10.1093/jnci.dnj045.
15. Land CE, Bouville A, Apostoaei J, et al. Projected lifetime cancer risks from exposure to regional radioactive fallout in The Marshall Islands. Health Phys. 2010;99(2):201–15. https://doi.org/10.1097/HP.0b013e3181dc4e84.

16. Kamite Y. Prejudice and health anxiety about radiation exposure from second-generation atomic bomb survivors: results from a qualitative interview study. Front Psychol. 2017;8:1462. https://doi.org/10.3389/fpsyg.2017.01462.
17. Russo MT, DeLuca G, Degan P, et al. Accumulation of the oxidative base lesion 8-Hydroxyguanine in DNA of tumor-prone mice defective in both the Myh and Ogg1 DNA glycosylases. Cancer Res. 2004;64(13):4411–4. https://doi.org/10.1158/0008-5472.CAN-04-0355.

Chapter 16
Lessons Learned from the Management and Prevention of Clinical Radiation Late Effects

As advances in the care of cancer patients continue to be reported, there are many patients living longer and these survivors unfortunately are experiencing the delayed/late side effects of cancer including radiation therapy [1–8]. Nowhere has the accumulation of side effects been more evident than that with pediatric patients, who were treated decades ago when they were in early childhood and now are adults [1, 9–13]. In the decades 1980–2000, there was a push to add more components to the combination regions. That chemotherapy drugs were supplemented with a fourth drug, then with a fifth [4, 14–17]. Then in the decades of 2010, there was a move to eliminate drugs that did not add to cure, but there were still side effects [18, 19]. The regimen ABVD (Adriamycin, Bleomycin, Vinblastine, and Dacarbazine) for lymphomas was changed to eliminate the "B" (Bleomycin) [3].

With respect to cancer patients and the other rare instances in which therapeutic radiation was used as part of the medical care program, there are numerous examples of late side effects of radiotherapy, many of those were either not considered or not reported [20–33]. Radiation therapy was prescribed with consideration of toxicity to some, but not all organs. A history of the use of ionizing irradiation in patient care with emphasis on treatment of cancer now reveals the origin and in some cases the mechanism of many unexpected severe late effects [5, 9, 34].

Since the first use of therapeutic ionizing irradiation, several generations of radiation oncologists have been trained and each generation has had available more sophisticated radiation therapy delivery devices, but radiation biology has not changed [35–37]. It is useful to look at the review of the evolution of clinical radiotherapy and by so doing learn lessons in the management and, hopefully, the prevention of late effects of this treatment modality. The side effects of radiotherapy were initially thought to be a consideration that was only relevant to limited conditions limited dose constraints and with a limited number of organs. For example, decades of delivery of 36–40 Gy to the mantle field to treat Hodgkin's lymphoma assumed that the heart could tolerate the dose with little side effects. Blocks were placed to shield the left ventricle by largely learning there were no lymph nodes there, but late

J. Greenberger, *Radiation Oncology and Radiation Biology*, https://doi.org/10.1007/978-3-031-66300-0_16

Table 16.1 Radiation side effects that were initially unexpected and not considered relevant

Treatment paradigm	Unexpected side effects, not considered relevant	Modification of treatment picture
Mantle irradiation for Hodgkin's disease	Cardiac damage	Reduce radiation dose, eliminate radiotherapy
Para-aortic fistula from Hodgkin's disease	Pancreas cancer	Delete this treatment volume
Pelvic radiotherapy for Hodgkin's disease	Sterilization induction of leukemia/lymphoma	Eliminate this procedure.
Whole brain irradiation for pediatric lymphoma	Cognitive loss	Eliminate WBI except for few cases
Pediatric irradiation	Growth inhibition, second cancers	Reduce or eliminate dose
Adult brain irradiation—spare hippocampus	Spare hippocampus to preserve cognition	Change treatment field

cardiac toxicity is now a reality [2, 5, 9, 10]. The era of orthovoltage radiotherapy, followed by the introduction of cobalt 60 (1960–1965) megavoltage teletherapy machines, and then in the modern era of linear accelerators (1965-present day), there has evolved an increasing controversy about the use of radiotherapy [38, 39]. Surgery techniques have also changed to decrease toxicity [40], and now techniques are being developed to predict late effects [41].

In recent cancer treatment protocols radiotherapy is eliminated according to this controversy. At the present time, there are fewer patients with a variety of cancers, who are being referred for radiotherapy (Table 16.1). Clear directives for radiation dose reduction and a clear goal for the eventual replacement of radiotherapy with cancer prevention, earlier diagnosis, and, most importantly, the availability of systemic targeted therapies to treat both primary and metastatic cancers will prevail. In the current era of evidence-based medicine, it has become more difficult to justify the continued use of treatment protocols that include previously standard doses and treatment volumes of therapeutic radiation. This controversy is focused on randomized prospective clinical trials to treat patients without radiation or with lower doses and achieve the same clinical outcomes while avoiding the side effects of irradiation.

Side Effects of Radiotherapy Relate to the Basic Principles of Dose, Fraction Size, and Treatment Volume

Regardless of the technological advancements in clinical radiotherapy, the basic principles of radiation biology have not changed [7, 8, 32, 33, 35]. Notwithstanding are the monumental discoveries in understanding and modulating radiation-induced DNA double-strand breaks and organ systems biology. These discoveries will lead to great advances in radiation biology, ameliorating human radiation damage effects, but they are not here yet.

Since the original radiation biology experiments with animal models and the pioneering clinical studies [30, 37], it has been confirmed that there are four basic principles, which apply to nearly every form of the delivery of ionizing irradiation as radiotherapy, namely (1) irradiation dose; (2) fraction size; (3) treatment volume; and (4) treatment course duration [33, 35]. These basic principles include some nuances, which are important, such as dose rate, quality of the beam (LET of particles), oxygenation of tissues, and some other modulators of the basic principles, but these main principles continue to guide radiation oncologists to plan treatment strategies by which to control cancer.

Radiation Acute and Late Effects

The greatest body of data on late effects is that associated with the outcomes with patients, who have been cured of head and neck cancer [2] and gynecologic cancers [7]. The pioneering clinical studies [7] revealed the dose-response curves for human cancers and the normal tissue damage effects. The clinical trials for treating these volumes of normal tissue in the head and neck and pelvic regions, respectfully, strived for the goal of getting long-term local control of the cancer without causing severe damage to surrounding tissues and organs. The clinical trials of the 1950s and 1960s clearly revealed that there were dose and volume constraints, which indicated that a radiation dose could be "too low" to control cancer, and other radiation doses were "too high" to allow the necessary cancer control but caused serious and, in some cases, irreparable deleterious side effects [8]. Once the appropriate dose range was established, once the safe fractionation schemes were developed (safe dose delivered per day and time required for tissue recovery between doses) [33], and once it was recognized that there was a huge effect of increasing the size of the treatment field volume, then generations of radiation oncologists were trained to understand these basics of clinical radiotherapy. Any further modifications of treatment plans that deviated from the lessons learned from the results of clinical trials in the 1960s have been modest [32]. In fact, modifications have focused mostly on reducing the volume of normal tissue in the target volume with more advanced radiation delivery devices that could allow better avoidance of the spinal cord and brainstem in the treatment field; there were attempts to increase radiation dose. These clinical studies uncovered two new lessons: (1) there was no advantage in increasing the radiation dose to the cancer above a certain level (for example, in nonsmall cell lung cancer) and esophagus cancer [18, 19, 29], and (2) there were unrecognized damage effects of higher radiation doses to several unexpected organs including the heart [9].

The parameters, guidelines, and pathways for the now standard of care in clinical radiotherapy, therefore, have been established. Accordingly, the most recent reports of randomized prospective clinical trials have been focused on ways to add additional modalities (new drugs) to radiotherapy. Protocols now seek to de-escalate (lower) the prescribed radiation dose. We are in a new era. In the past, radiation side effects were deemed to be acceptable at a time when cancer control was the overwhelming goal. Women receiving postoperative radiotherapy, after mastectomy for breast cancer resection were found to have residual cancer in the postoperative chest wall [31]. Radiotherapy was prescribed, and there was accepted chest wall redness, dry, and moist desquamation (weeping lesions of lymph and swelling of tissue). There were reported additional cases of the more significant side effects of lymphedema of the arm (arising from treating the axilla with radiation, causing initial blockage of lymph drainage from the extremity due to swelling, and the late effects of fibrosis of the axilla and the chest wall muscles [31]. This acceptance of radiation side effects occurred for several decades, not only with breast cancer patients, but with patients treated at nearly every anatomic site. The goal was to control the cancer.

With the advent of modern linear accelerators and, most recently, with the technique of intensity-modulated radiotherapy (IMRT), women no longer were required to accept the side effects of chest wall irradiation in order to receive acceptable radiation doses that eliminated any residual cancer cells. Patients were no longer required to expect and accept the acute or late side effects as part of the treatment program [10]. IMRT allowed dose distributions to the chest wall that eliminated or reduced irradiation to the lung and heart and reduced the high-dose regions, so-called hot-spots with the skin and muscles underneath the entry points of the medial and lateral tangent field entry points for fields treating the chest wall irradiation [10]. IMRT is a technique, where multileaf collimators shape the radiation beam and the placement of the leaves on the collimator changes as the gantry position changes, and the machine moves across the patient. The dose delivered at a specific position can be higher or lower depending on how long the machine stays in that position. In essence, IMRT changes the shape of the field, and time that each position is held to minimize normal tissue exposure. Not only did IMRT significantly reduce chest wall radiation damage in postoperative breast cancer patients, it allowed the treatment of patients, who had an intact breast, namely those who had removal of the cancer only "lumpectomy" and sampling of axillary nodes to prove the absence of metastasis without dissection of axilla and "cleaning out" all nodes.

Breast cancer patients were some of the first to benefit from the surgical advances in introduction of minimally invasive surgical specialties. There is a focus on decresing normal tissue damage in cancer patient management. Great advances in many patient categories have followed. Examples include in urology doing prostate resections for prostate cancer without removing the pudendal nerve, thus allowing men to maintain penile erections [40] and, in thoracic surgery, the development of minimally invasive thoracoscopic and laparoscopic esophagectomy for lung and esophagus cancers [29]. Patients no longer required weeks of postoperative hospitalization to allow healing of thoracic surgery wounds.

The focus of radiation oncologists on reducing normal tissue late effects was dramatic in breast cancer patients. The concept of cosmesis was brought to the forefront in the 1970s [30]. The goal was to treat the breast after lumpectomy and axillary node sampling in a way that delivered the appropriate radiation dose and left the cosmetic effect on normal skin and breast tissue to be minimally altered from its pre-irradiation condition.

The "hanging-block" [30] technique for linear accelerators was implemented to prevent an overlap of the chest wall tangents with the supraclavicular field, for the reason of reducing any overlap of fields and the band of fibrosis at the margins of these two fields. These clinical reports of outcomes with this technique beginning in 1970s emphasized the importance of reducing radiation late side effects. One can evaluate this body of literature as a triumph of clinical radiation oncologists to change their focus from control of the cancer to overall welfare of the patient.

In other efforts to eliminate the side effects of whole-brain irradiation for a variety of cancers, there was a recognized understanding that the hippocampus could be spared (Table 16.1) from the treatment volume and, thereby, decrease the severity of the cognitive decline that was observed in long-term survivors of whole-brain irradiation [38, 39]. While reports of the deleterious late effects of brain irradiation were with pediatric patients, who received whole-brain irradiation for the prophylaxis of sanctuary sites of residual leukemia cells, the adaptation of whole-brain radiation was also being extended to use in those adult patients getting this treatment for prophylaxis of tumor metastasis in the brain after chemotherapy of small-cell lung cancer [38, 39]. The goal of therapy for these patients was then the same as for breast cancer patients during this era of radiation oncology, namely eliminating the cancer and not focusing on any unsuspected side effects. The goal was to eliminate multiple microscopic metastasis, where a large field was required.

Thus, similar to the change in chest wall radiation treatment planning, whole-brain radiation changed its focus to side effects, rather than the initial goal, which was to control cancer or prevent recurrence.

In the current era, radiation oncology protocols now focus on minimizng total dose to be delivered in treatment protocol. There must be a clear description of the dose per fraction/treatment and clear focus on reducing the volume of tissue treated for each radiotherapy treatment field, the revised focus is based upon the desire to eliminate both acute and chronic side effects. The radiation dosimetrist is the person, who designs the treatment technique. The radiation oncologist fills out a prescription showing the dose that he/she wants each normal tissue to receive, not just the cancer. The dosimetrist has a list of currently accepted doses for each tissue or organ. If the prescribed dose to the tumor cannot be delivered without exceeding the maximum allowable dose as defined on the list of each normal tissue on the form, the radiation oncologist must change the prescription to make a decision—either agree to exceed the allowable dose for that normal tissue/organ or change the treatment plan to change the tumor target volume that is to receive 100% of the prescribed dose [30, 37]. These rules are in place and followed by most radiation oncology departments. The acceptable maximum dose for each normal tissue is the result of data in the current literature and is based upon hundreds of reports of acute and late effects. The volume of each organ getting each accepted dose must also be indicated in the prescription. For example, in treating lung cancer, the volume of lung receiving 20% on the prescribed tumor dose is shown (V20). Also, the V5 is shown [30].

Different radiation oncology departments may add additional data points and constraints. Another updated data entry form is the required margin around the tumor volume as sometimes defined by PET scan or CT scan or MRI scan. For a lung metastasis near the esophagus, the margin may be 3 mm, and for one in distal peripheral lung, it may be 5 mm—owing to the need to prevent too high a dose to the esophagus. In addition, the volume of esophagus receiving the V20 or V5 may be indicated. All of these data can be entered into the treatment plan and the prescription, because the treatment planning software allows the mapping (contouring/drawing) of every anatomic structure by the physicians and then entered into a computerized treatment planning program. The software print-out of each plan includes a dose/volume histogram and graph showing the volume of tumor and each normal argan getting each % or total dose of each fraction. The focus is on knowing what each normal organ receives as dose and what volume of each organ receives that dose. Very focused compared to the treatment plans of the 1970s, but all involved the need to recognize that the basic radiation biology of the cancer and the normal tissues has not changed. All of this published experience is based upon the principle of irradiating normal tissue in the least-volume and to the lowest dose, while still delivering 100% of the prescribed dose to the cancer.

The physician, nurse, and all care providers in radiation oncology departments are aware of the individuality of every patient. Some may develop acute symptoms of radiation injury quite early, and treatment must be halted to allow for normal tissue recovery. Concomitant chemotherapy may increase side effects and the speed of first observation and rapid progression of side effects; then, a treatment break must be instituted. For example, a patient receiving a planned course of 5 weeks radiotherapy for lung cancer (25 treatments/5 per week) may develop difficulty swallowing after 2 weeks, whereas this symptom would not be expected until week 4, even using a perfect IMRT plan or an even more sophisticated VMAT plan (moving of the gantry and multileaf collimators in real time rather than with multiple fixed position fixed fields), the individual patient may exhibit symptoms of toxicity earlier than expected. This is why the radiation biology, which is taught to radiation oncology residents, is still critical to patient care, no matter how sophisticated the machine and computer delivering the radiation [19].

The above considerations describe two of the three basic principles: dose and volume. The third issue of fraction size has recently been addressed by analysis of the results with different programs of hyperfractionation, and, recently, hypofractionation. What is fraction size? The dose that is delivered per treatment. Why is fraction size relevant? There has been an acceptance of the fact that normal tissues recover from radiation after each dose. The clinically accepted time for this recovery has been 4–6 h [11, 36]. The number is based on cell culture studies with cell lines and with irradiation of animal models. The cancer also recovers between fractions. Modern radiotherapy practice requires that the time between fractions is determined by the normal tissue, not the cancer. The fractionation schemes are based on the so-called 4 Rs of fractionation [24]: (1) reoxygenation; (2) repopulation; (3) redistribution; and (4) repair [35].

Whether these metrics are logical and whether they apply to all tissues and all cancers are the subjects of continued discussion, but the origin of each is based upon real data. Hypoxic tumors are radioresistant, so it makes sense to allow blood flow to bring oxygen to the treatment volume. Tumor cell lines that were synchronized for growth/cell doubling showed more radiation killing immediately before and during miosis, so it made sense to allow time for tumor cells to re-enter other phases of the cell cycle. The tumors contain some cells that are resting and not dividing, so-called quiescence, so it makes sense to allow them time to start growing to repopulate the tumor. Finally, the concept of repair is confusing to some, because one wants to allow the normal tissue to repair, but not the tumor. Nevertheless, the 4–6 h between fractions do not seem to significantly allow cancers to complete all radiation DNA double-strand break repair, while the normal tissues tolerated the next radiation dose better if the time was 4–6 h before the next dose.

Changes to treatment fractionation approaches to fraction size were based on shift in attitude from cancer control to that of quality of life for patients, which means decreasing side effects. Initial hyperfractionation protocols in which lower radiation fraction sizes were delivered twice a day separated by four (recently changed to six) hours. This change in number of treatments per day was carried out to obtain the same local control that comes with decreased side effects. While initial studies of hyperfractionation were focused on giving total higher doses, the ultimate goal of such protocols was to decrease side effects.

In contrast, the hypofractionation protocols currently still being tested are designed to limit the number of treatments and move patients through their radiotherapy course in a more efficient fashion. The standard fractionation schemes, which were developed by radiation oncologists in the 1940s and 1950s, were based on the concept of one treatment per day, 5 days a week, and moving patients through the process in an efficient manner. However, the idea of increasing the fraction size and limiting the number of treatments came into use for different reasons. In the United Kingdom, hypofractionation was initially used for prostate cancer to move patients through the treatment programs more quickly [25]. One theory as to the reason for this change in protocol was that there were too few linear accelerators available and more patients requiring radiotherapy for prostate cancer. With the change over the last decades in referral patterns for prostate cancer, there have been fewer referrals based upon the elimination of some patients with lower risk categories [25]. Conclusions were that there was no need to move more patients through a treatment program more quickly and free up the machine time for other patients. This is a theory. There is a new potential reason to explain the use of hypofractionation protocols. If the side effects of a larger fraction such as 3 Gy or 4 Gy per fraction can be used under conditions in which the treatment volume is defined more precisely, using IMRT and VMAT, why not move the patients through the treatment program more quickly and eliminate the need for multiple trips to the radiation therapy department? Initial randomized prospective clinical trials using the "short course" compared to the conventional way of treating prostate cancer led to observations that there was no significant increase in side effects and the outcomes were the same. More and more radiation therapy protocols are going to a hypofractionation protocls. These protocols are feasible and safe, largely, because of the experience with stereotactic radiotherapy (SBRT) and stereotactic ablative radiotherapy (SABR), respectively.

Very effective patient immobilization techniques are now available for SBRT, and the use of multileaf collimators [25] and improved three-dimensional treatment planning including four-dimensional treatment planning for patients with lung cancer in which respiratory gating [26] can be used (The machine turns off when the tumor volume in the lung moves out of the field.) made it possible to give higher fraction sizes to smaller volumes with no increase in the acute side effects. Nowhere is the importance of reducing the volume treated more evident than in the case of the hypofractionation regimens used for SBRT. The pioneering work of Ralph Weichselbaum, M.D., at the University of Chicago on oligometastasis [38, 39] and that at the U. Texas Southwestern determined and publicized the now standard and safe dose fractionation schemes for SBRT, which are now being used throughout the country to treat primary brain tumors and metastasis [39].

Reduction or Elimination of Clinical Radiotherapy

The pediatric radiotherapy population provided the most convincing evidence that any radiation dose can be deleterious. Recent reports from St. Jude Children's Hospital, Philadelphia Children's Hospital, and others indicate that even modest doses of radiotherapy should be avoided if possible [24] (Table 16.1). In the treatment of Wilms' tumor for prophylaxis of lung metastasis, in craniospinal irradiation for medulloblastoma, and in use of radiotherapy for thoracic or abdominal tumors, there has been a continuing evolution of protocols in which radiation dose has been decreased [24]. Radiotherapy has been virtually eliminated for preparation of children as the recipient for bone marrow transplantation. The chemotherapy preparation of the recipient using the drugs Busulfan and Cytoxan has replaced radiation for some cancers [13]. Whole-brain irradiation is no longer a general practice for prophylaxis of sanctuary sites harboring lymphocytic leukemia, and use of radiation in patients with Ewings sarcoma, rhabdomyosarcoma, and other pediatric tumors in which radiation was routinely used in the 1970s Pediatric Radiotherapy has continually decreased. Multiple publications on the late effects of radiotherapy have documented that essentially any radiation dose that is delivered to children may have side effects that can be measured decades later (Table 16.1).

An Evolving Understanding of the Spectrum of Radiation Late Effects

The greatest evidence for radiation late effects comes from those patients, who have been cured of head and neck cancer [2], and gynecologic cancers [33]. In these two categories, patients have the same common experience. Radiotherapy doses were escalated to provide the greatest chance for local control and cure, and in the 1970s and 1980s, with the introduction of IMRT and sophisticated treatment planning, radiation doses could be delivered to primary tumors and regional lymph nodes. The head and neck cancer patients provide the most convincing examples of the importance of understanding late effects.

Head and neck cancers of the oral cavity, oropharynx, base of tongue, floor of the mouth, tonsillar fossa, hypopharynx, nasopharynx, and other local sites provided treatment volumes that could be managed in treatment planning that avoided the critical structures of the brainstem and spinal cord [2]. The larynx and pharyngeal constrictor muscles in many of the treatment volumes were not considered (originally) as normal tissues that could suffer severe late effects [2]. However, the pioneering work on late effects [14, 15] revealed that radiation late effects had a significant onset beginning in a great number of patients at 12–18 months after completion of radiation doses of 60–70 Gy [19, 29].

Progressive radiation fibrosis in the larynx and in pharyngeal constrictors provided the concept of the "trajectory of side effects." This concept has gained great relevance in the survivorship clinics that are maintained in most cancer centers. The concept of survivorship is one, which is happily very common. Patients with head and neck cancer are, indeed, cured, including those who have had surgery only, surgery plus radiation, or surgery, radiation, and adjuvant chemotherapy. Hundreds of patients are alive at 10–20 years or longer after curative therapy for head and neck cancer. These patients are presenting with radiation side effects and provide a great resource for understanding radiation late effects and also for providing a strategy to both manage and prevent these late effects.

There are biomarkers for the onset of late radiation fibrosis in head and neck cancer patients. Measurement of plasma protein levels for inflammatory cytokines can be carried out using the Luminex assay [34]. MicroRNA measurement in the plasma can quantitate the increase in activation of genes for the inflammatory cytokines [41]. Therefore, following patients with not only clinical examination but also measurement of these biomarkers of the onset of fibrosis can provide ways in which new antifibrotic therapies can be tested. There are clinical trials in which several categories of drugs have been used to attempt to reverse fibrosis or prevent the onset of fibrosis. Pentoxifylline, antioxidants such as Vitamin C, and physical therapy approaches including ways to increase the flexibility of tissues and prevent the onset of fibrosis have been implemented in many survivorship clinics [14, 22]. Once patients are in a category of long-term survival/cure, they are not just simply followed for cancer recurrence, but are now followed for early biomarkers of the onset of fibrosis.

Attempts to reduce or decrease fibrosis from irradiation have followed similar programs in management of patients with thermal burn-induced fibrosis, postsurgical fibrosis, and situations in chemical burns. Physical therapy approaches to maintain tissue flexibility have been implemented. These include deep tissue massage, exercise programs including swimming and stretching, and clinical trials of antifibrosis drugs [23]. The trajectory of late effects including fibrosis, as described by Nilsen, may be very relevant to understanding the radiobiology of late effects. The clinical observations indicate that total radiation dose, fraction size, and volume treated are just as important for understanding late effects, as for the acute effects. Therefore, the continued evolution of treatment planning techniques including better immobilization, reducing the target volume based not only on PET/CT fusion images at the time of treatment planning, and use of multileaf collimators to limit normal tissue radiation exposure are now being increasingly used in head and neck cancer patients. The reduced volume focus led to the development of the PTV approach. PTV1, PTV2, and PTV3 have been used as planning treatment volumes to give larger doses to the earlier treatment plan, and then, reducing the volume of tissue treated until the final smallest dose is used [18, 19]. The GTV is the gross tumor volume and is considered to be the target for where the highest dose is given, but that high dose need not be delivered to regional lymph nodes or places, where there is not gross tumor. While less available for rapid observable clinical diagnostic examination, the late effects observed in gynecologic cancer patients have also been approached with great interest.

The concept of curative radiation doses for cervix and endometrial cancers led to the optimization of a combination of intracavitary radioisotope brachytherapy (radium replaced by cesium sources) and external beam radiation [21]. The addition of an external beam dose to a brachytherapy dose led to the concept of a total cumulative dose. In patients, who receive intracavitary or interstitial brachytherapy implants, it was clear that reducing the external beam dose could decrease side effects. Side effects of this combination of treatment modalities were measured in bladder fibrosis as frequency and urgency, and reduced volume of urine having decreased bladder capacity, rectal stricture, and, most importantly, in the acute periods after radiotherapy, vaginal and vulvar fibrosis leading to dyspareunia. The initial treatment of radiation late effects was associated with Premarin vaginal cream to keep tissues flexible. However, with a greater number of survivors of gynecologic cancers living for decades, the focus has been on bladder and rectal strictures. Sophisticated treatment planning and minimizing the target volume led to a decrease in side effects, but with the advent of adjuvant chemotherapy, there is clear evidence that radiotherapy side effects are increased if there is also a delivery of chemotherapy.

The Importance of Combined Injury in Radiotherapy Late Effects

Postoperative radiotherapy is associated with an increased risk for radiation fibrosis [38]. The timing of when to initiate radiotherapy after surgery has been an evolving concept. Thoracic surgeons frequently suggested that radiotherapy should not begin after resection of a lung cancer including patients with segmentectomy, lobectomy, or pneumonectomy, until surgical wounds had healed usually at 4–6 weeks. However, analysis of radiation late effects has evolved as decreased total radiation dose and decreased volume have been part of the protocols for postoperative management of patients with lung cancer. The same holds true for those patients treated after minimally invasive esophagectomy, who had positive resection margins or lymph nodes detected at the time of surgical excision of the tumor. The same concept of waiting for weeks for tissue healing to occur after surgery before starting radiotherapy has been closely watched in combined modality management of most cancer patients.

When to initiate adjuvant chemotherapy has also been a concept and focus of research. The concept of a neoadjuvant chemotherapy or starting the chemotherapy before surgery and radiotherapy is one which is closely followed to determine the effect on side effects [3–5]. The use of preoperative radiotherapy led to postoperative has also been a focus of intense investigation. In patients with a rectal cancer, preoperative radiotherapy was often used with the argument that this could decrease the magnitude of surgical excision and the total volume of tissue removed. However, physicians reported that at the time of resection, it was difficult to determine the volume of tumor that needed to be removed and the associated normal tissue that would be in the resection volume [17]. The movement toward postoperative radiotherapy for rectal cancer focused on the need for surgeons to observe the PET/CT volume relevant to the gross pathological appearance of the tumor in the surgical field. Postoperative radiotherapy was then commonly used. The arguments on both sides have continued. Proponents of preoperative radiotherapy suggested that a smaller treatment volume including less normal tissue could be included. Proponents of postoperative radiotherapy suggested that the original treatment volume could be included in the target volume and that postoperative radiotherapy provided more information from the surgeon's report as to what nodal areas needed to be treated. Clinical trials are still in progress, particularly, with the addition of new chemotherapy drugs for colorectal cancer. The main concepts continue to be a focus in all of these areas: reduced total dose, reduced fraction size, and minimum possible treatment volume.

Does Proton Radiotherapy or Carbon Ion Radiotherapy Reduce Late Effects Compared to X-Rays?

The analysis of the quality of life of survivors of proton radiotherapy, particularly, in the pediatric population in which craniospinal irradiation is delivered by protons, compared to historical match with patients treated with X-ray photon irradiation is providing the best evidence for understanding that protons may have an advantage [20]. Initial reports from St. Jude indicated that there was no significant decrease in the incidence of second cancers in pediatric patients, who receive craniospinal irradiation [20], but at the time of that presentation, there was insufficient evidence of the analysis of late effects. There are studies now reporting a potential decrease in late effects/fibrosis in patients receiving proton irradiation for head and neck cancer, lung cancer, and pelvic malignancies. The concept of total dose, fraction size, and tissue volume may be in favor of proton irradiation to reduce the magnitude of fibrosis and, potentially, also delay the onset of fibrosis. These studies are in progress. The major point remains the importance of total volume treated, fraction size, and total dose. Carbon ion radiotheray is in development and analysis of outcomes is in progress.

Knowledge of Clinical Radiotherapy Late Effects Helps Direct Development of Radiation Countermeasures

With clinical radiotherapy outcomes analysis, relevant data are available to help design radoaion countermeasures. For other indications, for NASA and the upcoming Mars Mission, it will be possible to compare clinical TBI effects with the data obtained from the limited number of individuals, who have been exposed to total body, sporadic space irradiation. Thankfully, the small number of individuals, who have had radiation exposure from nuclear reactor accidents or from working in plutonium plants (Colorado/Wyoming) are in numbers too small for evaluation at the present time [42]. Radiation dose-response curves for both astronauts exposed to space irradiation and workers in nuclear reactor or nuclear weapons production facilities are small in number, and the analysis is ongoing. There is a major concern in these research areas whether the side effects of irradiation will lead to cancer and neurodegenerative disease. However, radiation fibrosis remains a consideration in nearly all forms of radiation exposure. The exciting data from the Wake Forest Nonhuman Primate (NHP) Center is leading the way to understand the spectrum of radiation late effects beyond what is learned from human cancer survivors [34]. The NHP experiments with Rhesus Macaque monkeys exposed to TBI, partial body irradiation (5% marrow sparing), and thoracic irradiation have revealed late effects on organs not previously thought to be vulnerable to late radiation injury. These include pancreas/diabetes, brain blood vessels/multiple mini-strokes, and osteomalacia/bones and joints [34]. The data from clinical radiotherapy outcomes are indeed being supported by experimental models of space radiation and military and civilian radiation weapon systems. Much new information is becoming available and will be needed to plan for protection of our military personnel and our astronauts.

References

1. Bitsko MJ, Cohen D, Dillon R, et al. Psychosocial late effects in pediatric cancer survivors: a report from the Children's Oncology Group. Pediatr Blood Cancer. 2016;63(2):337–43. https://doi.org/10.1002/pbc.25773.
2. Nilsen ML, Mady LJ, Hodges J, et al. Burden of treatment: reported outcomes in a head and neck cancer survivorship clinic. Laryngoscope. 2019;129(12):E437–44. https://doi.org/10.1002/lary.27801.
3. Stamatoullas A, Brice P, Bouabdallah R, et al. Outcome of patients older than 60 years with classical Hodkin lymphoma treated with front line ABVD chemotherapy: frequent pulmonary events suggest limiting the use of bleomycin in the elderly. Br J Haematol. 2015;170(2):179–84. https://doi.org/10.1111/bjh.13419.
4. Mariotto A, Feuer EJ, Harlan LC, et al. Trends in use of adjuvant multi-agent chemotherapy and tamoxifen for breast cancer in the United States: 1975–1999. J Natl Cancer Inst. 2002;94(21):1626–34. https://doi.org/10.1093/jnci/94.21.1626.
5. Hahn E, Jiang H, Ng A, et al. Late cardiac toxicity after mediastinal radiation therapy for Hodgkin lymphoma: contributions of coronary artery and whole heart dose-volume variables to risk prediction. Int J Radiat Oncol Biol Phys. 2017;98(5):1116–23. https://doi.org/10.1016/j.ijrobp.2017.03.026.
6. Baclesse F. Five-year results in 431 breast cancers treated solely by Roentgen Rays. Ann Surg. 1965;161(1):103–4. https://doi.org/10.1097/00000658-196501000-00017.
7. Thames HD Jr, Withers HR, Peters LJ, et al. Changes in early and late radiation responses with altered dose fractionation: implications for dose-survival relationships. Int J Radiat Oncol Biol Phys. 1982;8(2):219–26. https://doi.org/10.1016/0360-3016(82)90517-x.
8. Fletcher GH. Elective irradiation of subclinical disease in cancers of the head and neck. Cancer. 1972;29(6):1450–4. https://doi.org/10.1002/1097-0142(197206)29:6<1450::aid-cncr2820290605>3.0.co;2-q.
9. Heidenreich PA, Kapoor JR. Radiation induced heart disease: systemic disorders in heart disease. Heart. 2009;95(3):252–8. https://doi.org/10.1136/hrt.2008.149088.
10. Wang H, Wei J, Zheng Z, et al. Radiation-induced heart disease: a review of classification, mechanism, and prevention. Int J Biol Sci. 2019;15(10):2128–38. https://doi.org/10.7150/ijbs.35460.
11. Chan S, Rowbottom L, McDonald R, et al. Does the time of radiotherapy affect treatment outcomes? A review of the literature. Clin Oncol (R Coll Radiol). 2017;29(4):231–8. https://doi.org/10.1016/j.clon.2016.12.005.
12. Jeraj M, Robar V. Multileaf collimator in radiotherapy. Radiol Oncol. 2004;38(3):235–40.
13. Chou RH, Wong GB, Kramer JH, et al. Toxicities of total-body irradiation for pediatric bone marrow transplantation. Int J Radiat Oncol Biol Phys. 1996;34(4):843–51. https://doi.org/10.1016/0360-3016(95)02178-7.
14. Nilsen ML, Clump DA II, Kubik M, et al. Prevision of multidisciplinary head and neck cancer survivorship care during the 2019 novel coronavirus pandemic. Head Neck. 2019;42(7):1668–73. https://doi.org/10.1002/hed.26256.
15. Nilsen ML, Johnson JT. Potential for low-value palliative care of patients with recurrent head and neck cancer. Lancet Oncol. 2017;18(5):e284–9. https://doi.org/10.1016/S1470-2045(17)30260-7.

16. Davis AM, O'Sullivan B, Turcotte R, et al. Late radiation morbidity following randomization to preoperative versus postoperative radiotherapy in extremity soft tissue sarcoma. Radiother Oncol. 2005;75(1):48–53. https://doi.org/10.1016/j.radonc.2004.12.020.
17. Zagars GK, Ballo MT, Pisters PWT, et al. Surgical margins and reresection in the management of patients with soft tissue sarcoma using conservative surgery and radiation therapy. Cancer. 2003;97(10):2544–53. https://doi.org/10.1002/cncr.11367.
18. Bradley JD, Hu C, Komaki RR, et al. Long-term results of NRG oncology RTOG 0617: standard-versus high-dose chemoradiotherapy with or without cetuximab for unresectable stage III non-small-cell lung cancer. J Clin Oncol. 2020;38(7):706–14. https://doi.org/10.1200/JCO.19.01162.
19. Bernard ME, Glaser SM, Gill BS, et al. Results of a single institution experience with dose-escalated chemoradiation for locally advanced unresectable non-small cell lung cancer. Front Oncol. 2017;7:1. https://doi.org/10.3389/fonc.2017.00001.
20. Hall EJ. Intensity-modulated radiation therapy, protons, and the risk of second cancers. Int J Radiat Oncol Biol Phys. 2006;65(1):1–7. https://doi.org/10.1016/j.ijrobp.2006.01.027.
21. Holschneider CH, Petereit DG, Chu C, et al. Brachytherapy: a critical component of primary radiation therapy for cervical cancer: from the Society of Gynecologic Oncology (SGO) and the American Brachytherapy Society (ABS). Brachytherapy. 2019;18(2):123–32. https://doi.org/10.1016/j.brachy.2018.11.009.
22. Straub JM, New J, Hamilton CD, et al. Radiation-induced fibrosis: mechanisms and implications for therapy. J Cancer Res Clin Oncol. 2015;141(11):1985–94. https://doi.org/10.1007/s00432-015-1974-6.
23. Westbury CB, Yarnold JR. Radiation fibrosis—current clinical and therapeutic perspectives. Clin Oncol (R Coll Radiol). 2012;24(10):657–72. https://doi.org/10.1016/j.clon.2012.04.001.
24. Paulino AC. Treatment strategies to reduce radiotherapy late effects in children. J Radiat Oncol. 2013;2:121–8.
25. Kupelian PA, Willoughby TR. Short-course, intensity-modulated radiotherapy for localized prostate cancer. Cancer J. 2001;7(5):421–6.
26. Kazda T, Jancalek R, Pospisil P, et al. Why and how to spare the hippocampus during brain radiotherapy: the developing role of hippocampal avoidance in cranial radiotherapy. Radiat Oncol. 2014;9:139. https://doi.org/10.1186/1748-717X-9-139.
27. Rose MA, Olivotto I, Cady B, et al. Conservative surgery and radiation therapy for early breast cancer. Long-term cosmetic results. Arch Surg. 1989;124(2):153–7. https://doi.org/10.1001/archsurg.1989.01410020023002.
28. Olivotto IA, Rose MA, Osteen RT, et al. Late cosmetic outcome after conservative surgery and radiotherapy: analysis of causes of cosmetic failure. Int J Radiat Oncol Biol Phys. 1989;17(4):747–53. https://doi.org/10.1016/0360-3016(89)90061-8.
29. DeFoe SG, Pennathur A, Flickinger JC, et al. Retrospective review of patients with locally advanced esophageal cancer treated at the University of Pittsburgh. Am J Clin Oncol. 2011;34(6):587–92. https://doi.org/10.1097/COC.0b013e3181f942af.
30. Mitchell RA, Wai P, Colgan R, et al. Improving the efficiency of breast radiotherapy treatment planning using a semi-automated approach. J Appl Clin Med Phys. 2017;18(1):18–24. https://doi.org/10.1002/acm2.12006.
31. Krueger EA, Fraass BA, McShan DL, et al. Potential gains for irradiation of chest wall and regional nodes with intensity modulated radiotherapy. Int J Radiat Oncol Biol Phys. 2003;56(4):1023–37. https://doi.org/10.1016/s0360-3016(03)00183-4.
32. Overgaard J. Fractionated radiation and hyperthermia: experimental and clinical studies. Cancer. 1981;48(5):1116–23. https://doi.org/10.1002/1097-0142(19810901)48:5<1116::aid-cncr2820480512>3.0.co;2-j.
33. Thames HD Jr, Peters LT, Withers HR, et al. Accelerated fractionation vs hyperfractionation: rationales for several treatments per day. Int J Radiat Oncol Biol Phys. 1983;9(2):127–38. https://doi.org/10.1016/0360-3016(83)90089-5.

34. Olson JD, Schaaf GW, Elgohari BA, et al. Radiation-induced pulmonary fibrosis in non-human primates (NHPs) is preceded by cellular senescence and upregulation of tyrosine kinase Fgr, which is detectable by bronchial alveolar (BAL) gavage. Radiat Res. 2024. In press.
35. Withers HR. The four R's of radiotherapy. Adv Radiat Biol. 1975;5:241–71.
36. Wheldon TE, Deehan C, Wheldon EG, et al. The linear-quadratic transformation of dose-volume histograms in fractionated radiotherapy. Radiother Oncol. 1998;46(3):285–95. https://doi.org/10.1016/s0167-8140(97)00162-x.
37. Giraud P, Houle A. Respiratory gating for radiotherapy: main technical aspects and clinical benefits. Bull Cancer. 2010;97(7):847–56. https://doi.org/10.1684/bdc.2010.1143.
38. Pitroda SP, Chmura SJ, Weichselbaum R. Integration of radiotherapy and immunotherapy for treatment of oligometastases. Lancet Oncol. 2019;20(8):e434–42. https://doi.org/10.1016/S1470-2045(19)30157-3.
39. Bergsma DP, Salama JK, Singh DP, et al. Radiotherapy for oligometastatic lung cancer. Front Oncol. 2017;7:210. https://doi.org/10.3389/fonc.2017.00210.
40. Catalona WJ, Bigg SW. Nerve-sparing radical prostatectomy: evaluation of results after 250 patients. J Urol. 1990;143(3):538–43. https://doi.org/10.1016/s0022-5347(17)40013-9.
41. O'Reilly S. MicroRNAs in fibrosis: opportunities and challenges. Arthritis Res Ther. 2016;18:11. https://doi.org/10.1186/s13075-016-0929-x.
42. Thorne MC. Responding to radiation accidents: what more do we need to know? J Radiol Prot. 2022;42(3) https://doi.org/10.1088/1361-6498/ac8c4c.

Chapter 17
Radiation Countermeasures: An Emerging Scientific Field Based Upon Concerns for Nuclear Reactor Accidents and Radiation Terrorism

The concept of radiation mitigators by its very nature presents a challenge. The difference between a radiation protector [1] and a radiation mitigator is significant [2, 3]. Administering a radiation protector occurs before exposure to ionizing irradiation [4–33]. By its very nature, a radiation protector is given before a person enters an area likely to place the person at risk for exposure to ionizing irradiation [1]. Such would be the case with a nuclear reactor worker, who was entering a "hot zone" after a radiation spill. It would also apply to a situation in which military personnel were entering an area that had been exposed to radiation fallout, and where there were known radioisotopes in the environment. In contrast, a radiation mitigator is delivered after radiation exposure that has already occurred [3]. It is designed by definition to reduce the effects of irradiation. What is not immediately clear is how a radiation mitigator differs from a treatment of radiation injury. The definition of a mitigator is one that is given after radiation exposure but before the appearance of symptoms or signs of radiation exposure [2, 3, 22, 23]. This situation is unique to ionizing irradiation, because there is a gap between the time of radiation exposure and the appearance of symptoms and signs. Unlike a situation in which there has been thermal burn, concussion, or penetrating wounds, the ionizing irradiation does not present an immediate sign of exposure, but rather there is a lag between the exposure and the appearance of symptoms or signs of the exposure.

Symptoms of an exposure include the experience by the patient/victim of the exposure. With respect to ionizing irradiation that would be nausea and vomiting, diarrhea, redness of the skin, or in the case of very high doses of irradiation, a headache and the consequences of brain swelling. Signs of radiation exposure are already those, which indicate ionizing irradiation has induced changes in cells, tissues, and organs, such as swelling, vascular dilation (erythema reddening of the skin), and changes in the physical appearance. There has been a great effort to discover radiation mitigators [22–24] (Table 17.1), which has accelerated since the events of 9/11 and the clear terrorist attack on the United States territory. The United States military, as well as the military of other nations, has considered the importance of the

J. Greenberger, *Radiation Oncology and Radiation Biology*,
https://doi.org/10.1007/978-3-031-66300-0_17

Table 17.1 Categories of radiation countermeasures: both FDA approved (+) and under development (d)

Category	Specific agents	FDA approved for use as a radiation countermeasure
Growth factor	G-CSF	+
Cytokine	GM-CSF	+
Repurposed pharmaceutical	Captipril	d
Human growth hormone hGH	hGH	d
Small molecules	GS-nitroxides,	d
	Nitroxide—triphenyl phosphonium,	d
	Necrostatin	d
	Baicalein,	d
	Anti-pyroptosis drug	d
Cell therapies	Endothelial cells	d
	Adipocyte stem cells,	d
	Bone marrow stem cells,	d
	Bone marrow stromal cells	d
Genetically engineered		
Lactobacillus reuteri	LR-IFN-β	d
	LR-IL-22	d

d = in review/evaluation

radiation mitigator since the first atomic bomb testing in 1945. In the years after the Hiroshima and Nagasaki atomic bomb events, there was heightened fear of the use of tactical nuclear weapons on the battlefield of a then future war. Therefore, the military did consider the importance of radiation mitigators, but because of the sparse available scientific evidence that there could be such a pharmaceutical, there was more of a focus on radiation protectors since military personnel would enter a contaminated zone and would require the protection before exposure to irradiation [1–3].

Radiation mitigators assumed heightened importance when the threat of a thermonuclear war or radiation terrorist event including a fission-type bomb became a major concern [34–44]. Therefore, the Rad-Nuc program of the National Institutes of Allergies and Infectious Disease (NIAID) began to direct its resources toward establishing programs for the discovery and development of radiation mitigators. The Center for Medical Countermeasures Against Radiation (CMCR) Program, which initiated around 2009 and moved toward a consortium of funded centers in the Center for Medical Countermeasures Against Radiation Consortium (CMCRC) focused attention on discovering and developing mitigators [3, 45, 46]. Also, a mission of the CMCRC Program was the discovery of better biological dosimeters [47, 48], as well as physical dosimeters [34–36] to be able to define those victims/patients, who had been exposed to a dose of radiation that might require administration of mitigators. Faced with the possibility of thousands or tens of thousands of exposed victims in the case of a nuclear bomb detonation and attendant fallout, the focus of the program was also the concept of operations (Con-Ops). Administering a radiation mitigator to an individual, who had been exposed to a dose of radiation likely to cause symptoms and signs in the future, the administration would have to be streamlined and available to large numbers of individuals. An oral delivery would be ideal [49–52], but not possible if people were vomiting [53]. Cellular therapies are exciting but limited at present [34–57]. Given that some exposed individuals would already be experiencing symptoms and signs of exposure (nausea and vomiting included), the administration of an oral mitigator would not be suitable for such people. Therefore, there was a focus on topical skin administration or each injectable administration such as found in the epi-pen administration of epinephrine in the case of an anaphylactic reaction.

Since 9/11, there has been a great expansion of knowledge regarding radiation injury and how a radiation mitigator could be discovered and developed to a stage where it could be part of the National stockpile. Since the CMCR Program and other NIAID-related agencies began the search for mitigators, there have been additions to the National stockpile including, granulocyte colony-stimulating factor (G-CSF) and granulocyte macrophage colony-stimulating factor (GM-CSF). Both of these cytokines have been in clinical use in bone marrow transplant centers for decades since both targeted the Hematopoietic Acute Radiation Syndrome (H-ARS) (Table 17.1). G-CSF and GM-CSF were given to patients during the days—weeks after total body irradiation for bone marrow transplantation, and application of these drugs was also in clinical use for patients, who had severe neutropenia (drop in white blood cell counts) from chemotherapy agents.

Decades of use of these pharmaceuticals (G-CSF, GM-CSF) in clinical medicine provided significant background information to facilitate FDA approval of these agents for the National stockpile as radiation mitigators in the event of a nuclear accident or radiation terrorist event. Because these agents are cytokines and perishable, a program was put into effect in which the pharmaceutical companies that produced these drugs would be able to call them back from bone marrow transplant centers and deliver them to a site of distribution to an area of a rad-nuc event. The federal agencies that would be alerted to supply radiation countermeasures, including G-CSF and GM-CSF would be mobilized initially through the CDC (Center for Disease Control), and then through FEMA, the agency that would deliver the agents as part of the push-pak through airlift, or ground transportation to a site of a nuclear disaster, where thousands of individuals might need a radiation mitigator.

There remains one challenge with respect to the current availability of G-CSF and GM-CSF; namely, that it must be an injectable mitigator. This requires syringes and needles and personnel at a site that could draw the material from vials into syringes and inject each individual. There would also be a requirement for dose delivery depending on the relative age of the victim/patient, body weight, and injection site. Accordingly, the CMCRC Program focused in recent years on the discovery and development of mitigators that could be more easily distributed, and perhaps, have a longer shelf life, such as "freeze-dried" preparations or lyophilization and have a longer shelf life.

Practical issues regarding radiation mitigators provided another challenge to those scientists working on this problem. The classic radiation biology had to be modified to include a more focused approach to understanding the response of the human body to ionizing irradiation. The basic principles of radiation biology were the same; namely, the total dose of radiation sustained, dose rate, the volume of tissue irradiated, fraction size (in this case, a single fraction from a bomb detonation or nuclear accident), and the concept of the condition of the individual before radiation exposure. While the concept of radiation mitigators began to take hold with respect to radiation biology, there was continuing development of treatments for radiation injury. For individuals already exposed to radiation and exhibiting signs and symptoms of such exposure, treatments were administered based on what was available at the time. In the irradiated, epilated survivors of the Hiroshima and Nagasaki atomic bombing, there was some availability of radiation treatments. Blood products including transplant of whole blood and plasma had been developed during World War II, and if available, these could be administered to individuals, who had a falling peripheral blood count. Also, treatments for thermal burn include the administration of antibacterial agents to the skin and materials to cover burned areas. Radiation burns appeared at the time to be similar to thermal burns and were treated as such. Based on animal experiments, and dose-response relationships, there was already an appreciation of the Hematopoietis Acute Radiation Syndromea (H-ARS) and the Gastrointestinal Acute Radiation Syndrome (GI-ARS), the latter a clinical presentation that could not be reversed by bone marrow transplantation.

The pioneering work on marrow transplantation in experiments with total body irradiated dogs, led to clinical bone marrow transplantation [54]. It was acknowledged that certain doses and dose rates of irradiation could not be rescued by bone marrow transplantation. These observations in animals and the atomic bomb survivors led to an understanding of different syndromes of radiation exposure, which would follow such exposure. Using a mitigator by definition would be delivered before the time the patient/victim exhibited the symptoms and signs of that exposure. Therefore, the basic physics of radiation exposure was applied in the early design of mitigators. Where were the individuals relative to the hypocenter of the exposure? What if they had visible combined injuries such as thermal burn and concussion injuries? If radiation exposure was the only suspected insult, then the distance from the radiation event would be used to predict whether this individual was at risk for the H-ARS (in humans doses between 3 and 4.5 Gy) or received a higher dose and would be susceptible to the GI-ARS. Individuals closer to the hypocenter would be at risk for the central nervous system—acute radiation syndrome (CNS-ARS), and would likely already be presenting with the symptoms and signs of brain swelling. They might be triaged to a facility where they would receive intravenous fluids and other supportive care. Since individuals presenting with a CNS-ARS would be close to the hypocenter, then combined injury would also likely be apparent including thermal burn, penetrating wounds, injury from flying glass, and debris in addition to irradiation. How would such a CNS-ARS victim appear and under what conditions? Discussions about neutron irradiation from a fission bomb or fusion bomb would come into play since neutrons could penetrate high-molecular weight materials including concrete and still deliver a high enough radiation dose to cause the CNS-ARS. Accordingly, in NIAID programs over the last 20 years have focused on developing mitigators for the hematopoietic system and gastrointestinal system. Also, there has been a focus on mitigators that would be of use in cutaneous irradiation such as that from fallout, and recently a concern for discovering and developing mitigators that could be administered safely to "vulnerable populations" including the unborn fetus, pediatric patients, the elderly, and the infirm including those with a comorbid disease. Therefore, the practical nature of radiation mitigators came into play and is still a primary focus of research. There are threats from inhaled radiation-emitting particles [58, 59, 69] and rare, but deadly isotopes delivered orally [60]. Chelator drugs to remove inhaled or swallowed isotopes are a major area of research [61]. Drugs to target each of several radiation-induced death pathways are needed [2, 22, 23, 62–66].

As it relates to the discovery and development of radiation mitigators, the molecular mechanism of radiation injury has been a focus of renewed interest [63, 64]. The basic kinetics of ionizing irradiation injury have been known for decades: immediate ionization of oxygen and water producing free radicals, immediate effect of indirect irradiation (radical oxygen species including ionized water and oxygen) on inducing DNA strand breaks in the cell nucleus, and direct effects of high linear energy transfer particles such as neutrons causing direct DNA strand breaks. What was not appreciated until the recent decades has been the importance of the kinetics of DNA repair in the nucleus [63, 64] and the subsequent events that follow this initial injury; namely, transport to the cellular mitochondria of mediators of multiple different radiation-induced cell death pathways [22, 23, 62]. The first pathway to be elucidated was that of apoptosis or programmed cell death [2]. The cascade of events occurring in the mitochondria was elucidated and is still being studied. Each event represents a target for the discovery of a mitigator that would inhibit that step. Several other cell death pathways have been discovered including those that did not involve the same molecular biologic events such as apoptosis. These include necroptosis, ferroptosis, parthanatos, pyroptosis, intramitotic cell death, and others yet to be defined [22, 23, 62]. Radiation mitigators were discovered that could be delivered after radiation exposure and to target each of these cell death pathways. Furthermore, the timing of initiation of each distinct pathway could be used to optimize the time of delivery of a mitigator for each pathway [67]. After individual cell responses to radiation including each of the cell death pathways, there became a great focus on the communication of injury from irradiated cells to unirradiated cells (or cells that had received the lower radiation dose than that, which had induced the cell death pathways in highly irradiated site). Different tissues release cytokines and other biological response modifiers in response to cell death that occurred from the above cell death pathways. The elevation in inflammatory cytokines and the "master regulator" molecules involved in inflammation came into focus. These were also quickly recognized as potential targets for radiation mitigation. The use of steroids is highly controversial, because of the likelihood of rebound of injury when the drug is withdrawn [67]. Age and gender differences in response are factors [68]. Psychological factors are also a factor in the distribution of mitigators [47].

Finally, there was a renewed interest in radiation late effects as a target for development of radiation mitigators. Late effects had been known for decades before 9/11, principally, through the long clinical experience of radiotherapy for cancer [15, 66]. Patients cured of head and neck cancer and gynecologic neoplasm lived for decades and experienced late effects of irradiation. Therefore, there became a new focus on the discovery and development of mitigators to target late effects.

Before the 9/11 terrorist attacks on the World Trade Center, Pentagon, and the attempted attack on the White House, which was foiled by the brave passengers on the hijacked flight and led to its crash in rural Pennsylvania, there was already ongoing research to develop radiation countermeasures [3]. These countermeasures were then called radiation protectors [1].

Definitions were changed to reflect the human clinical conditions: (1) Protectors are given before irradiation; (2) Mitigators are given after irradiation exposure, but before detectable symptoms of injury; and (3) Treatments are delivered when victims are displaying symptoms and signs of damage from irradiation. These first radiation protectors were part of an already emerging field of research to address the need in clinical cancer patient management of new strategies by which to protect normal tissues during clinical radiotherapy. One of the most successful agents developed during this "Pre-9/11" era was the plasmid liposome delivery of the transgene for the radiation protector enzyme, Manganese Superoxide Dismutase (MnSOD) [2–4]. MnSOD is one of three enzymes in all mammalian cells that neutralize the free radical superoxide that is generated by ionizing irradiation [2]. Unlike the other two superoxide dismutases, which are metalloenzymes that utilize copper/zinc in their activation (SOD1 and SOD3, as they are called [5–7]). MnSOD (also called SOD2) utilized manganese for its activation [9]. All three SODs are part of the cellular defense system against oxidative stress from all sorts of damaging agents in the body's natural physiologic functioning and against environmental threats including ionizing irradiation exposure.

Elegant studies with cell lines that were either naturally deficient in MnSOD or genetically engineered to express high levels of the added transgene for MnSOD showed that mitochondrial targeting of the enzyme was required for radioprotection [9]. These cell culture studies clearly showed that this mitochondrial naturally localized enzyme was one of the most prominent radiation-attenuating agents in cells [9]. Moving on to preclinical studies in rats and mice, the data showed that the administration of the transgene for MnSOD was radioprotective when delivered before irradiation [10–12]. A transgene is a sequence of bases for the naturally occurring enzyme that is placed in a transmitting vehicle or "vector." To prepare for clinical use in patients, who were receiving radiotherapy and suffering organ-specific side effects, the transgene for MnSOD was delivered to experimental systems first in an adenovirus vector [13], Herpes virus, and in plasmid-containing lipid particles called liposomes that were also tested as a vector [14, 15]. Each of these vectors delivered the transgene for MnSOD to cells in culture or in vivo quite effectively and decreased the magnitude of subsequent ionizing irradiation damage.

The clinical application of this MnSOD as a radiation protector first was tested as part of an FDA-approved Phase I/II Clinical Trial for patients with nonsmall cell lung cancer, who were planned to receive multifield radiotherapy and chemotherapy for their locally advanced nonsmall cell lung cancer [16].

The clinical trial [16] was FDA approved in part, because the then standard of care for these patients, who had cancer that was unresectable because of known positive regional lymph node spread and/or invasion of adjacent tissues, suffered severe esophagitis [16]. These patients were part of a then standard protocol to use radiotherapy and chemotherapy to control the growth of the cancer and provide a symptom-free increase in survival. By the fourth week of a 7-week radiotherapy protocol, nearly all patients were suffering from severe radiation-induced esophagitis (inflammation of the esophagus leading to dysphagia or difficulty swallowing) as a side effect of the chemoradiotherapy [16]. This clinical trial used MnSOD-PL as a radiation protector. It was a preventative drug against dysphagia.

In the clinical trial, patients swallowed MnSOD-plasmid liposomes (MnSOD-PL) in a 30-ounce tablespoon size liquid volume every third day during their 6–7 week course of chemoradiotherapy. This radioprotector drug was targeted to deliver the MnSOD-PL to the epithelial cells in the esophagus. Multiple preclinical studies were based on the FDA animal rule. The animal rule then required a demonstration of effectiveness in a single animal model that was reflective of the actual clinical problem [3]. The animal model studies in mice were confirmed [16]. A second species, Rabbits, were used to confirm distribution in tissue. The drug was shown to provide significant prevention of dysphagia in some patients. The Phase I Clinical Trial was published [16]. Other radioprotector drugs were being developed and some were tested in clinical trials [53]. The strategy for such radioprotection in clinical radiotherapy patients was associated with a technique of organ-specific delivery.

In other model systems, swallowed MnSOD-PL delivery to protect the oral cavity and esophagus [18, 19] or intravessel instillation (delivery to the bladder by catheter insertion) to prevent cystitis [20]. Other proposed applications suggested intestinal delivery or intrarectal delivery to prevent radiation-induced proctitis [14]. There were other developments of medical radiation countermeasures, then called radioprotectors that were not associated with gene delivery or targeting specific transgenes, but rather drugs designed to ameliorate already existing symptoms [5]. Such drugs were also being delivered to patients to decrease the side effects of radiotherapy on tissues during a course of clinical radiotherapy. Drugs were locally delivered to anatomic sites including the rectum, bladder, oral cavity, oropharynx, and esophagus [17–21].

The nomenclature for radiation countermeasures has since changed the categories of such agents to separate them into three classifications: protectors—delivered before radiation exposure; mitigators—delivered after radiation exposure, but before symptoms of radiation are detected; and treatments—treatments—which are agents that ameliorate the symptoms of ionizing irradiation exposure. At present, the primary focus in the development of radiation countermeasures is overseen by the RAD/NUC program of the National Institutes of Allergy and Infectious Diseases (NIAID) [36] and is for radiation mitigators. The program is currently developing agents that will have either a focus on the hematopoietic acute radiation syndrome (H-ARS) or gastrointestinal syndrome (GI-ARS), as well as a systemic effect on all organs and organ systems. There are new programs focused on skin damage, gender differences, and vulnerable populations like pregnant women and the fetus.

Why is the funding for RAD/NUC events managed by NIAID and not the National Cancer Institute (NCI)? After the World Trade Center attacks on 9/11/01, the United States Congress appropriated funding for counter-terrorism research. The primary focus at that time was the fear of willful release of infectious agents, and, thus, a significant budget was delivered to the National Institutes of Health targeting the NIAID (National Institutes of Allergy, and Infectious Diseases), since this was the institute that dealt with infectious agents. There were requests for proposals (RFAs) for studies focused on using air surveillance instruments to detect any possible distribution of tularemia, anthrax spores, Ebola virus, influenza, smallpox, and other possible airborne infections. There was a definite fear of terrorism using anthrax spores. There were reports of using the mail to deliver a white powder in envelopes to members of Congress or to other government officials or to members of the military during this time, which was in the weeks/months immediately after the 9/11 terrorist events [36]. In one instance, a U.S. Post Office was evacuated, all windows sealed, and the entire building filled with Sodium Azide aerosol to kill anthrax spores [37]. That year, there was a shortage of masking tape in hardware stores, as people were rushing to seal their windows against aerosolized anthrax spores and other infectious agents [37].

The congressionally appropriated funding that was delivered to the NIAID included a budget for solutions to counter-terrorism against radiation. While delivery of radiation-emitting isotopes such as would be the case with a "dirty bomb" [69] was considered to be a real threat, there was also some concern about a fission bomb, such as that used in Hiroshima or Nagasaki [3]. At that time after the "Cold War," the former Soviet Union nuclear weapons were being inventoried, and there was less concern about global thermonuclear war. But there was concern that the fission core of a thermonuclear weapon might fall into hands of a terrorist group and be detonated somewhere in the U.S. that would produce a ten kiloton fission bomb like that at Hiroshima and Nagasaki in 1945.

There was also fear over the accidental or willful dispersal of radioisotopes to the general population. This fear led to organizations including hospitals placing radiation detectors near supplies of milk, drinking water, and other public access materials. There were warnings promulgated about so-called weakly defended "soft targets" for terrorists such as football stadiums, churches, and concerts. Any collection of large numbers of people were considered a "soft target" for radiation terrorism. One focus of the first available funding for radiation countermeasures was for NIAID to develop Centers for Medical Countermeasures against Radiation (CMCR). This program led to several potentially seminal and quite resourceful discoveries.

The first CMCR funding was distributed to seven academic institutions, including some that were in partnerships with American corporations. Each center was charged to either develop new radiation countermeasures or new radiation exposure detection systems. The University of Washington at Seattle and the Fred Hutchison Cancer Center focused on a canine model of hematopoietic stem cell transplantation to mitigate radiation injury and looked at both placenta and umbilical cord blood as a source for delivering hematopoietic reconstituting stem cells in a dog model system. (In subsequent years, another cell therapy using endothelial cells was developed by the Albert Einstein Medical Center in Bronx, New York.) The University of Wisconsin received funding to study their use of ACE-inhibitors like Captopril (a blood pressure medicine) to mitigate radiation damage to the kidneys and lungs [3]. The Columbia University program focused on developing novel biomarkers for the detection of radiation injury from both radioisotopes and external radiation. Columbia University developed a novel technology for using peripheral blood collected in small volumes (capillary tubes) for automated quantitation of single-cell DNA double-strand breaks and chromosomal aberrations, which were the then most reliable indicators of ionizing irradiation injury. Dartmouth University was tasked with developing novel approaches to the detection of changes in bones and teeth as biomarkers of prior or recent radiation injury. The University of Pittsburgh, University of California at Los Angeles, Harvard University/Dana Farber Cancer Institute, and Rochester University, New York, each were tasked with developing small molecule radiation mitigators (drugs).

From the time of initiation of the Center for Medical Countermeasures Program at NIAID, there were initially seven research groups. In subsequent years, the individual groups were then merged into a consortium called the Centers for Medical Countermeasures Against Radiation Consortium (CMCRC). The consortium allowed for efficient transfer of new data, new resources, and the sharing of research discoveries between these institutions.

The CMCRC Program is in its 19th year in 2024. During these years, there evolved an entirely new research field of science focused on radiation countermeasures (Table 17.1). There was a shift from developing radiation protectors (delivered before planned clinical radiotherapy) to radiation mitigators (countermeasures delivered after radiation exposure, but before the onset of symptoms). The change in focus to mitigators was logical, since warning of a terrorist event was unlikely, and there would be little opportunity for practical administration of a radiation protector. One exception was that military and civilian first responders, who would know about a radiation-contaminated zone or a battlefield or after a terrorist event, respectively, would be able to prepare for radiation exposure by receiving a radiation protector agent. However, the main focus of the research in the CMCRC was radiation mitigators. The defined area of research in radiation mitigators was distinct from other research into the development of "radiation injury treatments." Radiation injury treatments are those agents delivered after the individuals, who have been exposed to irradiation and are already experiencing symptoms of injury.

Since, 2001, there have been hundreds of publications on a multitude of radiation countermeasures, mostly mitigators. An analysis and summary of these types of mitigators have evolved and expanded into a huge discipline, as a subcategory of Radiobiology [5]. In some instances, new radiation damage mitigators have been determined to apply to other forms of terrorism events using chemicals or infectious agents, but also to other forms of injury that could involve large segments of the population [41, 46].

Radiation Countermeasures Target Different Phases of the Normal Organisms' Response to Ionizing Irradiation

Collections of new radiation countermeasures have been reported to focus on the initial event of DNA double-strand breaks following exposure to ionizing irradiation [63, 64]. With the development of practical countermeasures that would be delivered after irradiation exposure, it made little sense to focus on events before DNA damage. There was knowledge from studies in basic radiation chemistry that some events occurred within cells within seconds or fractions of a second after radiation exposure [10, 11]. There was no way to deliver a countermeasure to prevent events in radiation chemistry including ionization of water and oxygen. These radiation chemistry events produced the chemical structures called free radicals that cause DNA double-strand breaks. In contrast, many radiation countermeasures were developed that targeted the next phase of the cellular response to ionizing irradiation; namely, DNA double-strand breaks [63].

One of the first centers for countermeasures against radiation at Harvard/Dana Farber Cancer Institute involved the pioneering work of Alan D'Andrea, M.D. with finding the structure of the DNA repair scaffold of proteins that are defective in patients with Fanconi Anemia [64]. This novel approach to radiation mitigators led to the development of drugs that would not only prevent DNA double-strand breaks was logical. However using drugs that could rapidly repair these breaks before they initiated the next phases in the radiation damage response was a challenge. The DNA double-strand breaks and also the single-strand breaks, the importance of which has been relatively little studied [2], occur within seconds after radiation exposure. There follows a cascade of new DNA double-strand breaks after the radiation exposure has ended. How can this cascade happen? The answer is that after radiation, there follows the so-called "cytokine storm" of inflammation [22, 23]. The inflammatory response, which is common to other forms of tissue injury causes further and sometimes even more massive tissue injury and cellular DNA double-strand breaks. Inflammatory cytokines and inflammatory cells (including neutrophils and monocytes in the circulation and resident within each tissue) release oxidants that are used to kill infectious agents like bacteria. Therefore, giving drugs that targeted elements in the FA pathway [64], specifically, those associated with the DNA double-strand break repair mechanisms of homologous recombination and nonhomologous end-joining was a logical approach to discovering new radiation countermeasures [57]. But next steps were important. It was not too late, even 24 h after irradiation exposure, to give an agent that counteracted the cascade of DNA double-strand breaks. Several innovative approaches to targeting DNA double-strand breaks have been reported. Commercialization of such DNA double-strand break mitigators is being investigated.

Once, DNA double-strand breaks have begun to occur, both the direct radiation-induced breaks and those from the subsequent cascades of inflammation-induced "indirect" breaks, the so called 'cytokine storm' follows.

There is a next step in the radiation response of single cells that follows the initial direct DNA double-strand breaks. This next step is the translocation from the nuclear DNA sites of injury of signals to sites outside the cell nucleus specifically to the cellular cytoplasm, and, primarily, to the mitochondria [10, 11]. Mitochondria are the engines of survival of oxygenated cells and facilitate oxidative metabolism without which there can be no sustained life of mammals including humans. The signals from the nucleus to mitochondria include molecules that either directly cause or initiate pathways in the mitochondrial membrane that lead to oxidative stress. Oxidative stress reactions in the mitochondria destroy the structure of the mitochondrial lipid membrane components, cause lysis of the mitochondria, and loss of their function. Once, enough mitochondria are lysed or their membranes lose integrity and leak their contents including cytochrome C, into the cytoplasm, then the cell dies by apoptosis or other forms of cell death.

Thus, mitochondrial oxidative stress is a logical target for irradiation mitigation.

The use of antioxidants as radiation mitigators was an early discovery, but targeting them to the mitochondria is a relatively new approach. Delivering ascorbic acid (Vitamin C), Vitamin E, and other components of antioxidant/chemopreventive diets were approaches and all were tested in animal model systems of radiation mitigation (Table 17.1) [3]. Mitochondrial targeting of radiation countermeasures was innovative [55, 56, 62]. There was a remarkable discovery that the time from nuclear DNA double-strand breaks to the detectable delivery to the mitochondrial outer membrane of the signaling molecules that started membrane oxidation was measurable and in some cell phenotypes could take hours [10, 11].

Importance of the Mitochondria for Radiation Countermeasures

Mitochondrial outer membrane binding of these signaling molecules from the nucleus included p53, p21, pro-apoptotic proteins BAX and BAD, and others [9]. These nucleus to mitochondria translocation events could be measured in irradiated cells in culture, and the time first detectable delivery of these signaling molecules to mitochondria was determined to be minutes, but was not peak until hours later. While this time frame may seem to be a short interval, it is much longer than the time for radiation-induced ionization of water and oxygen (fractions of a second) and much longer than the first detectable DNA double-strand breaks themselves in the nucleus (seconds) [63, 64]. Mitochondrial-targeted antioxidants presented an innovative and clever way to develop radiation mitigators. By delivering drugs that brought to the mitochondria antioxidants including molecules that would neutralize superoxide, nitric oxide, and hydrogen peroxide (products of dismutation of superoxide), there appeared to be an extremely innovative and effective strategy for radiation mitigation. Because the concentrations of these small molecule antioxidants at the mitochondria were found to be increased compared to the total cellular levels (between 30-fold and 600-fold) and depending on the length of the mitochondrial targeting attachment structure to the antioxidant [9], there was a clear way to get these new radiation mitigators to the proper site to preserve mitochondrial function, and, thus, prevent cell death (Fig. 17.1).

Two strategies were reported as effective ways to deliver radiation mitigators to the mitochondria. These strategies included using triphenyl phosphonium to tag the nitroxide molecule and direct it to the mitochondria [2, 22, 23]. Another strategy was that of attaching a component of the hemigramacidin antibiotic molecule to the small molecule. This strategy was particularly clever because mitochondria were thought to have evolved from billions of years ago, as the product of a primitive cellular engulfment of early archeobacteria.

In the first chapter, this book dealt with the evolution of life on the planet Earth including the evolution of single cells to those that contained mitochondria. There must have been two types of single cells at that time, one of which could not utilize oxygen. The mitochondria having an origin archeobacteria suggest that these bacteria may have also been anaerobic and like the earliest nucleus-containing cells could not utilize oxygen. Once, cells engulfed archeobacteria, and these became cytoplasmic organelles, there evolved a communication system between these two structures. The bacteria had their own DNA, which controlled cell division. The cells had nuclear DNA of their own, but no oxidative metabolism. Once this stable entry of archeobacteria into the cell cytoplasm occurred, there had to evolve cooperation but also preservation of the independence of each—both for replication and function. The subject of interaction of the cell nucleus to mitochondria is a separate and fascinating topic and one that deserves more attention. But the mitochondria do replicate and the numbers of mitochondria per cell do change depending on cell function and need for oxygenation. For example, cardiomyocytes, which require huge consumption of oxygen to maintain heart contraction, have large numbers of mitochondria while resting hematopoietic bone marrow stem cells have relatively few. Furthermore, the mitochondria within individual cells move within the cells depending upon local energy needs. In neurons, mitochondria reside in clusters near the nucleus but will move down the axon to the distal signal transduction region with

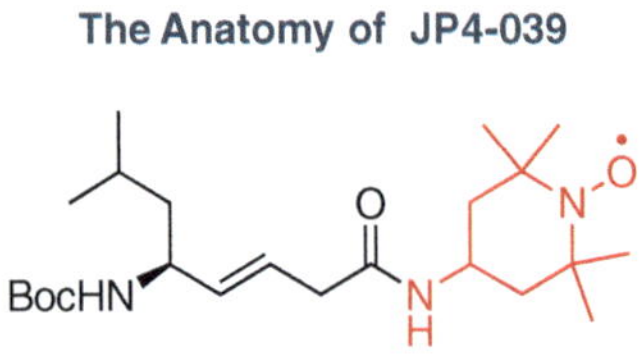

Fig. 17.1 Mitochondrial targeting nitroxides as radiation mitigators: structure of JP4–039 is shown

proximity to other neurons if the latter is damaged such as in an ischemic event or where oxygen may be needed [9]. These facts concerning the importance of mitochondria to cell and tissue survival suggested that an antibacterial drug to target archeobacteria that happened to be residing in the cell cytoplasm under a different name—mitochondria could be used to target a radiation mitigator drug to the mitochondria. This strategy was indeed a clever idea and is the product of innovative thinking by an innovative chemist, Peter Wipf, Ph.D. [2, 22, 23]. Mitochondrial-targeted nitroxides were designed by attaching a peptide from the hemigramacidin antibiotic to the 4-amino-tempol antioxidant nitroxide (Fig. 17.1). The other strategy for antioxidant targeting to mitochondria used tri-phenyl-phosphonium as a molecule that when attached could target a carried nitroxide to the negatively charged outer mitochondrial membrane. Attaching this structure to an antioxidant was also extremely innovative [2]. Both mitochondrial-targeted drugs were highly effective radiation mitigators for cells in culture and in animal models in vivo (Fig. 17.1).

Why Was 24 h Chosen as the Time for Effective Radiation Mitigator Delivery?

The scientists at NIAID and their consultants worked closely with members of the Radiation Injury Treatment Network (RITN) [41] during the years after the 9/11 terrorist attacks for practical approaches developing a policy that could be rolled out to the general public in the event of a radiation terrorist attack. Such policies could also apply to a nuclear reactor accident, or the combination of these events in which there was a radiation terrorist attack on a nuclear reactor resulting in leakage into the environment of radiation isotopes. The 24-h time point was chosen based on the technicality of the first responders. It was determined that it would require at least 24 h from the time the event was detected, to the arrival on the scene of first responders. There were tests carried out using modified ambulances that were developed in the United States that would carry radiation detectors and equipment capable of analyzing the types and strengths of radioisotopes [34–36]. The ambulance delivery system of radiation detectors was associated with the development by companies including Thermo Fisher Corporation of small handheld radiation detectors, which could be placed on the walls or on the ceiling of an ambulance allowing first responders to detect radiation-emitting isotopes on or in the first victims [34–36]. The timing was critical, and a final analysis was that it would take at least 24 h for radiation countermeasures to arrive at the scene of an event.

A test of the hypothesis of a 24-h window for delivering radiation mitigator countermeasures was that of the Boston Marathon bombing event [36, 69]. Explosives were placed in a pressure cooker and left by the side of the road, where marathon runners would be coming by. The explosion created a cloud of dust that engulfed not only the runners but also spectators on the sides of the road. The first ambulances to arrive on the scene for evacuation of victims transported these victims to area hospitals, and provided valuable data on the reality of the 24-h time point. Thankfully, there were no radioisotopes in the pressure cooker bombs. Modeling was carried out to test the scenario of "What if there had been aerial dispersal of radioisotopes in that cloud of dust."

The evaluation of the prevailing winds at the time of the Boston Marathon bombing led to the visualized spread of the dust cloud. This visualization allowed investigators to determine the "what-if" of these pressure cookers contained radioiodine, radioactive cesium, powder found in Cobalt 60 teletherapy sources, or the neutron-emitting Uranium compounds including Plutonium 239. While the "dirty bomb" concept was always in the minds of those investigators, who were developing countermeasures, the analysis of the spread of clouds of dust and how respirable particle size would deliver these radioisotopes deep into the lungs of people suddenly became a new focus of research. Respirable particles focus of the original counterterrorism research at Lovelace Laboratories [58, 59, 69] shortly after 9/11, reported that the human airway is designed to prevent delivery of particulate material deep into the lungs and the cilia in the bronchi move particles centrally for coughing and expulsion. In contrast, aerosol drug delivery such as those in inhaled steroids, and beta-agonists that are used in patients with asthma provided a basis by which theoretical terrorists could use this technology to develop ways to attach radioisotopes to very small droplets or particles that could penetrate deep into the lungs. Significant research was carried out on ways to combat this form of terrorism using countermeasures for inhaled radioisotopes.

A separate area of research was then developed within the overall program of radiation countermeasures and focused on chelators. A chelator is an agent, which grabs a target and holds on to it until it can be cleared from the system by either the kidney or liver, or in some cases delivered to a site, where it can be eliminated from the body. Research has evolved rapidly, and there have been a number of commercially developed chelators. The pioneering work at Lawrence Livermore Laboratory [46, 51] developed the first chelator compounds that could target Uranium 235 and Plutonium 239. While these elements were thought to be the primary ones in an aerial dispersal of a dirty bomb, the extremely long half-life of Plutonium 239 (1000 years) and Uranium 235 (over 100,000 years [43]) posed a definite hazard and strategy for developing radiation countermeasures. While Trans-Uranium compounds [43] would not likely cause acute injury, the deposition of these elements by an aerosol terrorist event that attached the molecules to very small particles that could reach the distal alveoli posed a significant threat. The clearance of such particles containing the radioisotopes into the central lymphatics in the lungs and to lymph nodes posed a real problem since the only way to remove such centralized particles would be through either bronchopulmonary lavage or surgical removal of the lymph nodes.

The Challenge of Inhaled or Swallowed Radioisotopes

The scenario of having hundreds or thousands of people with these isotopes in their lungs produced a theoretical public health crisis of significant magnitude. Detection of such inhaled isotopes that emit gamma-ray photons or beta-irradiation/electrons would be more easily detectable than the detection of neutrons or alpha particles (helium nuclei).

The work at Lawrence Livermore Laboratory showed that the Trans-Uranium compounds followed the calcium biochemistry in the body and were rapidly deposited in bone [43]. Furthermore, the time required after such isotopes were deposited in bone (in rat models) suggested that the administration of a chelator after the isotopes had arrived in the bone would require months or even years of continuous administration of the chelators as the isotopes left the bone and entered the blood along with calcium that was in this calcium cycle. Bone deposition and reabsorption is a natural process in the human body involving osteoblasts and osteoclasts, and calcium is required for the osteogenesis component of this cycle. If such radioisotopes were using the same transport systems as calcium, then it is obvious that a competition by giving huge quantities of calcium to such exposed individuals to combat the deposition of Trans-Uranium compounds or a rapidly deployed chelator would be required. Chelators were developed that could remove Trans-Uranium compounds from the blood, but the immediate concern was that these had to be administered within 1 h to be able to remove such elements from getting from the theoretical deposition in alveoli in the lung into the circulation. This timeline makes a practical delivery of chelators that would be therapeutic then clearly impossible. The development of chelators did focus on an orally administered drug rather than intravenous injection of chelators [43, 61]. In general, the radiation countermeasures field focused on feasible and practical delivery, which would be either through microneedle injection, such as that used for epi-pen to deliver epinephrine for those people in an allergic reaction, an oral administration (although, this was impractical for individuals, who had nausea and vomiting), a patch of either skin absorption or microneedle delivery, or intramuscular injection.

Since 9/11 and since the Boston Marathon bombings, the available radiation detectors have been modified to detect neutrons. Knowing that respirable particles were in the lungs of large numbers of people, even in relatively low concentrations would produce a public health crisis and panic. The idea that a chelator drug administration soon after the recognized/diagnosed inhalation of such a terrorist vehicle was a focus of new radiation countermeasures research.

Another radiation terrorist scenario involves Polonium 210. The event of poisoning Alexander Litvenko [60] with the alpha emitter radioisotope Polonium 210, then called attention to the need to add alpha particle detection to the available monitoring device. The then current detection of Polonium 211 required the collection of liters of urine and sending this sample to one of two laboratories that could detect this alpha irradiation at the time of the Polonium poisoning. It took weeks to make the diagnosis of what caused the anemia, hair loss, and death of this victim. The concept/idea that a time of at least 24 h became established. That time would be required before a feasible reasonable delivery of radiation countermeasures to the site of a terrorist event.

How do radiation countermeasures get delivered to the victims? Depending upon the magnitude of the terrorist event and the accessibility of the roadways, the delivery could be by air or by road. Also, the number of casualties would determine the structure of the response. FEMA has "push-packs" [44] that are both specific for radiation injuries and general response structures that contain the necessary medical therapeutics. What about chelators for radioisotopes?

All of the radiation countermeasures under development also focus on delivery vehicles and methods that must be designed to replace the impractical intravenous administration to 100–1000 victims of a countermeasure. Intraperitoneal injection, which was a practical way to do basic science research in rodents, was also not practical for humans since the thickness of the abdominal wall varied between adults, and the delivery through the intraperitoneal route was impractical given the potential length of the needle required.

With external x-ray or neutron irradiation, as well as radioisotope dispersal—a combined threat could involve both. For fission bombs, there are relatively short-lived isotopes. Prussian blue neutralized radioactive Cesium, radioiodine can be removed by overloading individuals with Potassium Iodide capsules (regular iodine) and outcompeting the radioisotope of iodine receptors. Other radioprotectors must be identified to target urine or feces, and then countermeasures delivered.

Radiation Countermeasures that Target Distal Steps Including Inflammation

After significant radiation damage has occurred, and after an estimation can be made of the percent of the body that had been irradiated (some individuals will have been shielded by having a portion of their body behind concrete walls or geographic location at a distance from the hypocenter of a nuclear fission bomb) was determined, before delivery of a countermeasure could be calculated. Depending on the radiation dose sustained and the percent of the body irradiated, the triage process focused on the basic three-by-three rule. Based on evaluable data from radiation accidents in nuclear power plants, estimations from Hiroshima and Nagasaki data, and other information, the RITN and other first responders were educated to follow the three-by-three rule. If the victim had experienced or was experiencing nausea and vomiting within 3 h of the event (nuclear explosion, radiation dispersal), then that person received a dose over 3 Gy of total body radiation [44]. This was an estimate but allowed first responders to have some basis for determining urgency of administering countermeasures.

A confounding variable for all strategies of medical triage and for determining when to administer radiation countermeasures is that of "combined injury." Victims exposed to irradiation close to the detonation site would also likely experience thermal burns, concussion, penetrating wounds, and other treatable conditions, which affect the analysis of the radiation dose. Evaluating the dose-response of humans was only possible in cases of total body administration for therapeutic use. This protocol was limited to those patients, who received single fraction or fractionated irradiation to prepare them as recipients for bone marrow transplantation. Under these conditions, data was available as to the time of the inflammatory response to irradiation and that, thus, this information was available and potentially useful for the design of radiation countermeasures.

It was known for years since the first delivery of TBI for bone marrow transplantation [54], that humans have the first symptoms of TBI according to radiation delivery (if the dose rate was lowered to 3–5 Roentgen per minute requiring a treatment time in excess of 1 h) or in the case where patients were receiving conventional dose rate of 1.8–2 Gy per minute, and the literature on TBI suggested that the first symptoms would be those of nausea and vomiting from the G.I. Syndrome, and this might occur during the administration of TBI at low-dose rate or in the 24 h after completion of the treatment. The first bone marrow transplant clinical trials involved a latent period between the TBI and the delivery by intravenous injection of the donor bone marrow. This allowed clinicians to observe the 24 h after TBI exposure and provided some information as to the ways to treat symptoms, but also provided valuable information on the development of radiation countermeasures. It was clear that one of the first symptoms after irradiation exposure was the inflammatory response. Increased plasma levels of IL-1, TNF-α, TGF-β, and others are associated with irradiation-induced death of circulating peripheral blood lymphocytes, which are very radiosensitive [58]. These cytokine elevations led to symptoms very similar to a flu-like syndrome of acute infection from a virus. Amelioration of these symptoms was possible with nonsteroidal anti-inflammatory drugs or administration of steroids [67]. Administration of cytokines or other systemic anti-inflammatory response molecules followed the body's response to such inflammation. Accordingly, radiation countermeasures included the discovery of anti-inflammatory drugs, and administration of cytokines that would be likely to neutralize the inflammatory response (Table 17.1 lists some of these countermeasures that have been developed). Very few are FDA approved as a radiation countermeasure. An overriding principle is that of "triage." In the military, approach to the management of mass casualties and in the current emergency room, patients are first screened for the severity of injury and separated into groups that require fast or delayed attention. The concept of combined injury, which involves radiation leads to the need to add to the triage process, another factor in addition to the current standard list of factors to access. Currently, patients are screened for vital signs, and then for the magnitude of injury. Concussion and burn injury and penetrating wounds can be assessed, but now triage medical personnel will need to include "distance from the radiation-emitting device" and Geiger Counter survey of their clothing for radioactive dust, and then after clothing removal for evidence of radiation emission by isotopes on the skin or in the lungs or GI tract [34–36].

Benefits and Problems with Polypharmacy

The development of radiation countermeasures has also focused on the reality of the medical conditions of the population in the exposed environment [2, 22, 23]. People take medications routinely for the control of hypertension and diabetes, and many are treated for acute conditions including infections (taking antibiotics), and acute treatments for autoimmune reactions including osteoarthritis. How would these drugs interact with the introduction of a radiation countermeasure? It would be a negative effect of assuming that all people could receive the same countermeasure. Differences in the response to radiation of males and females are becoming an important area to consider. Available evidence from animal models indicates that females are relatively radioresistant, in part, because of the effects of estrogen and progesterone. However, studies indicate that only gender bias does not apply until females are of reproductive age. Pediatric and elderly females do not appear to be relatively radioresistant [68]. Another recognized factor was the concept of weight and age of individuals. A single dose of a radiation countermeasure had to consider the fact that only one injection was likely feasible, since the first responders would arrive on the scene 24 h or later after the terrorist event. Furthermore, adjusting the dose for the weight or age of the patient was probably impractical since hundreds or thousands of people needed to have an administration. Therefore, a very narrow dose-response effect of any radiation countermeasure had to be avoided.

There would now be a potentially serious problem of delivering "too little" of a drug, or "too much" of a drug. The difference between individuals, not only with respect to what drugs they are already taking for medical conditions had to be considered. Therefore, a drug needed to be effective as a radiation countermeasure, but over a dose range that was not narrow. The concept of safety must now include not only its unlikely cause of untoward toxicity in children and the elderly but also the extremely unlikely interaction of the drug with a medication that the individual is taking. The dose of a countermeasure delivered must be safe over a wide range and the concept of giving too much should not be an issue. Pharmacokinetics and pharmacodynamic studies on every new radiation countermeasure must precede any clinical trials, and ensure its safety in people of all ages, genders, and those taking other medications [69, 70, 71].

References

1. Greenberger JS. Radioprotection. In Vivo. 2009;23(2):323–36.
2. Fink MP, Macias CA, Xiao J, et al. Hemigramicidin-TEMPO conjugates: novel mitochondria-targeted antioxidants. Biochem Pharmacol. 2007;74(6):801–9. https://doi.org/10.1016/j.bcp.2007.05.019.
3. Stone HB, Coleman DN, Moulder JE, et al. Models for evaluating agents intended for the prophylaxis, mitigation, and treatment of radiation injuries. Report of an NCI workshop, December 3–4, 2003. Radiat Res. 2004;162(6):711–28. https://doi.org/10.1667/rr3276.

4. Greenberger JS, Kagan VE, Pearce L, et al. Modulation of redox signal transduction pathways in the treatment of cancer. Antioxid Redox Signal. 2001;3(3):347–59. https://doi.org/10.1089/152308601524 09004.
5. Greenberger JS, Epperly MW, Gretton J, et al. Radioprotective gene therapy. Curr Gene Ther. 2003;3(3):183–95. https://doi.org/10.2174/1566523034578384.
6. Greenberger JS, Epperly MW. Radioprotective antioxidant gene therapy: potential mechanisms of action. Gene Ther Mol Biol (GTMB). 2004;8:31–44.
7. Greenberger JS, Epperly MW. Pleiotrophic stem cell and tissue effects of ionizing irradiation protection by MnSOD-plasmid liposome gene therapy. In: Columbus F, editor. Progress in gene therapy. Nova Science Publications; 2005. p. 110–8.
8. Epperly MW, Guo HL, Bernarding M, et al. Delayed intratracheal injection of manganese superoxide dismutase (MnSOD)-plasmid/liposomes provides suboptimal protection against irradiation-induced pulmonary injury compared to treatment before irradiation. Gene Ther Mol Biol. 2003;7:61–8.
9. Epperly MW, Gretton JE, Bernarding M, et al. Mitochondrial localization of copper/zinc superoxide dismutase (Cu/ZnSOD) confers radioprotective functions in vitro and in vivo. Radiat Res. 2003;160:568–78.
10. Epperly MW, Osipov AN, Martin I, et al. Ascorbate as a "redox-sensor" and protector against irradiation-induced oxidative stress in 32D cl 3 hematopoietic cells and subclones overexpressing human manganese superoxide dismutase. Int J Radiat Oncol Biol Phys. 2004;58(3):851–61. https://doi.org/10.1016/j.ijrobp.2003.10.022.
11. Epperly MW, Bray JA, Esocobar P, et al. Overexpression of the human MnSOD transgene in subclones of murine hematopoietic progenitor cell line 32D cl 3 decreased irradiation-induced apoptosis, but does not alter G_2/M or G_1/S phase cell cycle arrest. Radiat Oncol Investig. 1999;7:331–42.
12. Epperly MW, Epperly LD, Zhang X, et al. Overexpression of MnSOD transgene product protects cryopreserved bone marrow hematopoietic progenitor cells from ionizing irradiation. Radiat Res. 2007;168(5):560–6. https://doi.org/10.1667/RR1071R.1.
13. Zwacka RM, Dudus L, Epperly MW, et al. Redox gene therapy protects human IB-3 lung epithelial cells against ionizing radiation-induced apoptosis. Hum Gene Ther. 1998;9(9):1381–6. https://doi.org/10.1089/hum.1998.9.9-1381.
14. Guo HL, Wolfe D, Epperly MW, et al. Gene transfer of human manganese superoxide dismutase protects small intestinal villi from radiation injury. J Gastrointest Surg. 2003;7(2):229–35. https://doi.org/10.1016/s1091-255x(02)00186-5.
15. Epperly MW, Bray JA, Kraeger S, et al. Prevention of late effects of irradiation lung damage by manganese superoxide dismutase gene therapy. Gene Ther. 1998;5(2):196–208. https://doi.org/10.1038/sj.gt.3300580.
16. Tarhini AA, Belani C, Luketich JD, et al. A phase I study of concurrent chemotherapy (paclitaxel and carboplatin) and thoracic radiotherapy with swallowed manganese superoxide dismutase (MnSOD) plasmid liposome (PL) protection in patients with locally advanced stage III non-small cell lung cancer. Hum Gene Ther. 2011;22(3):336–42. https://doi.org/10.1089/hum.2010.078.
17. Stickle RL, Epperly MW, Klein E, et al. Prevention of irradiation-induced esophagitis by plasmid/liposome delivery of the human manganese superoxide dismutase (MnSOD) transgene. Radiat Oncol Investig. 1999;7(4):204–17. https://doi.org/10.1002/(SICI)1520-6823(1999)7:4<204::AID-RO12>3.0.CO;2-S.
18. Epperly MW, Travis EL, Sikora C, et al. Manganese [correction of magnesium] superoxide dismutase (MnSOD) plasmid/liposome pulmonary radioprotective gene therapy: modulation of irradiation-induced mRNA for IL-1, TNF-α, and TGF-β correlates with delay of organizing alveolitis/fibrosis. Biol Blood Marrow Transplant. 1999;5(4):204–14. https://doi.org/10.1053/bbmt.1999.v5.pm10465100.
19. Guo HL, Seixas-Silva JA, Epperly MW, et al. Prevention of irradiation-induced oral cavity mucositis by plasmid/liposome delivery of the human manganese superoxide dismutase

(MnSOD) transgene. Radiat Res. 2003;159(3):361–70. https://doi.org/10.1667/0033-7587(2003)159[0361:porioc]2.0.co;2.
20. Epperly MW, Kagan VE, Sikora CA, et al. Manganese superoxide dismutase-plasmid/liposome (MnSOD-PL) administration protects mice from esophagitis associated with fractionated irradiation. Int J Cancer. 2001;96(4):221–31. https://doi.org/10.1002/ijc.1023.
21. Kanai A, Epperly MW, Pearce L, et al. Differing roles of mitochondrial nitric oxide synthase in cardiomyocytes and urothelial cells. Am J Physiol Heart Circ Physiol. 2004;286(1):H13–21. https://doi.org/10.1152/ajpheart.00737.2003.
22. Steinman J, Epperly M, Hou W, et al. Improved total-body irradiation survival by delivery of two radiation mitigators that target distinct cell death pathways. Radiat Res. 2018;189(1):68–83. https://doi.org/10.1667/RR14787.1.
23. Thermozier S, Hou W, Zhang X, et al. Anti-ferroptosis drug enhances total body irradiation mitigation by drugs that block apoptosis and necroptosis. Radiat Res. 2020;193(5):435–50. https://doi.org/10.1667/RR15486.1.
24. Epperly MW, Bray JA, Krager S, et al. Intratracheal injection of adenovirus containing the human MnSOD transgene protects athymic nude mice from irradiation-induced organizing alveolitis. Int J Radiat Oncol Biol Phys. 1999;43(1):169–81. https://doi.org/10.1016/s0360-3016(98)00355-1.
25. Epperly MW, Defilippi S, Sikora C, et al. Intratracheal injection of manganese superoxide dismutase (MnSOD) plasmid/liposomes protects normal lung, but not orthotopic tumors from irradiation. Gene Ther. 2000;7(12):1011–8. https://doi.org/10.1038/sj.gt.3301207.
26. Epperly MW, Epstein CJ, Travis EL, et al. Decreased pulmonary radiation resistance of manganese superoxide dismutase (MnSOD)-deficient mice is corrected by human manganese superoxide dismutase-plasmid/liposome (SOD2-PL) intratracheal gene therapy. Radiat Res. 2000;154(4):365–74. https://doi.org/10.1667/0033-7587(2000)154[0365:dprrom]2.0.co;2.
27. Epperly MW, Gretton JA, DeFililppi SJ, et al. Modulation of radiation-induced cytokine elevation associated with esophagitis and esophageal stricture by manganese superoxide dismutase-plasmid/liposome (SOD-PL) gene therapy. Radiat Res. 2001;155(1 Pt 1):2–14. https://doi.org/10.1667/0033-7587(2001)155[0002:morice]2.0.co;2.
28. Epperly MW, Travis EL, Whitsett JA, et al. Overexpression of manganese superoxide dismutase (MnSOD) in whole lung or alveolar type II (AT-II) cells of MnSOD transgenic mice does not provide intrinsic lung irradiation protection. Int J Cancer. 2001;96(1):11–21. https://doi.org/10.1002/1097-0215(20010220)96::1<11::aid-ijc2>3.0.co;2-r.
29. Epperly MW, Sikora C, DeFilippi S, et al. Manganese superoxide dismutase (SOD2) inhibits radiation-induced apoptosis by stabilization of the mitochondrial membrane. Radiat Res. 2002;157(5):568–77. https://doi.org/10.1667/0033-7587(2002)157[0568:msdsir]2.0.co;2.
30. Guo H, Epperly MW, Bernarding M, et al. Manganese superoxide dismutase-plasmid/liposome (MnSOD-PL) intratracheal gene therapy reduction of irradiation-induced inflammatory cytokines does not protect orthotopic Lewis lung carcinomas. In Vivo. 2003;17(1):13–21.
31. Epperly MW, Sikora CA, DeFilippi SJ, et al. Pulmonary irradiation-induced expression of VCAM-1 and ICAM-1 is decreased by MnSOD-PL gene therapy. Biol Blood Marrow Transplant. 2002;8(4):175–87. https://doi.org/10.1053/bbmt.2002.v8.pm12014807.
32. Pearce LL, Epperly MW, Greenberger JS, et al. Identification of respiratory complexes I and III as mitochondrial sites of damage following exposure to ionizing radiation and nitric oxide. Nitric Oxide. 2001;5(2):128–36. https://doi.org/10.1006/niox.2001.0338.
33. Epperly MW, Sikora C, DeFilippi S, et al. Plasmid/liposome transfer of the human manganese superoxide dismutase (MnSOD) transgene prevents ionizing irradiation-induced apoptosis in human esophagus organ explant culture. Int J Cancer. 2000;90(3):128–37. https://doi.org/10.1002/1097-0215(20000620)90:3<128::aid-ijc2>3.0.co;2-u.
34. Dickson R, Kim JO, Huq MS, et al. Interceptor and phantom trials of EDNS at UPMC. Health Phys. 2013;105(5 Suppl 3):S199–208. https://doi.org/10.1097/HP.0b013e31828356b6.
35. Kim JO, Huq MS, Novotny J Jr, et al. Performance characteristics of a novel radioactive isotope detection and notification system designed for use in hospitals. Health Phys. 2011;100(Suppl 2):S71–8. https://doi.org/10.1097/HP.0b013e3181fa370f.

36. Dickson R, Kim JO, Huq MS, et al. A mobile alert system for preparing the delivery of radiation mitigators. In Vivo. 2015;29(5):505–13.
37. Riedel S. Anthrax: a continuing concern in the era of bioterrorism. Proc (Bayl Univ Med Cent). 2005;18(3):234–43. https://doi.org/10.1080/08998280.2005.11928074.
38. Singh VK, Romaine PLP, Seed TM. Medical countermeasures for radiation exposure and related injuries: characterization of medicines, FDA-approval status, and inclusion into the strategic national stockpile. Health Phys. 2015;108(6):607–30. https://doi.org/10.1097/HP.0000000000000279.
39. Waselenko JK, MacVittie TJ, Blakely WF, et al. Medical management of the acute radiation syndrome: recommendations of the strategic National Stockpile Radiation Working Group. Ann Intern Med. 2004;140(12):1037–51. https://doi.org/10.7326/0003-4819-140-12-200406150-00015.
40. Williams JP, Brown SL, Georges GE, et al. Animal models for medical countermeasures to radiation exposure. Radiat Res. 2010;173(4):557–78. https://doi.org/10.1667/RR1880.1.
41. Ross JR, Case C, Confer D, et al. Radiation Injury Treatment Network (RITN): healthcare professionals preparing for a mass casualty radiological or nuclear incident. Int J Radiat Biol. 2011;87(8):748–53. https://doi.org/10.3109/09553002.2011.556176.
42. Coleman CN, Hrding C, Bader JL, et al. Medical response to a radiologic/nuclear event: integrated plan from the Office of the Assistant Secretary for Preparedness and Response, Department of Health and Human Services. Ann Emerg Med. 2009;53(2):213–22. https://doi.org/10.1016/j.annemergmed.2007.12.021.
43. Goriely S, Pinedo GM. The production of transuranium elements by the r-process nucleosynthesis. Nucl Phys A. 2015;944:158–76.
44. Veenema TG, Moran TP, Schneider-Firestone S, et al. Radiation injury treatment network medical and nursing workforce radiation: knowledge and attitude assessment. Disaster Med Public Health Prep. 2022;16(1):170–6. https://doi.org/10.1017/dmp.2020.253.
45. Flynn DF, Goans RE. Nuclear terrorism: triage and medical management of radiation and combined-injury casualties. Surg Clin North Am. 2006;86(3):601–36. https://doi.org/10.1016/j.suc.2006.03.005.
46. DiCarlo AL, Hatchett RJ, Kaminski JM, et al. Medical countermeasures for radiation combined injury: radiation with burn, blast, trauma, and/or sepsis. Report of an NIAID workshop, March 26–27, 2007. Radiat Res. 2007;169(6):712–21. https://doi.org/10.1667/RR1295.1.
47. Russ E, Fatanmi OO, Wise SY, et al. Serum microRNA profile of rhesus macaques following ionizing radiation exposure and treatment with a medical countermeasure, Ex-Rad. Sci Rep. 2024;14(1):4518. https://doi.org/10.1038/s41598-024-54997-8.
48. Li K, Epperly M, Greenberger J, et al. Longitudinal fecal microbiome study of total body irradiated mice treated with radiation mitigators identify bacterial associations with survival. Front Cell Infect Microbiol. 2021;11:715396. https://doi.org/10.3389/fcimb.2021.715396.
49. Zhang X, Fisher R, Hou W, et al. Second generation probiotics producing IL-22 increase survival of mice after total body irradiation. In Vivo. 2020;34(1):39–50. https://doi.org/10.21873/invivo.11743.
50. Hamade DF, Espinal A, Yu J, et al. *Lactobacillus reuteri* releasing IL-22 (LR-IL-22) facilitates intestinal radioprotection for whole-abdomen irradiation (WAI) of ovarian cancer. Radiat Res. 2022;198(1):89–105. https://doi.org/10.1667/RADE-21-00224.1.
51. Espinal A, Epperly MW, Mukherjee A, et al. Intestinal radiation protection and mitigation by second-generation probiotic *Lactobacillus-reuteri* engineered to deliver Interleukin-22. Int J Mol Sci. 2022;23(10):5616. https://doi.org/10.3390/ijms23105616.
52. Hamade DF, Epperly MW, Fisher R, et al. Release of interferon-β (IFN-β) form probiotic *Limosolactobacillus reuteri*-IFN-β (LR-IFN-β) mitigates gastrointestinal acute radiation syndrome (GI-ARS) following whole abdominal irradiation. Cancers (Basel). 2023;15(6):1670. https://doi.org/10.3390/cancers15061670.
53. Wu K, Bergman KL. Dose selection in a pandemic: a framework informed by the FDA animal rule. Clin Transl Sci. 2021;14(1):5–7. https://doi.org/10.1111/cts.12936.

54. Peters LJ, Withers HR, Cundiff JH, et al. Radiobiological considerations in the use of total-body irradiation for bone-marrow transplantation. Radiology. 1979;131(1):243–7. https://doi.org/10.1148/131.1.243.
55. Rafii S, Ginsberg M, Scandura J, et al. Transplantation of endothelial cells to mitigate acute and chronic radiation injury to vital organs. Radiat Res. 2016;186(2):196–202. https://doi.org/10.1667/RR14461.1.
56. Ejaz A, Epperly MW, Greenberger JS, et al. Adipose-derived stem cell therapy ameliorates ionizing irradiation fibrosis (RIF) via hepatocyte growth factor-mediated TGF-β downregulation and recruitment of bone marrow cells. Stem Cells. 2019;37(6):791–802. https://doi.org/10.1002/stem.3000.
57. Weimar IS, Miranda N, Muller EJ, et al. Hepatocyte growth factor/scatter factor (HGF/SF) is produced by human bone marrow stromal cells and promotes proliferation, adhesion, and survival of human hematopoietic progenitor cells (CD34+). Exp Hematol. 1998;26(9):885–94.
58. Finch GL, McNeill KL, Hayes TL, et al. In vitro interactions between pulmonary macrophages and respirable particles. Environ Res. 1987;44(2):241–53. https://doi.org/10.1016/s0013-9351(87)80233-5.
59. Finch GL, Hoover MD, Mewhinney JA, et al. Respirable particle density measurements using isopycnic density gradient ultracentrifugation. J Aerosol Sci. 1989;20(1):29–36.
60. Harrison J, Fell T, Leggett R, et al. The polonium-210 poisoning of Mr Alexander Litvinenko. J Radiol Prot. 2017;37(1):266–78. https://doi.org/10.1088/1361-6498/aa58a7.
61. Choi TA, Furimsky AM, Swezey R, et al. In vitro metabolism and stability of the actinide chelating agent 3, 4, 3-LI(1,2-HOPO). J Pharm Sci. 2015;104(5):1832–8. https://doi.org/10.1002/jps.24394.
62. Yu P, Zhang X, Liu N, et al. Pyroptosis: mechanisms and diseases. Signal Transduct Target Ther. 2021;6(1):128. https://doi.org/10.1038/s41392-021-00507-5.
63. Nelson WG, Kastan MB. DNA strand breaks: the DNA template alterations that trigger p53-dependent DNA damage response pathways. Mol Cell Biol. 1994;14(3):1815–23. https://doi.org/10.1128/mcb.14.3.1815-1823.1994.
64. Grompe M, D'Andrea A. Fanconi anemia and DNA repair. Hum Mol Genet. 2001;10(20):2253–9. https://doi.org/10.1093/hmg/10.20.2253.
65. Abbotts R, Wilson DM III. Coordination of DNA single strand break repair. Free Radic Biol Med. 2017;107:228–44. https://doi.org/10.1016/j.freeradbiomed.2016.11.039.
66. Kalash R, Epperly MW, Goff J, et al. Amelioration of irradiation pulmonary fibrosis by a water-soluble bi-functional sulfoxide radiation mitigator (MMS350). Radiat Res. 2013;180(5):474–90. https://doi.org/10.1667/RR3233.1.
67. Evans ML, Graham MM, Mahler PA, et al. Use of steroids to suppress vascular response to radiation. Int J Radiat Oncol Biol Phys. 1987;13(4):563–7. https://doi.org/10.1016/0360-3016(87)90072-1.
68. Patterson AM, Vemula S, Plett PA, et al. Age and sex divergence in hematopoietic radiosensitivity in aged mouse models of the hematopoietic acute radiation syndrome. Radiat Res. 2022;198(3):221–42. https://doi.org/10.1667/RADE-22-00071.1.
69. Bass SB, Greener JR, Ruggieri D, et al. Attitudes and perceptions of Urban African Americans of a "dirty bomb" radiological terror event: results of a qualitative study and implications for effective risk communication. Disaster Med Public Health Prep. 2015;9(1):9–18. https://doi.org/10.1017/dmp.2014.158.
70. Barbosa SCM, Pereira VBM, Wong DVT, et al. Amifostine reduces inflammation and protects against 4-fluorouracil-induced oral mucositis and hyposalivation. Braz J Med Biol Res. 2019;52(3):e8251. https://doi.org/10.1590/1414-431X20188251.
71. Molinar-Inglis O, Price LN, DiCarlo AL. Highlighting the NIAID Radiation and Nuclear Countermeasures Program's commitment to training and diversifying the radiation workforce. Radiat Res. 2024;201(4):330–7. https://doi.org/10.1667/RADE-23-00207.1.

Chapter 18
Medical Consequences of Exposure to Ionizing Irradiation, High Dose Rate Fission or Fusion Bomb, Isotopic Fallout, and the Effects of Radiation Countermeasures

Depending upon the magnitude of the explosion and range of dispersal of both ionizing irradiation and radioisotopes, the management of casualties from a nuclear reactor accident, detonation of a fission bomb, detonation of a dirty bomb, or willful dispersal of radioisotopes may each produce a significant public health crisis [1–16]. The information from the atomic bomb casualties in Hiroshima, Japan, has provided much information on casualty management, but in the setting of a war-torn country in 1945. The work of pioneer William C. Maloney, M.D. in the aftermath of the bombings provided a great basis for current casualty management approaches [1–3] (Fig. 18.1). His publications on the analysis of casualties are seminal [2–5]. The management [15, 16] of radiation casualties must be preceded by knowing if there has been a radiation dispersal of isotopes, as well as a blast [17–21]. Management of radiation-exposed casualties follows several sets of guidelines [22–28] and then distribution of countermeasures [29–44]. This meeting includes presentations by experts in recent approaches to casualty management and discussion of issues including the triage of patients to different hospitals and managing hospitals that have been contaminated by radioisotopes [17–19]. The meetings ongoing address the challenges of coordination of first responders, hospital personnel, and healthcare professionals as to how to manage with the "worried-well," who are terrified and in shock sometimes with no evidence of direct exposure to themselves [8]. There are many issues regarding the acute effects, but also there are considerations of the long-term effects of administration of radiation mitigators and the expected need for long-term medical consequences of individuals, who survive the event and its immediate aftermath [33–44].

In the case of a limited radiation dispersal, such as that in the nuclear reactor accident in Chernobyl/Ukraine in 1986 [9] and the nuclear reactor melt-down in Fukushima/Japan in 1911 [10], there was initially limited available information on the magnitude of the event and the results of the intervention by first responders and medical personnel. There continues to be more available information disseminated about these events and the results of the first management decisions, casualties, and

J. Greenberger, *Radiation Oncology and Radiation Biology*,
https://doi.org/10.1007/978-3-031-66300-0_18

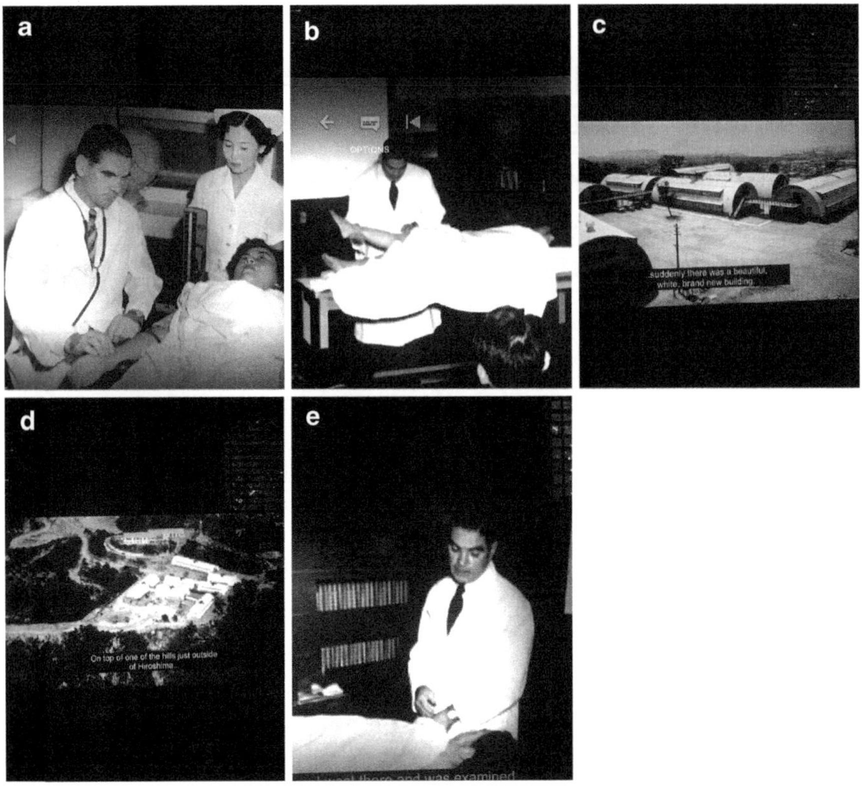

Fig. 18.1 The Atomic Bomb Casualty Center: Hiroshima, Japan. The pioneering work of Dr. William C. Moloney (Panels **a**–**e**)

outcomes. There is also additional information from nuclear accidents involving both military and civilians, which led to exposure of limited numbers of people to ionizing irradiation [11–15]. The international as well as U.S. medical communities are becoming more educated about the challenges of dealing with patients/victims, who have sustained radiation exposure. The issues of managing individual hospital emergency rooms and more broadly, the geographic networks of hospital systems, will be a challenge. Hospitals will be tasked with accommodating potentially large numbers of patients. The concept of "surge capacity" in disaster management has assumed real meaning [17–19]. The surge capacity is defined as the extent to which a given hospital can safely manage an increasing number of emergency patients. Considering that each patient/victim must receive a medical evaluation and diagnosis, the number of individuals seeking help at any facility may overwhelm that facility's resources at any one time. Since the events of "9/11," there have been several approaches to preparation for a radiation nuclear disaster including the use of new radiation detectors suitable for hospitals and ambulances [17–19]. Some radioisotopes present specific challenges, particularly, if long-lived isotopes were inhaled or swallowed [45–49], or if there was significant neutron exposure [50].

In one reported approach to handling victims of a radiation terrorist event, the scenario was that for a hospital of 300 beds in a moderate size American city [18]. This hospital would be identified as one of several proximate sites for evacuation of casualties from the detonation of a fission bomb (Hiroshima/Nagasaki type bomb 10 kiloton TNT equivalent magnitude of explosion). Under these conditions, a centralized disaster management (CDM) facility would accumulate, evaluate, and disperse the first immediate information. The CDM might be the emergency monitoring office in the executive floor of a hospital system network. This CDM would obtain information from local, county, and state police personnel, who arrive near the scene. Also, information on the size of the destructive diameter of blast, closure of roads, and bridges due to direct blast damage, and other first assessments of the size of the detonation, not immediately available, but soon to follow would be the expected area of contamination from fallout, based on prevailing winds and the height of the cloud of dust and debris. Data will be collected by police and military personnel, including as soon as possible, the identification of the radiation device and radiation isotopes that are detectable [17–19].

After the terrorist events of 9/11, there was rapid expansion of the already available research activities, which were tasked with cataloging each element of the disaster plan for such a scenario. One of the most important discussions was that of how to manage the triage of patients from the site of the detonation to each of several local hospitals. Communication systems were developed including both those of limited access and general public access to information would be updated and made available on a real-time basis [17–19].

As first responders would enter the region near a blast zone (later to be designated a nuclear contamination zone), the first to arrive might not be immediately aware of whether there was ionizing irradiation and/or radioisotopes involved. Also, not immediately available would be the types of isotopes detected and the types of protection needed. Protective clothing for the first responders would be essential, particularly, as they helped to evacuate patients/victims and move them into ambulances and other transportation vehicles to get them out of the blast zone and to hospitals. Protocols have been developed [8] to be distributed to first responders and hospital emergency departments in real time [19].

Hospital Preparedness for Radiation Casualties

Since 9/11, many hospitals now have radiation detection devices both in their ambulance bay and in the emergency rooms. Geiger Counters are now available to screen patients as they enter for use, primarily, to determine whether a patient's clothing is contaminated with dust that may be radioactive. Identification of the kinds of isotopes on the patients may not be readily available to all hospital personnel, particularly, those at facilities, which are close to the detonation site. Radiation Safety officers and radiologists on staff at hospitals will likely be those called in as the hospital personnel most likely to be called in for an investigation. These personnel have been educated and will be updated with just in time information coming from the CDM on how to assess whether the isotope contamination of patients that was diagnosed by initial Geiger Counter or new radiation detectors [17–19] used in screening. Are the contaminating isotopes releasing X-rays, beta radiation, gamma irradiation and of what energies [17–19]? Is the contamination by that of detected radioiodine, cesium, or other isotopes [17–20]?

One hospital policy that has been implemented by some is to remove clothing from patients, who are positive by Geiger Counter reading scans and then reassess them again. The skin can be washed, and the contaminated clothing is stored in a "hot" room. Then, determining whether individuals with washed skin have had inhalation or oral ingestion of contaminated material would be carried out. In the case of patients with combined injuries such as those with penetrating wounds, thermal burns, concussion, and other forms of injury that require immediate attention due to blood loss, shock, cardiac arrest, respiratory arrest, and spinal cord damage. It may not be possible to immediately obtain all the information on the type of contamination with isotopes with radiation emitting isotopes before the patients are moved to X-ray machines and CAT scanners to handle immediate life-threatening components of the combined injury. Thus, there is danger of radioisotope contamination of hospital equipment. There are discussions about how hospitals that are contaminated with radioisotopes would continue to manage patients, or whether such hospitals would be isolated and limited to only radioactive patients. Clearly, in the case of patients/victims, who present with combined injury, those non-irradiation, but potentially fatal injuries would be managed first. Hospital personnel, who handle these victims, would potentially be exposed to contaminated clothing, and the situation for first responders as well as hospital personnel. Their challenge would be very similar to that in the early stages of the COVID-19 pandemic [15, 16]. Hospital personnel must wear gloves, masks, and gowns that can be shed and discarded to the "hot" zones as soon as feasible [17–19]. However, the precautions against radiation exposure would be different from those in the case of communicable infectious diseases. Many radiation casualty management policies for hospitals have been developed and physicians, nurses, and other healthcare providers would have to follow these policies. Most important would be gown, mask, and glove precautions for all hospital workers.

The issue of the "surge capacity" of hospitals [17–19] has been introduced, but must be understood and managed. Real-time communication with ambulance drivers would determine to which facility patients would be evacuated. The more that is known about each patient before he/she is loaded into the ambulance, and then after more information is accumulated when in the ambulance, but not yet enroute to the hospital, the better the triage and management can be [18]. If one hospital is already exceeding its surge capacity—is overloaded with patients—ambulances would divert from that location and travel to other possible sites. Of great concern in the case of a large nuclear detonation, many highways, bridges, and transport routes to a hospital would be impassible and this fact would be communicated by the CDM to ambulance drivers [22]. There would be concern for traffic jams to be avoided. Civilians evacuating their own casualties in their own vehicles would be occurring and could clog highways. Radio stations would communicate real-time information to civilians about the necessity to strictly adhere to and follow guidance plans.

How to Manage Radiation-Exposed Casualties

Integrating the local-scale reaction (in the vicinity of the bomb—5 mile radius) must establish the considerations for evacuation and triage, but the communication with regional and National agencies that will have information coming in from many sources will be important. Within minutes–hours after the detonation of a fission bomb (Plutonium Pit/Fission core/Hiroshima scale explosion that would be of the order of 100 kilotons of TNT) [24] (Fig. 18.1) or a fusion bomb detonation (which would be a much greater megatons of TNT type explosion similar to the Marshalese island [11] and Nevada atmospheric testing events of the 1950s), such an event would be communicated worldwide and the United States agencies that would deal with this situation would be activated and take charge. These agencies include FEMA (Federal Emergency Management Association) [23] that would distribute medical materials to the site, and the CDC (Communicable Disease Center) [25, 26], which would have ready for delivery by FEMA the "push-packs" containing medical equipment. Both the CDC and FEMA have resources ready to deploy to respond to the reported specific geographic location. Determining radiation dose sustained by each victim is important [15, 16].

FEMA has available—push-packs, which are specific and relevant to a radiation incident. These radiation response push-packs contain materials that would be used at the site of a detonation. If it is known that the event is one of radiation and isotope dispersal, the radiation contamination zone would be determined. Then, a specific radiation countermeasure push-pack would be directed to that location. If the scope or the types of components of the disaster are not known, other general disaster push-packs have a broader distribution of inventory. Transportation of the "push-packs" to the site of the terrorist event or nuclear reactor accident will be critical to determine. All of these push-packs would be delivered to the site of the event by air, likely to a local military or civilian airport or to multiple airports [25]. Some push-packs might be delivered by trucks and other land vehicles. Push-packs for a radiation event would contain both surgical and medical equipment. But the key elements would be medicines for burns, pain, I.V. fluids, and the available radiation countermeasures, such as potassium iodide, Prussian blue, G-CSF, or GM-CSF, and chelator drugs [25].

Local hospitals would contribute all available on-site inventory of these and other medical supplies until push-packs arrived. Components of the general disaster push-pack would also include intravenous fluids, the medical agents used to manage burns, intubation kits, portable oxygen, and both adult and pediatric emergency equipment. In the case of a known radiation event, the available radiation countermeasures would be delivered [31–33]. There are many new radiation countermeasures that are being evaluated and going through the FDA approval process, so the current list will likely expand to include new agents [36–44]. The kind of weapons that could be used are devastating to comprehend [45–49].

If radioiodine is a component of the fallout contamination, potassium iodide [25] for oral administration would now be delivered. The strategy is to outcompete with "cold" Iodine for thyroid uptake, any radioactive iodine that has been ingested or inhaled or is in the skin in the form of radioactive dust. In the case of Cesium contamination, Prussian Blue [25] will be delivered to chelate the radioactive Cesium and move it to metabolism into the urine and there would be likely delivery of all available countermeasures rather than delay administration until samples from the detonation site were evaluated.

The components of a dirty bomb would be difficult to analyze rapidly, since any of a large list of potential radioactive isotopes, including those that could have been obtained from a medical or research facility. A combination of isotopes could be packaged in an explosive device, which could distribute these radioactive materials over a wide range. Analysis of the cloud of dust dispersal from the Boston Marathon bomb illustrates the potential challenge [22, 28].

In the United States, hospital workers and emergency responders are who will be tasked with managing radiation terrorist victims will treat them as patients, but there must not be a priority that most often ignore their own safety. Therefore, education, preparation, and "just-in-time" communication of instructions must be part of the training process. Since 9/11, the training has increased [7, 27]. There is a new awareness of radiation terrorism. There is also experience from the COVID-19 patients has had transformed most hospital emergency rooms into more dynamic systems that can handle large numbers of patients that require healthcare providers to wear precautions including gowns, gloves, and masks [22]. The faster the communication from a DMC "Disaster Medical Command Center" command center can be delivered to local hospitals, the more knowledgeable hospital workers will be with managing their own safety. The concept of delivering to hospital personnel instructions for management would be by the Just-In-Time approach. Local transmission of just in timed information to emergency rooms and hospitals of video assisted instructions will also be made available.

Until a wider variety of radiation countermeasures are available [36, 37], those that have already been approved would be considered. While first responders and medical personnel are dealing with the first casualties, physicists, and radiation chemists within each hospital system in the geographical area would be evaluating the scope of the exposed population [22, 28, 29], meteorologists will analyze the current and expected prevailing winds for likely direction and magnitude of dispersal of radioisotopes in the blast cloud and begin to give reports to local hospitals, including prediction of the sites likely to be contaminated by aerial dispersal of isotopes [35]. If the region around the blast is experiencing rain or snow, the fallout area at risk would be more geographically limited in scope.

One potential scenario for a fission or fusion bomb detonation that has recently been modeled to analyze the potential scope of radioactive fallout has been that of a nuclear explosion at one of the 450 ICBM (Intercontinental Ballistic missile) silos that are known to be located in Colorado, Wyoming, Nebraska, and North Dakota [45–48]. In a recent report [51], a review of the approximately 450–500 silos for ICBM Missiles, which are located primarily in Wyoming, Colorado, Nebraska, and North Dakota, is known to contain approximately 1000–2000 warheads, each of which has a fission core called a "plutonium pit." These Plutonium pits are the nuclear fission devices that are approximately the size of a ten-pin bowling ball and contain Plutonium 259 in a powder or liquid state that is surrounded by an array of shaped charges that will simultaneously implode centrally to push the Plutonium to critical mass and generate a nuclear fission event similar to that which occurred with the "fat-man" bomb that was dropped over Nagasaki, Japan, in 1945. The Plutonium pit detonation is the first stem in generating the heat required for the nuclear fusion reaction that follows within fractions of a second. The fusion reaction of the thermonuclear bomb generates the megaton explosion of this weapon.

Regarding these plutonium pits, which number 1000–2000, they are, in fact, fission bomb detonation core components of the thermonuclear warhead. There has been a United States military program initiated to replace all of these Plutonium pits with new ones. The strategy of having multiple Plutonium pits per missile is that of the MIRV (Multiple Independently Targeted Re-Entry Vehicles) concept that was developed during the "Cold War" in the 1970s. The missile leaves its silo and enters the Earth's orbit, then upon re-entry, the warhead releases multiple subcomponents each of which targets a different geographic location and each carrying with it a Plutonium pit surrounded by its own components of the nuclear fusion event to follow [48]. The 450–500 ICBM missile sites in the USA are currently being refurbished in sequence. Congress has recently approved a 1.2 trillion budget over the next 10 years [22] to replace the Plutonium pits in all of these sites. Three issues are evident from this update on the United States missile defense program.

The Condition of Radioactive Fallout

The first is that the missile sites are known to all countries that could potentially launch an attack on the United States, so there is ongoing concern that these areas would be targeted as a way to limit the possible U.S. retaliation. Not only would targeting the ICBM silos be a strategic decision to limit, but not prevent a retaliation, the explosions would result in massive aerial contamination of the environment by the dispersal of the Plutonium. Notwithstanding the fact that such a pre-emptive strike against the United States, ICBM missile silos would fail to prevent a horrific retaliation (The land-based arsenal represents one-third of the U.S. arsenal since nuclear missile armed submarines and airplanes (bombers) would surely retaliate). The result of such an attack would create devastating nuclear fallout in the USA. Depending upon the time of year and prevailing winds, there have been reports of the likely geographic distribution of the fallout and number of individuals, who might be exposed, which might total in the millions. If such an event were to occur, individuals in the fallout risk area would be instructed to shelter at home, stay indoors, or in places, in which dust or other radioactive material could fall from the sky on their geographic area. A separate issue would be the aerial fallout contamination of agriculture and water supplies, as well as, farm animals and other food sources.

Prior to this recent update on the likely targets for producing massive environmental contamination from nuclear weapon components, there have been precise model systems experiments of the number of individuals, who would be exposed, types of casualties, and other medical consequences of a nuclear bomb detonation in a large city [29, 45]. The information to construct model systems has been derived largely from detailed studies of Hiroshima and Nagasaki, and now nearly 70 years since the use of nuclear weapons in Japan, it has become clear that there is much more sophisticated information now available even from these historically remote events. For example, the survivors of the Japanese nuclear weapons exposure have reported the location where they were at the time of the detonation, whether there was partial body exposure (lower body was behind concrete or steel), and other precise information. In analysis of Hiroshima and Nagasaki, it has become clear that calculation of radiation doses based on the distance from the hypocenter of detonation can be quite precise [49]. The data have been re-analyzed, with the knowledge that the bomb detonation, which occurred above ground level in the case of those bombs, would be very different from that associated with a nuclear explosion at ground level, for example, in the missile silos in the United States. The closer the detonation would be to the ground, the greater the depth of the explosion crater and also the likely greater atmospheric delivery of greater weight of radioactive dust and radioactive particles from the materials in the crater and these materials would reach higher altitudes in the atmosphere, where prevailing winds would carry the dust hundreds or over thousands of miles away [27, 48]. Historical accounts of the Hiroshima and Nagasaki bombs report detonation at around 1000 meters above the ground level, and the severe sphere of both bomb zones and movement of the radiation clouds from each initial detonation site have been modeled [46].

The second issue is the 1000–25,000 new plutonium pits that are being produced by breeder reactors in Wyoming, at the U.S. Nuclear Weapons Production Facility [51, 52]. The third issue is what to do with the 1100–2000 plutonium pits that are being retired. That is 2000–4000 plutonium pits—fission bombs that will be transported throughout the United States over the 10 years of the military upgrade program.

A challenge in the analysis of the Hiroshima and Nagasaki nuclear weapons was that documentation of the casualties by types of injury was incomplete, sometimes sporadic and not all the data were collected by the same metrics that would be used today [1–8]. In the case of the willful detonation of a nuclear weapon in the United States or anywhere in the globe at the present time, more precise information would be collected. The blast area, radiation dose sustained, quality of irradiation, and, most importantly, the specifics of the atmospheric dispersal and complete analysis of each of the multiple radioisotopes would be more precisely calculated, sophisticated, and more available. This is an event that we all hope never happens!

Management of Large Numbers of Irradiated Victims: Radiation Casualties

Most victims of a nuclear weapon attack, or a radiation terrorist event, or even a nuclear reactor explosion would be managed by triage of patients on an individual basis, and there would be identification of the obvious effects of combined injury: concussions, burns, bone fractures, and penetrating wounds. These visible and obvious consequences of a radiation weapon would be immediately handled by hospitals and, more specifically, by emergency rooms. The individuals, who had suffered radiation exposure alone, would be very large in number depending upon the size of the blast and the distance of individuals from the blast site. A distance that was far enough away from the detonation site to escape flying glass, rubble, and the blast overpressure that would cause concussion, would still potentially deliver lethal or sublethal irradiation [30].

Calculations on the distance of each individual from the blast site could determine their need for immediate administration of radiation countermeasures against the hematopoietic syndrome (3–5 Gy total body dose) or the gastrointestinal syndrome (5–10 Gy) [15, 16]. The "three by three" rule is still used to triage patients, who are suspected to have been irradiated [15, 16]. Most emergency room personnel have been educated, but will also be advised in real time about the triage of radiation casualties. The "three by three" rule is as follows: If patients present with nausea and vomiting within 3 h of the detonation, they are triaged as having been determined to have received 3 Gy total body irradiation or higher. The physiological basis of this rule is based upon the known radiation-induced gastric and intestinal release of inflammatory mediators, such as serotonin from the argetiffin cells of the small intestine. The data come from bone marrow transplant patients, who received TBI as preparation for a marrow infusion, but the data from the transplant patients do not take into account the much higher dose rate of irradiation from a fission or fusion bomb, nor the very high dose rate in the case of a bomb blast. The high dose rate radiation from a fission bomb would likely make patients" symptomatic at lower radiation doses compared to those dose rates used in clinical transplant patients. Furthermore, a nuclear bomb might be releasing up to 40% of the total radiation by neutrons with a much higher RBE (relative biological effect) [50]. High dose rate irradiation-exposed humans, who present with nausea and vomiting, include data form examples supplied from nuclear accidents, radiation workers, and rare other reported events. Individuals who present with nausea and vomiting might be candidates for the available quantities of G-CSF, GM-CSF, or other limited FDA-approved drugs that have been designated for use in cases of radiation counterterrorism [36, 37]. In the absence of any new FDA-approved drugs, these would be the only radiation countermeasures now available.

Once, more radiation countermeasures are available, there will be an even greater need to evaluate the potential side effects of delivery of a countermeasure to each individual candidate for treatment. In a previous chapter on radiation countermeasures, the FDA approval of a drug for use as a radiation countermeasure must be cleared for use by fulfilling the concept of safety first. It might not be possible in the case of mass casualties to determine whether each individual was taking other medicines and whether there was a suspected deleterious effect of adding the radiation countermeasure to the patient's existing polypharmacy. There would be concern for any potential effect of drug interaction. It may also not be possible in a mass casualty event to assess peripheral blood counts in each person twice over 12–24 h to allow physicians to calculate the radiation dose of exposure by the fall in percent of lymphocytes in the blood over a 6- to 18-h interval (another accepted metric for determining radiation dose).

Therefore, the administration of a radiation countermeasure would have to be approved for use based upon data showing that it is safe in individuals with a spectrum of possible other conditions that could not be readily measured in everyone. Depending on the number of casualties, triage procedure for delivery of available G-CSF and GM-CSF would be determined by the DMC command center and each individual would receive the drug according to a schedule that had been developed at a national level. The schedule would be transmitted in real time to each hospital facility that is managing casualties in real time [15, 16, 36, 37].

Triage of Irradiated Victims

The "worried-well" will comprise a large number of individuals [15, 16]. People will come to emergency rooms and report that they were either at a distance from the explosion, which had been judged to be "relatively safe" based on calculation of the radiation dose likely received. These individuals would be triaged by instruction to shelter at home and wait for further instructions. Triage at hospitals would be extremely important. At the present time, hospital emergency rooms are well prepared and skilled in triage. For example, during COVID-19, individual coming in with upper respiratory symptoms only and no evidence of pneumonia were triaged to areas separate from those who were having clear breathing difficulties and required oxygen. During this entire time, emergency cases unrelated to COVID-19 would be triaged and in some cases jump ahead of the COVID-19 victims. For example, multiple gunshot wounds, stabbing, or trauma from automobile accidents would be grounds for moving patients into a different triage area. In the case of nuclear weapons or willful dispersal of radioisotopes, the situation would be much more difficult. Each hospital emergency room would have its own general guidelines, but there would be individual protocols that would direct hospital personnel as to how to triage patients [15, 16].

What Would Be the General Medical Consequences of Radiation Exposure and After Administration of Radiation Countermeasures?

In the case of aerial dispersal of radioisotopes or exposure of individuals, who were several miles from the hypocenter of a detonation, radiation dose calculations would be made based on where they were at the time of the initial detonation. People, who were inside or had partial body shielding, could report this to their healthcare providers and radiation dose calculations would be made. The question of who gets a radiation countermeasure would be a local decision. One of the missions of the Radiation Injury Treatment Network (RITN) [33] was to provide a system in which hospitals in all geographic areas would be designated as radiation casualty systems. These hospitals would have available the network for distribution of G-CSF and GM-CSF [34–37].

One strategy that has been discussed is for patients in bone marrow transplant centers and in cancer centers in which these drugs are routinely given to cancer patients, would receive notice that a disaster has happened. All elective cases would be delayed, and the hospital supplies of these radiation countermeasures (only FDA-approved drugs at the present time) would be delivered to the site of the detonation. Triage programs at each site would determine, who gets these radiation countermeasures. Based on the number of casualties, it may be possible to determine whether individuals are taking other medicines that might conflict or be a problem for their radiation countermeasures. Whether people taking multiple medications would be disqualified from receiving G-CSF or GM-CSF is not known. However, individual hospital personnel would have to rely on their own triage policies [15, 16, 36, 37].

What Are the Expected Long-Term Consequences of Administration of a Radiation Countermeasure?

The long-term effects of delivering a radiation countermeasure must be clearly documented. At present, the data that are available for radiation countermeasures come from medical uses of G-CSF and GM-CSF and from the radiation accident victims at Chernobyl and Fukushima [9, 15, 16]. There were three radiation reactor accidents of note that led to the current catalog and the evolution of safety measures/policies and improvements in nuclear reactor design: Three Mile Island in 1979; Chernobyl 1986, and Fukushima Daiichi 2011. In the future, if there is a nuclear reactor accident or radiation terrorist event, each radiation-exposed individual must be treated separately. Every person has his/her own medical history, which will influence both medical management and the expectations of outcome [15, 16].

There are multiple disease states in which individuals take a medication chronically for years or months or their entire life. As with diabetics, who are constantly receiving insulin usually by auto-injector based on their blood sugar levels, people can live an entirely normal life taking this medication for decades. The same is true for antihypertensive drugs and for patients who have chronic renal or liver disease medications can be delivered for decades, and patients can live relatively normal lives. There are more available drugs to treat chronic conditions: autoimmune diseases, hemophilia, chemotherapy drugs, targeted therapies, monoclonal antibodies, and others; each medication has its own potential side effects and instructions for delivery. In the case of delivery of radiation countermeasures, there will be a clear need to document every patient's needs and response to the therapies. But, if there are mass casualties and no history can be obtained, the decision must be made regarding who gets the countermeasure administration, pregnant women, the elderly, children, the unconscious? The policy of each hospital must be considered as well as real-time information coming from a National source [33].

What Are the Known Long-Term Medical Consequences of Irradiation Exposure and Administration of Radiation Countermeasures

The best available recent evidence to predict how the lives of radiation-exposed individuals would change comes from the available information on patients, who receive total body irradiation and bone marrow transplantation for cancer management. Recovery from acute radiation exposure usually occurs within months after exposure, blood counts return to normal levels, physiologic functioning of most organ systems returns to normal, and patients focus on management of their cancer, close follow-up, and close interaction with their physicians regarding management of other medical conditions, which they had prior to the need for total body irradiation.

The same timeline will likely be the case in those individuals, who were far from the blast zone of a nuclear detonation. It will also be the case with those, who have been in an environment of radioactive fallout. In the latter category, patients may be candidates for protocols to receive chelators [35], and others may be triaged to sites in which total body burden of radioisotopes could be collected.

In the 1970s, the Brookhaven Hospital facility, in preparation for the nuclear event of a Cold War nuclear detonation, had devices for measuring total body burden of radioisotopes [35]. This estimation of total body burden of radioisotopes can still be carried out. However, facilities are not equipped to analyze mass casualties. As we previously described, patients will be placed into a scanner and the total body burden of radioisotopes would be assessed. Collections of feces, urine, and peripheral blood would be made. The individuals, who inhaled respirable particles containing radioisotopes, would be the most challenging. Depending on the number of casualties, individuals could receive bronchoalveolar lavage and removal of fluid, measurement of the types of isotopes, and periodic long-term follow-up. Some long-lived isotopes such as Plutonium 239 or Uranium 235 would require individuals to be followed routinely over their lifetime. Others who had inhaled radioiodine or Cesium or other isotopes with shorter half-lives might be managed for a shorter term.

The long-term medical consequences of delivering radiation mitigators, particularly (in the case of new mitigators likely to be added to the national stockpile in the next years), will be dependent upon the known pharmacokinetics and pharmacodynamics of each of these drugs. Administration of G-CSF or GM-CSF has been well studied [36, 37]. The need for multiple injections has been studied. Pegylated drug with longer half-life [37], if available, to be administered to patients with at risk for hematopoietic syndrome, would be managed by physicians, who are skilled at delivering these drugs to cancer patients.

New radiation mitigators will be more of a challenge for healthcare providers, who will be following their patients. For example, a drug that targets mitochondrial oxidative stress such as JP4–039 (a GS-nitroxide) has not yet been tested in clinical trials and is not FDA-approved [38]. This drug, while highly effective against H-ARS [38], would be one in which several administrations would be likely necessary. Since this drug would be given to people, who had a radiation dose above 3 Gy, therefore, new data would be collected, and available information on ways to assess patients is not yet available.

There are exciting new potential radiation countermeasures that are in varying stages of development. One promising approach is the oral administration of a genetically engineered bacteria that released a cytokine into the intestine and would prevent the acute gastrointestinal syndrome of irradiation, would be the same challenge [42–45]. Since no clinical trial has yet been reported for use of this agent in GI irradiation, a countermeasure based upon genetically engineered *Lactobacillus reuteri* (LR) is promising [39–42] as well as new small molecule countermeasures [43, 44]. These new drugs combine the known safety of swallowing LR, which is a major constituent of yogurt, with the engineered rapid release in the intestine of each of two cytokines (interleukin 22 (IL-22) and interferon-βeta (IFN-β)) that are known to heal intestinal crypt stem cells and prevent intestinal permeability that causes leakage of other bacteria into the blood, where they can cause sepsis [39–42]. New radiation countermeasures are being evaluated for addition to the National stockpile.

References

1. Moloney WC, Sharon J. Pioneering hematology: the research and treatment of malignant blood disorders, reflections on a life's work. Cannon, MA: Science History Publications/USA, Division of Watson Publishing International; 1997.
2. Moloney WC, Kastenbaum MA. Leukemogenic effects of ionizing radiation on atomic bomb survivors in Hiroshima City. Science. 1955;121(3139):308–9. https://doi.org/10.1126/science.121.3139.308.

3. Moloney WC. Leukemia in survivors of atomic bombing. N Engl J Med. 1955;253(3):88–90. https://doi.org/10.1056/NEJM195507212530302.
4. Inskip PD, Kleinerman RA, Stovall M, et al. Leukemia, lymphoma, and multiple myeloma after pelvic radiotherapy for benign disease. Radiat Res. 1993;135(1):108–24.
5. Curtis RE, Boice JD, Stovall M, et al. Risk of leukemia after chemotherapy and radiation treatment for breast cancer. N Engl J Med. 1992;326(26):1745–51. https://doi.org/10.1056/NEJM199206253262605.
6. Tomonaga M. The atomic bombings of Hiroshima and Nagasaki: a summary of the human consequences, 1945-2018, and lessons for Homo sapiens to end the nuclear weapon age. J Peach Nucl Disarm. 2019;2(2):491–517.
7. Ozasa K, Shimizu Y, Suyama A, et al. Studies of the mortality of atomic bomb survivors, report 14, 1950-2003: an overview of cancer and noncancer diseases. Radiat Res. 2012;177(3):229–43. https://doi.org/10.1667/rr2629.1.
8. Daugherty W, Levi B, Von Hippel F. Casualties due to the blast, heat, and radioactive fallout from various hypothetical nuclear attacks on the United States. In: Solomon F, Marston RQ, editors. Institute of Medicine (US) Steering Committee for the symposium on the medical implications of nuclear war. Washington (DC): National Academic Press (US); 1986.
9. Moller AP, Nishiumi I, Suzuki H, et al. Differences in effects of radiation on abundance of animals in Fukushima and Chernobyl. Ecol Indic. 2013;24:75–81.
10. Yoschenko V, Ohkubo T, Kashparov V. Radioactive contaminated forests in Fukushima and Chernobyl. J For Res. 2018;23(1):3–14.
11. Dainiak N. Hematologic consequences of exposure to ionizing radiation. Exp Hematol. 2002;30(6):513–28. https://doi.org/10.1016/s0301-472x(02)00802-0.
12. Dainiak N, Waselenko JK, Armitage JO, et al. The hematologist and radiation casualties. Hematology Am Soc Hematol Educ Program. 2003;2003:473–96. https://doi.org/10.1182/asheducation-2003.1.438.
13. Waselenko JK, MacVittie TJ, Blakely WF, et al. Medical management of the acute radiation syndrome: recommendations of the strategic national stockpile radiation working group. Ann Intern Med. 2004;140(12):1037–51. https://doi.org/10.7326/0003-4819-140-12-200406150-00015.
14. Dainiak N, Gent RN, Carr Z, et al. First global consensus for evidence-based management of the hematopoietic syndrome resulting from exposure to ionizing radiation. Disaster Med Public Health Prep. 2011;5(3):202–12. https://doi.org/10.1001/dmp.2011.68.
15. Lopez M, Martin M. Medical management of the acute radiation syndrome. Rep Pract Oncol Radiother. 2011;16(4):138–46. https://doi.org/10.1016/j.rpor.2011.05.001.
16. Goans RE, Holloway EC, Berger ME, et al. Early dose assessment in criticality accidents. Health Phys. 2001;81(4):446–9. https://doi.org/10.1097/00004032-200110000-00009.
17. Kim JO, Huq MS, Novotny J Jr, et al. Performance characteristics of a novel radioactive isotope detection and notification system designed for use in hospitals. Health Phys. 2011;100(Suppl 2):S71–8. https://doi.org/10.1097/HP.0b013e3181fa370f.
18. Dickson R, Kim JO, Huq MS, et al. Interceptor and phantom trials of EDNS at UPMC. Health Phys. 2013;105(5 Suppl 3):S199–208. https://doi.org/10.1097/HHP.0b013e31828e56b6.
19. Dickson R, Kim JO, Huq MS, et al. A mobile alert system for preparing the delivery of radiation mitigators. In Vivo. 2015;29(5):505–13.
20. Greenberger JS. Emergency management system. 2012. U.S. patent application no. 60/820,115, refiled as no. 11/780,042. 06-0059-02, University of Pittsburgh, 6/30/12, 10/15/12 issued #8, 289, 152.
21. Greenberger JS, Yealy DM. What if the Boston bombings contained radioactive materials? Are you ready? Fast facts for the radiologist. PA Radiological Society Newsletter. May issue. 2013.
22. Matsuoka Y, Nishi D, Nakaya N, et al. Concern over radiation exposure and psychological distress among rescue workers following the Great East Japan earthquake concern over radiation exposure and distress. BMC Public Health. 2012;12:249. https://doi.org/10.1186/1471-2458-12-249.

23. Arooj A, Farooq MS, Umer T, et al. Cognitive internet of vehicles and disaster management: a proposed architecture and future direction. Trans Emerg Telecommun Technol. 2019;33(7):e3625. https://doi.org/10.1002/ett.3625.
24. Peterson PF. Long-term safeguards for plutonium in geologic repositories. Sci Glob Secur. 1996;6(1):1–29.
25. Coleman CN, Sullivan JM, Bader JL, et al. Public health and medical preparedness for a nuclear detonation: the nuclear incident medical enterprise. Health Phys. 2015;108(2):149–60. https://doi.org/10.1097/HP.0000000000000249.
26. Coleman CN, Blumenthal DJ, Casto CA, et al. Recovery and resilience after a nuclear power plant disaster: a medical decision model for managing and effective, timely, and balanced response. Disaster Med Public Health Prep. 2013;7(2):136–45. https://doi.org/10.1017/dmp.2013.5.
27. Whitcomb RC Jr, Ansari AJ, Buzzell JJ, et al. A public health perspective on the U.S. response to the Fukushima radiological emergency. Health Phys. 2015;108(3):357–63. https://doi.org/10.1097/HP.0000000000000198.
28. Gates JD, Arabian S, Biddinger P, et al. The initial response to the Boston marathon bombing: lessons learned to prepare for the next disaster. Ann Surg. 2014;260(6):960–6. https://doi.org/10.1097/SLA.0000000000000914.
29. Singh VK, Seed TM. A review of radiation countermeasures focusing on injury-specific medicinal and regulatory approval status: part I. Radiation sub-syndromes, animal models, and FDA-approved countermeasures. Int J Radiat Biol. 2017;93(9):851–69. https://doi.org/10.1080/09553002.2017.1332438.
30. Cullings HM, Fujita S, Funamoto S, et al. Dose estimation for atomic bomb survivor studies: its evolution and present status. Radiat Res. 2006;166(1 Pt 2):219–54. https://doi.org/10.1667/RR3546.1.
31. Singh VK, Seed TM. Repurposing pharmaceuticals previously approved by regulatory agencies to medically counter injuries arising either early or late following radiation exposure. Front Pharmacol. 2021;12:624844. https://doi.org/10.3389/fphar.2021.624844.
32. Schleipman AR, Gerbaudo VH, Castronovo FP. Radiation disaster response: preparation and simulation experience at an academic medical center. J Nucl Med Technol. 2004;32(1):22–7.
33. Ross JR, Case C, Confer D, et al. Radiation injury treatment network (RITN): healthcare professionals preparing for a mass casualty radiological or nuclear incident. Int J Radiat Biol. 2011;87(8):748–53. https://doi.org/10.3109/09553002.2011.556176.
34. Checker R, Patwardhan RS, Jayakumar S, et al. Chemical and biological basis for development of novel radioprotective drugs for cancer therapy. Free Radic Res. 2021;55(5):595–625. https://doi.org/10.1080/10715762.2021.1876854.
35. Taha MT, Morsi T. Estimation of the total body burden for some individuals using whole body counter. J Radiat Res Appl Sci. 2022;15(3):353–6.
36. Lapidari P, Vaz-Luis I, Meglio AD. Side effects of using granulocyte-colony stimulating factors as prophylaxis of febrile neutropenia in cancer patients: a systematic review. Crit Rev Oncol Hematol. 2021;157:103193. https://doi.org/10.1016/j.critrevonc.2020.103193.
37. Morris ES, MacDonald KPA, Rowe V, et al. Donor treatment with pegylated G-CSF augments the generation of IL-10-producing regulatory T cells and promotes transplantation tolerance. Blood. 2004;103(9):3573–81. https://doi.org/10.1182/blood-2003-08-2864.
38. Goff JP, Epperly MW, Shields D, et al. Radiobiologic effects of GS-nitroxide (JP4-039) in the hematopoietic syndrome. In Vivo. 2011;25(3):315–23.
39. Zhang X, Fisher R, Hou W, et al. Second generation probiotics producing IL-22 increase survival of mice after total body irradiation. In Vivo. 2020;34(1):39–50. https://doi.org/10.21873/invivo.11743.
40. Hamade DF, Epperly MW, Fisher R, et al. Genetically engineered probiotic *Limosilactobacillus reuteri* releasing IL-22 (LR-IL-22) modifies tumor cells microenvironment enabling irradiation in ovarian cancer. Cancers (Basel). 2024;16(3):474. https://doi.org/10.3390/cancers16030474.

41. Espinal A, Epperly MW, Mukherjee A, et al. Intestinal radiation protection and mitigation by second-generation probiotic *Lactobacillus-reuteri* engineered to deliver Interleukin-22. Int J Mol Sci. 2022;23(10):5616. https://doi.org/10.3390/ijms23105616.
42. Hamade DF, Espinal A, Yu J, et al. *Lactobacillus reuteri* releasing IL-22 (LR-IL-22) facilitates intestinal radioprotection for whole-abdomen irradiation (WAI) of ovarian cancer. Radiat Res. 2022;198(1):89–105. https://doi.org/10.1667/RADE-21-00224.1.
43. Thermozier S, Hou W, Zhang X, et al. Anti-ferroptosis drug enhances total body irradiation mitigation by drugs that block apoptosis and necroptosis. Radiat Res. 2020;193(5):435–50. https://doi.org/10.1667/RR15486.1.
44. Leibowitz BJ, Wei L, Zhao G, et al. Interferon B drives intestinal regeneration after radiation. Sci Adv. 2021;7(41):eabi5253. https://doi.org/10.1126/sciadv.abi5253.
45. Martz JC, Schwartz AJ. Plutonium: aging mechanisms and weapon pit lifetime assessment. Actinides. 2003;55:19–23.
46. Taylor BC. Fat man and little boy: the cinematic representation of interests in the nuclear weapons organization. Crit Stud Mass Commun. 1993;10(4):367–94.
47. Lapp RE. Nuclear weapons: past and present. Bull At Sci. 1970;26(6):103–6.
48. York HF. Multiple-warhead missiles. Sci Am. 1973;229(5):18–27.
49. Wilson RR. Nuclear radiation at Hiroshima and Nagasaki. Radiat Res. 1956;4(5):349–59.
50. Cullings HM, Pierce DA, Kellerer AM. Accounting for neutron exposure in the Japanese atomic bomb survivors. Radiat Res. 2014;182(6):587–98. https://doi.org/10.1667/RR13663.1.
51. Scoles S. US continues push to restart plutonium pit production. Physics Today. 2021 Mar 5. https://doi.org/10.1063/PT.6.2.20210305a.
52. Gault M. The U.S. can't make enough plutonium triggers for its nuclear warheads. Trinity Audio, World News. 2024 Feb 15.

Chapter 19
Combined Injuries Added to Acute and Chronic Effects of Radiation Exposure: Both Medical Radiotherapy and Radiation Environmental Radiation Exposure

The concept of "combined injury" from the interaction between ionizing irradiation and other form of injury is not a new concept [1–31]. The trauma of surgery exacerbates radiation injury and time for healing must be observed before starting postoperative radiotherapy [3–10]. Chemotherapy also exacerbates radiation toxicity [11]. During the "Cold War" of the 1970s and 1980s, there was concern that the use of nuclear weapons in a thermonuclear war between the United States and then the Soviet Union might include a scenario in which a nuclear weapon was detonated followed by emission of an infectious agent, such as smallpox. This was a logical approach to dissemination of large numbers of "enemies" in civilian populations, because at the time of radiation exposure, white blood cell counts would fall, and the ability of individuals to respond to infection would be complete. Such a horrible example of combining two insults to human health initiated the section about "combined injury." Many new radiation countermeasures have been tested in combined injury models [18, 21, 31].

Now, the RAD-MUC Program of the Center for Medical Countermeasures Against Radiation, organized by the National Institutes of Allergies, Infectious Diseases of the National Institute of Health, has sent out notices about grant opportunities on studying ways to counteract combined injury. One of these most recent advertisements was for a request of applications to study interactions between ionizing irradiation-emitting weapons and chemical weapons. Chemotherapy for cancer includes toxic chemicals with respect to radiation therapy and is thus combined injury [11–13]. The initial understanding of the devastation caused by nuclear weapons came from the initial reports from the atomic bomb detonations at Hiroshima and Nagasaki. It was clear that the large number of casualties could not often be categorized as pure radiation to individuals since many people have also suffered penetrating wounds, concussions, thermal burns, and other forms of devastation from the blast injury. A very important understanding was that of "overpressure" injuries from the whole-body concussion events, blasts, and a subcategory of concussion to the brain and central nervous system (Fig. 19.1, Table 19.1). In the

J. Greenberger, *Radiation Oncology and Radiation Biology*,
https://doi.org/10.1007/978-3-031-66300-0_19

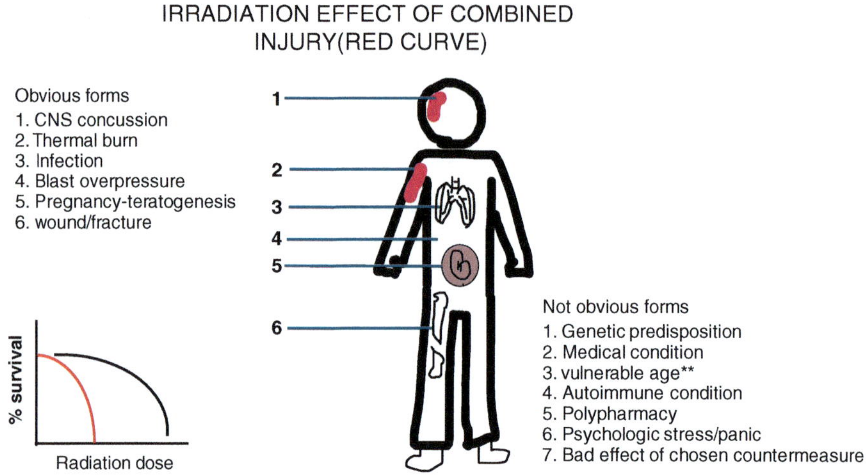

Fig. 19.1 Irradiation effect of combined injury (modification of radiosensitivity and radiation-induced damage). There are multiple forms of combined injury that could add to the deleterious effects of ionizing irradiation. Obvious forms are shown on the left and include blast or overpressure, thermal burn, infection, wound/fracture, pregnancy, which is itself a stress on the body, and the teratogenesis, which follows in the fetus, and CNS concussion (central nervous system, primarily the brain). Nonobvious effects, which would also add to the severity of radiation injury include genetic predisposition (radiosensitivity), a pre-existing medical condition, which would confound the effects of radiation. Having a vulnerable age, either very young, immunosuppressed, or elderly/aged, autoimmune condition, the polypharmacy of taking medications for other chronic diseases, such as diabetes or hypertension, and the psychological stress or panic reaction that would follow a radiation terrorist event. There is also the bad effect, potentially, deleterious effect of a chosen countermeasure, which in certain individuals, who have a genetic disposition to a deleterious effect, may suffer such an effect. Red line in figure in lower left shows that combined injury worsens survival at each radiation dose (total body irradiation shown)

years following the end of World War II, there was discussion about a radiation-emitting bomb that would kill large numbers of individuals, but not destroy buildings or property. This discussion focused around the knowledge that neutrons pass through steel and concrete and would only be attenuated by water or other small molecules. After World War II, nuclear reactors were used for nuclear power generation and breeder reactors were designed to produce Plutonium 239 by using the neutrons emitted from Uranium 235 to hit Uranium 238 and produce Plutonium 239. An understanding of the radiation biology of neutrons led to the concept of "neutron-bomb" in which theoretically a weapon could be used to generate neutrons, which would pass through the materials in tanks, armament, and even buildings and simply kill soldiers. Such a bomb was not tested, but the idea of a pure radiation injury led to discussions about combined injuries since most forms of weapons would have a component of blast and destruction of materials. Whenever a radiation-emitting bomb also caused large concussion events, there would be secondary flying glass, pieces of structure, and therefore combined injuries from these events as well as the radiation. The microbiome in humans is known to influence the

Table 19.1 Combined injury with ionizing irradiation

Category	Effect of combination
Thermal burn	Delays radiation healing
Concussion—CNS	Worse neurocognitive effect
Trauma	Delayed healing
Fracture	Delayed healing
Infection: Bacterial, viral, fungal	Prolonged infection, reduction of cellular immune response
Overpressure injury	Unconsciousness prolonged
Polypharmacy drugs that can exacerbate radiation damage: Adriamycin Cisplatinum Etopiside Taxol Corticosteroid withdrawal	Radiation sensitivity increased. Radiation sensitivity increased. Radiation sensitivity increased. Radiation sensitivity increased. Radiation sensitivity increased. Radiation sensitivity increased. Rebound pneumonia
Wound healing	Delayed
High fiber diet	GI toxicity of WAI
Chronic inflammatory disease	GI toxicity worse
Prior immunosuppression	Transplant patient

response to irradiation [32, 33], as immunosuppression [34–36] and infection [37]. While pregnancy puts a stress on females, radiation countermeasures may be effective and can help the fetus [38].

How to Assess Combined Injury Effects

There are two categories of combined injury those which are more obvious and include the combination of ionizing irradiation with second form of injury that could be evaluated and quantitated by first responders and all caregivers [39–46]. These include thermal burn, concussion to the head and brain, overpressure injury, which would cause rib fractures and difficulty breathing, penetrating wounds including fractures of bones, and the detection of infectious agents (Table 19.1, Fig. 19.1). Also included in such combined injuries would be the combination of ionizing irradiation and chemical weapons. There are other forms of combined injury, which should be also categorized as such but are not immediately obvious. Many of the ones listed in this category of combined injury are individual based. In the event of a nuclear weapon or nuclear reactor accident, those individuals in the area of radiation exposure would not be a uniform population. Many individuals would be on medications for the treatment of acute and chronic diseases, and any form of chemical pharmaceutical in their system could potentially interact with ionizing irradiation to form a combined injury. Much of the current Communicable Disease Center (CDC) outlined the potential sensitivity of individuals to Covid-19 virus exposure, including those that were immunosuppressed due to taking medications for other illnesses, and those who were elderly or infirm, and cautioned that such individuals should seek medical attention and a high priority for receiving antiviral medications; the categories of individuals, who have these conditions, would also count as those with a combined injury, in the event of an ionizing irradiation exposure. The elderly and children are populations that would be categorized as having a potentially worse outcome combined injury [47–50]. Ionizing irradiation increases the induction of senescent cells and leads to a phenomenon of accelerated aging [31]. Therefore, elderly individuals would be likely to have a greater sensitivity to each radiation exposure dose. Other groups in this "frailty" category would include newborn infants, children, and the unborn fetus. Recent research on fetal injury caused by maternal exposure to ionizing irradiation has led to some very inclusive evidence that the fetal state does reduce success of delivering medical countermeasures [38].

Perhaps, the most unobvious component of combined injury would be that caused by psychological stress, panic attack, and other psychosocial injuries that are a component of general medical approaches to all forms of disaster management, not only ionizing irradiation. There are numerous studies, which have indicated that experimental animals and humans exposed to conditions of stress [19] have an altered radiation survival curve, making them more susceptible to radiation lethality or other forms of acute radiation injury. Communication of the triage of patients in real time must occur [51].

As shown in Fig. 19.1, the categories of both obvious and unobvious components of combined injury indicate the complexity that will be associated with the triage of casualties in the event of a nuclear weapon detonation or nuclear reactor accident. Much of the work done on describing the effects of combined injury has been carried out with inbred strains of mice. These studies have led to the clear demonstration that female mice are more resistant to total body irradiation than males and have directed research towards the obvious differences: a difference in the intestinal microbiome of females compared to males and the presence of estrogen and progesterone levels in females. The other side of these differences includes the different microbiome in males and the effects of testosterone and androgenic hormones in males. However, studies with inbred mice even categorizing these animals for uniform age and genetic backgrounds must take into account the individual polypharmacy and history of other diseases that would be a component of managing human casualties. In this regard, the effect of diet [31], obesity, and other components of the overall health of humans must factor into the analysis of combined injury. Studies with inbred mouse strains are valuable, because of the concept of shift in the radiation dose-response curve. As shown in Fig. 19.1, basic radiobiology with in vivo experiments demonstrated usually alters the radiation dose-response curve. Whether studying gamma rays, X-rays, protons, high linear energy transfer (LET) particles, such as carbon 14 or the high LET particles of galactic cosmic irradiation, doses of irradiation can be quantitated by dosimeters that will precisely define the amount of radiation delivered in a total body radiation experiment. Dose-response curves show an increased killing of animals with an increased dose. The survival curve showing increased numbers of dead animals per radiation dose shifts to the left in the case of a combined injury. This means that a lower dose of radiation when sustained in the presence of another toxic agent in combined injury causes more death. These studies are the basis of the numerous publications from the Armed Forces Radiobiological Research Institute (AFRRI) and have led to excellent publications measuring the effect of radiation countermeasures in the setting of combined injury.

Radiation Countermeasures in Combined Injury

Radiation countermeasures have been the subject of another chapter in this book and remain a major focus of research worldwide. The possibility that a specific countermeasure against radiation may in fact be a form of combined injury in certain categories of radiation-exposed individuals has been suggested [21, 31]. While there are few agents that have been FDA-approved for the National Stockpile of radiation countermeasures, such as G-CSF and GM-CSF, and while these agents have been approved for distribution to casualties in the event of a radiation incident, there are places in which individuals have had an unexpected reaction to these drugs, and the dose-response curves that led to recommendation for specific quantities of drugs that can be safely distributed to humans were based upon animal studies. What led to approval by the FDA for inclusion of G-CSF and GM-CSF in the radiation countermeasures National Stockpile has been the plethora of published data on the use of these agents in clinical bone marrow transplantation. However, the clinical data have been generated in the setting of management of patients in a hospital setting with precise monitoring of the effects of the agents. In the case of a radiation countermeasure distribution to large numbers of individuals, there may be some who react to the radiation countermeasure with a toxic response. As research continues in the discovery and development of small molecule radiation countermeasures and the repurposing of drugs for use in this radiation countermeasure setting, there will be undoubtedly reports of untoward reactions and the possibility that a radiation countermeasure may prove to be toxic in some individuals. Thus, the programs in which new radiation countermeasures are being developed include a significant component of understanding efficacy and safety. Furthermore, the testing of radiation countermeasures in vulnerable or frail populations remains a new focus for discovery and development of new radiation countermeasures [48].

Much information about combined injury has been derived by the evaluation of the treatment of cancer patients, who at some point in their treatment history received radiation [1]. The current definition of "combined injury" comes from the literature on the development of radiation countermeasures [2]. As applied to a radiation terrorist event, in such a situation as a fission bomb or dirty bomb, there would be other non-irradiation injuries from the bomb (including thermal burns, overpressure injury from the blast, and penetrating wounds from flying glass and shrapnel) that would simultaneously affect victims (Table 19.1). However, the broad definition of combined injury includes an array of acute and chronic or existing conditions that the irradiated victim must also endure. There are multiple forms of injury, which can modulate or even counteract the mitigation of ionizing irradiation effects. Furthermore, irradiation can affect the treatment of the other injury conditions including wound healing and brain trauma (concussion). The concept of "combined injury" presents an ongoing challenge for management of radiation injuries.

Lessons from clinical radiotherapy provide valuable information about combined injury. For decades, surgeons in collaboration with radiation oncologists as part of the combined modality team for treating cancer have always insisted that the initiation of postoperative radiotherapy be delayed until an appropriate time for wound healing [3]. This is because of their experience that orthovoltage irradiation, which delivered a significant dose to the skin and subcutaneous tissue, delayed, and even prevented wound healing [4, 5]. In another example of the cooperation between medical specialty dealing with cancer patients, women, who have completed a course of postoperative radiotherapy for breast cancer, particularly, those who in past decades had a prior total mastectomy and positive resection margins in the chest wall often received a 4- to 5-week course of fractionated irradiation, usually 45–50 Gy, for postoperative radiation [6]. These women were followed closely, and many were observed to develop chest wall fibrosis as well as other complications including lymphedema of the ipsilateral arm [7] and brachial plexus nerve injury [8]. If the axilla had been dissected rather than sampled, the combined injury was worse [9].

A third example of lessons learned from the collaboration of medical specialties is that of radiation oncologists and surgeons. Radiation oncologists cautioned surgeons not to biopsy expected sites of local recurrence in an area of prior chest wall irradiation. The observation was that of a delayed combined injury. There was the risk that surgical manipulation to the irradiated field, even a biopsy, could contribute to the likelihood of incomplete healing of the biopsy site [10]. The radiation-damaged tissue from months or even years ago healed with respect to tissue integrity with respect to normal function, but the late effects of irradiation include the replacement of epithelial stem cells by fibroblasts causing tissue fibrosis in the fibrotic tissue, which is known to not facilitate normal wound healing.

There is the frequent example of combined injury effects in management of cancer patients, which involves medical oncology and radiation oncology. With the availability of new chemotherapy drugs, the addition of some of these to radiotherapy led to unsuspected injurious side effects. Such an example involved a then new drug in the 1970s, Adriamycin [11, 12]. The experience of adding Adriamycin to radiotherapy produced an example of a deleterious interaction. When the drug, Adriamycin, became available in the 1970s as a powerful new chemotherapy agent, which showed both in animal models and in clinical phase I toxicity trails, the drug showed a dramatic activity against previously uncontrollable aggressive soft tissue sarcomas [13, 14]. There was great excitement in the cancer treatment community. Combining Adriamycin treatment with concomitant with radiotherapy led to reports of severe skin reactions including redness and ulceration of the skin, breakdown, and in some cases injury to internal organs including the lung and heart [13, 14]. Furthermore, the toxicities observed with irradiation and Adriamycin, which constitute indeed a form of combined injury, were observed when the agents were delivered in sequence, as well as when delivered at the same time [14]. These toxic effects led to a now standard of care in which both agents are not given concomitantly. Furthermore, the standards of care include caution about administration of Adriamycin even weeks to months after completion of radiotherapy since it was observed that this protocol was associated with "recall" of radiation injury such that skin reactions were observed to appear in the previously irradiated field, which appeared to be well healed and normal until the Adriamycin was administered [14].

There is a very interesting and vivid example of the interaction between two forms of irradiation (ultraviolet irradiation and ionizing irradiation), which produce a "combined injury." In the therapeutic setting of delivery of a course of radiotherapy, patients are now cautioned to avoid prolonged sun exposure to the irradiated site. This is an example of interaction of ionizing irradiation with ultraviolet irradiation. Patients receiving a relatively large volume of clinical radiotherapy and with a large skin surface area in the treatment plan for example for the treatment of lung cancer or esophagus cancer were cautioned not to spend time in the sun, and with appropriate sun blocking ointment, because of the potential for severe sunburn [15]. While ionizing irradiation and ultraviolet irradiation deliver two very different forms of injury to the skin, there is caution of combined injury. While the molecular mechanism of cell killing by each form of irradiation is very different, there is the risk of combined skin injury under conditions, where one form of radiation alone would be safe. Ionizing irradiation damage differs from ultraviolet irradiation by its molecular mechanism of DNA damage in cells by double-strand breaks, while ultraviolet irradiation causes the formation of cyclobutene dimers at the DNA [16] and leads to cell death at the time of cell division. The additive effect on the skin can result in significant alterations, skin breakdown, and injuries.

Physical trauma is additive to ionizing irradiation. It is also known that tight fitting clothing such as elastic or containing coarse or harsh fiber material should not be worn during a course of fractionated radiotherapy, particularly, over the skin at places involving irradiated tissue. The friction of clothing movement causes early skin breakdown of irradiated skin [5, 17]. This scenario represents an example of this combined injury from irradiation and trauma. While these examples of medical management issues have led to changes in the standard of care for combined modality treatment of cancer patients, but they serve as examples of how other distinct agents can interact with ionizing irradiation to produce a deleterious effect on normal tissues.

The definition of "combined injury" needs to include many factors when discussing the response of the human body to ionizing irradiation. The Radiation Countermeasures Program of the NIH/NIAID defines "combined injury" as a condition, which is present at the time of exposure to ionizing irradiation such that it changes the dose-response curve of irradiation exposure for those individuals. Pioneering work in this area of research was carried out at the Armed Forces Radiation Research Institute (AFRRI) [18]. Dr. Pelmar defined several categories of combined injury (Table 19.1). These include (1) radiation plus bone fracture; (2) radiation plus infection (viral, fungal, or bacterial); (3) radiation plus thermal burns; (4) radiation plus overpressure/blast; (5) radiation plus brain concussion; and (6) radiation plus penetrating wounds. There is another category of combined injury, which should be considered including irradiation plus psychological terror/anxiety [19]. These combined injuries may occur at more than two categories at a time. The overpressure damage from an explosion (Table 19.1, Fig. 19.1) is of particular interest, because of the reality of how it will influence the triage of patients in an emergency room. Publications on each of these models of combined injury in rodents, rabbits, non-human primates, or other animal species have demonstrated that the presence of one or more of these non-ionizing irradiation factors can increase the morbidity and mortality of a given dose of ionizing irradiation and shift the radiation dose-response curve significantly such that death occurs after a radiation dose that should have been non-lethal [20]. Some of the forms of combined injury are obvious to emergency medical personnel and others are not so obvious. The examples from clinical management of cancer patients described above demonstrate the potential deleterious effect of systemic administration of a particular medication to irradiated individuals, which can produce a form of combined injury. The combination of ionizing irradiation plus surgery is very similar to that of the combined injury from penetrating wounds or bone fracture plus irradiation [21].

Other examples of combined injury from experiments with animal model systems have expanded the concept significantly. The conclusion from these studies with respect to protocols for administration of radiation countermeasures must address multiple factors in addition to knowing the calculated radiation dose sustained. In the caser of mass casualties, it may be difficult to fully consider the medical history of each individual. In addition, the notion of combined injury will apply differently depending upon the source and magnitude of the irradiation exposure.

In the case of a radiation terrorist event or nuclear reactor accident, hospitals and other care facilities will be tasked with caring for victims, who will present with many different combined injuries. The victims, who are involved in the local communities of civilian populations, will likely present a great spectrum in their medical histories of their polypharmacy (Table 19.1). Depending upon the number of casualties, it may not be possible to individualize care that is modified according to their medical histories. The general population will include individuals who are taking medications for chronic health conditions and those who are being treated for other unrelated acute conditions or diseases. Depending upon the number of casualties, the triage team at a hospital may have insufficient time to consider an individual's medical history.

In some other situations in which there is time to evaluate each person for their medical history, the administration of a radiation countermeasure may be individualized. In the case of NASA and the planned Mars Space Mission, each astronaut will be medically managed very precisely with respect to many factors in addition to the safest delivery of a medical radiation countermeasure. The astronauts will be managed with respect to diet [31], management of their microbiome, and any medications that they would be taking. In the case of military personnel, who might be exposed to ionizing irradiation, there will be a much more significant role for assessing the types and severity of combined injuries, since battlefield conditions will expose individuals to a greater spectrum of combined injury factors.

General Considerations on the Role of Combined Injuries

In the case of ionizing irradiation exposure, any condition, which produces a change in the cellular and tissue levels of oxidative stress, would be considered a combined injury (Table 19.1). Such conditions include inflammation and taking a medication for an inflammatory condition that is independent of irradiation exposure. Such a condition that requires administration of an anti-inflammatory drug would include ulcerative colitis, chronic colitis, rheumatoid arthritis, or any autoimmune condition [34]. This component of medical history must be considered as the prior condition and/or its medication can produce the potential for combined injury. In addition, a person, who was taking an anti-emetic or anti-diarrheal drug for acute viral gastroenteritis, might present a challenge for management (Table 19.1). For example, in the triage of irradiated individuals when following the three-by-three rule, a person presenting to a hospital at 2 h after detonation of a nuclear device with nausea and vomiting from a pre-existing condition might be triaged as having sustained a radiation dose above 3 Gy TBI and receive a radiation countermeasure that would not necessarily be required. This fact is why radiation countermeasures must be safe in multiple settings including that of a pre-existing medical condition.

Furthermore, if an individual is experiencing a significant stress reaction and has nausea and vomiting from fear may appear to be similar to another individual, who has a viral infection of the gastrointestinal tract causing nausea and vomiting. The condition of anxiety/fear may confuse the members of the triage team. Some infections, which may not appear at the time of presentation, such as chronic inflammatory bowel disease, osteoarthritis, rheumatoid arthritis, or any autoimmune disease in the background of an individual, would influence the outcome of a victim, who has been irradiated (Table 19.1). Not only would the presentation suggest that the individual has sustained a higher radiation dose, a medication that the individual is taking could interact with an administered radiation countermeasure.

Acute radiation exposure increases the levels of inflammatory cytokines in the circulation. It also decreases the number of circulating nucleated white blood cells and, specifically, decreases percentage of lymphocytes [34]. In individuals, who have a previous medical condition that may require intact immune response, the irradiation exposure will decrease their capacity to respond as planned. For example, an individual taking a course of antibiotic medications for the treatment of an infectious disease, such as pneumonia, who was just exposed to a source of ionizing irradiation may experience more severe symptoms of the now inadequately treated pneumonia. There will likely be an exacerbation of the incompletely treated infection. In addition, the presence of the pneumonia infection in an irradiated individual represents a combined injury [30], such that the irradiation dose that was actually sustained may appear to be higher. All of these considerations are taken into account by the FDA during review of the safety profile and effective dose of a new radiation mitigator that is being considered for addition to the national stockpile. An unknown at this time is the effect of COVID-19 late effects (long COVID) on the radiation response to lung irradiation for newly diagnosed lung cancer [30].

The Importance of Medical History in the Triage of Irradiated Victims/Patients

It may not be possible to obtain adequate medical history of the anticipated hundreds or thousands of victims of a fission bomb explosion, or even a dirty bomb that has caused the dispersal of radioisotopes. Therefore, the availability of a new radiation countermeasures, which has been vetted by the FDA, will necessarily have considered as very important the issue of safety. Some irradiated individuals who are presenting at an emergency room or medical care facility may not yet have symptoms of radiation exposure. In contrast, other individuals, who were completely shielded from exposure to irradiation and may not have been irradiated may present with fear and anxiety—the so-called "worried-well." Individuals will be asked to report where they were at the time of an explosion, and their calculated radiation dose will be available from the Disaster Management Center (DMC). However, if the individual was far from the site of a detonation or was completely shielded by having been behind a wall of dense concrete, the triage team of healthcare personnel would do their best to triage this individual to shelter at home and not receive necessary radiation mitigator drugs based on the anticipated low radiation dose. However, if the questions of location and shielding cannot be reliably resolved immediately, the administration of a radiation countermeasure may be appropriate. This countermeasure must be safe for that individual or receiver. A new mitigator must be safe to administration to people of all ages and over a broad spectrum of individuals including those with a non-reported chronic medical condition or those not displaying an obvious combined injury such as an infection. There are other factors, which can impact the delivery of emergency medical care to irradiated individuals.

Radiation countermeasures must be safe for children and the elderly. Infants and children may be candidates to receive a radiation countermeasure and the dose administered would be calculated based on age or body weight or the guidelines for delivery of that particular countermeasure. The countermeasure must be safe in pregnancy [38]. The currently available radiation countermeasures in the Push-Pack from FEMA may include Prussian Blue if there is a likelihood of cesium radiation exposure, potassium iodide if radioiodine I131 has been exposed, and after the individual has had evaluation of peripheral blood nucleated white blood cell, there may be a logical rationale for administration of G-CSF or GM-CSF to that person [39]. The medical history here would be critical, particularly, if the low white cell counts are explicable by another mechanism. For example, if that person is taking a drug that might be expected to lower blood counts, the low value should not be attributed to radiation exposure. There are some, but not many FDA-approved radiation countermeasures available [39]. The pipeline for drug development has many radiation countermeasures that are currently being tested. It is likely that there will be new agents available, and after FDA approval for one or more of these agents, they may be added to the radiation management Push-Pack. Healthcare professional must be advised in a just in time basis as to what countermeasures will be delivered and what doses, and, most importantly, what individuals should receive them, and under what conditions. The importance of combined injury in evaluating patients will be critical. Those individuals, who have overpressure/concussion injury, or are unconscious and known to have been in close proximity to the radiation source may be candidates for a radiation countermeasure even without obtaining a precise medical history. Other individuals, who present with obvious thermal burns, penetrating wounds, bone fractures, or combinations of injuries, can also be candidates for receiving radiation countermeasures. If an individual's location at the time of the radiation dispersal or bomb detonation cannot be confirmed, then in some cases; it may be difficult for emergency personnel to decide whether to deliver a radiation countermeasure.

The existence of another component of the combined injury may necessitate treatment of that non-radiation component first and defer any discussion about radiation countermeasures to a later date. For example, an individual with multiple fractures, thermal burns, and concussion may need surgical and medical management of these conditions independent of any calculated radiation dose sustained.

Psychological Stress as a Component of a Combined Injury: Three Mile Island, Chernobyl, and Fukushima Di-Ichi

In March of 1979, the Three Mile Island Nuclear Reactor accident in the region near Harrisburg, Pennsylvania, produced a situation in which psychological stress, and fear dominated the health of the people, who were living in the communities near the nuclear reactor site. Twenty years after the event, analysis of the local population and evaluation of medical conditions of everyone in the region revealed no significant increase in the incidence of cancer, nor was there evidence of any exposure of the general population to irradiation in excess of background levels [42]. Furthermore, the release into the atmosphere of Noble gasses including Krypton, Helium, Argon, and others was at an extremely low level and not significant with respect to any known adverse health effects [42]. However, at the time of the accident, there was a component of misinformation that was delivered to the public and there evolved a clear component of this fear factor, which caused a challenge for the healthcare community. Large numbers of individuals were reporting to emergency rooms and to their physicians terrified about radiation exposure levels. While it was clear that the cause of the accident was related to a valve in the water-cooling system for one of the two reactors, there was much concern about a more severe reaction. There was concern that there was a likelihood of a reactor meltdown releasing huge quantities of radioisotopes into the environment. While none of these events actually materialized, the fear factor in the community was intense.

If there had been a real significant dispersal of radioiodine, radioactive Cesium, Tritium, or other nuclear reactor-related isotopes, patients coming into emergency rooms would have presented with anxiety and fear-related changes in their laboratory results making it more difficult to assess any possible radiation exposure. Under such conditions, the dissemination of information from a disaster management center would be extremely important for hospital personnel to determine where the event occurred (nuclear reactor accident or dirty bomb explosion, or fission bomb explosion), and individuals would be required to report where they were geographically located at the time of the event. Administration of radiation countermeasures to large numbers of individuals, who are suffering from fear and anxiety, "worried well" would be extremely challenging.

By 1986, the Chernobyl nuclear reactor accident in Ukraine led to more severe damage and casualties. There was a large explosion and a large dust cloud containing radioactive isotopes including those products of nuclear fission: Cesium 137, Iodine 131, and Strontium 90. While there was much more available information for local populations, there was an initial delay in reporting the magnitude of the fallout from the reactor explosion. In fact, the radioisotopes were detected in Sweden before the information was disseminated to some of the countries that had the greatest dispersal, such as Belarus. There were some protocols for first responders and for the management of such a disaster. The measurement of the levels of isotopes in a very large cloud of radioiodine and Cesium that was released from Chernobyl site was possible at the time since monitoring devices were available in adjacent laboratories and in locations as far away as Germany, France, Greece, and other countries.

There was information disseminated rapidly concerning the contamination of agricultural products and food supplies such that people knew how to avoid consuming radiation-contaminated food. However, psychological and related comorbid diseases played a factor in the then available triage of casualties [44]. Those individuals, including firefighters and first responders, who were at the reactor site and were attempting to extinguish fires that were caused by fragments of the graphite rods that were fractured by the explosion, and flew onto the roof of the reactor building did suffer high doses of irradiation, estimated to be between 0.08 and 16 Gy total body dose [44]. These victims were treated with the then available protocols for managing radiation skin burns and trauma. The hospitalized personnel (over 100) led to around 30 deaths. There was the availability of bone marrow transplantation for some (Robert Gale, M.D.) and the limited available countermeasures at that time were administered [46]. The Chernobyl as well as the Fukushima accidents was categorized at level 7 disasters involving nuclear materials or those of international significance.

The most recent nuclear reactor disaster of international significance was the event at the Fukushima-Dai-Ichi nuclear reactor accident in 2011 [46]. This event was one in which much more detailed information was collected, although even at this time all of the information has not yet been released by Japan. The Fukushima accident was caused by an earthquake and subsequent tsunami, which delivered a wave to the reactor complex of buildings that was over 30 m high. The wave and its elevation deposited seawater into the reactor buildings and caused a complete electrical power failure. The water also led to failure of the back-up diesel generators so that there was no power for the cooling systems for the nuclear reactors. There followed a significant overheating of the water surrounding the reactors in each of the four buildings. The absence of a way to vent the reactor rooms led to pressure levels rising and finally explosions that produced large dust clouds containing nuclear fission products including Cesium 137, Iodine 131, and Strontium 90.

The explosions at the buildings at Fukushima led to powerplant failures and release of large quantities of radioisotopes into the environment and into the water. Of interest in the analysis of this event from 2011, the data reveal the importance of communication to the general population. Residents in the geographic area adjacent to the reactor were evacuated. Later others chose to re-enter the communities after analysis of radiation contamination was reported, and the population was informed that it was safe to return.

The population was monitored for appearance of the expected side effects of radiation isotope dispersal into the atmosphere and into the food supply. Individuals were monitored for thyroid nodules from the expected radioiodine contamination of food and were also monitored for general medical conditions. Of the significant number of thyroid nodules that were initially detected, the patients were followed, and the majority of these nodules were biopsied and on pathologic evaluation were benign [47]. However, there was a public health observation with respect to the residents near the reactor site, who returned home. There was an increase in obesity [48] for residents of the area near the nuclear reactor. These individuals were not leaving their homes and were sitting inside their homes and eating large quantities of food with no exercise. The data support the fact that several forms of psychological stress including fear and depression can follow any level of radiation exposure and should be considered a combined injury in the follow-up of these individuals.

Lessons Learned from the COVID-19 Pandemic with Respect to Planning for the Analysis of Combined Injury in Irradiation-Exposed Individuals

Once the cause of the COVID-19 pandemic was identified and the corona virus infection was being limited/managed by individuals wearing masks, gowns, and limiting transmission of the virus, the public health community turned its attention to other issues in disaster management. Much useful information should guide the medical establishment in managing a radiation disaster. Early in the pandemic, when individuals were presenting with severe pulmonary symptoms and pneumonia, the triage procedures in the United States and as reported in Italy as well were based upon standard criteria for evaluation of other opportunistic bacterial infections. There was limited availability of respirators in intensive care units [50]. The triage of patients to be candidates for respirators in intensive care units was managed by necessary new triage procedures. Prior to the availability of vaccines, the reported data indicated that the elderly and individuals with prior medical conditions were more vulnerable for rapid spread of the virus and these people were more likely to need intensive care and the available respirators. The high death rate in elderly patients and those with comorbid diseases, such as those who were immunosuppressed and being treated for cancer, was reported.

Many experimental treatments including the administration of high-dose steroids and antiviral drugs were tested. Once vaccines were available, there was a recognition that certain populations would be more vulnerable to COVID-19 exposure and should be triaged to receive vaccination more rapidly than others in the general population. Those included any individuals, who were immunosuppressed including cancer patients, the elderly, and the infirm. Once serial generations of vaccines were developed, these same vulnerable populations were candidates for the earliest administration of the new vaccines. These observations leading to policies that were established and then updated as new information became available within the medical communities would likely be followed for a situation in which there was radiation exposure to a large number of individuals.

Given the plethora of hospitals or medical care systems in most communities within the United States, hospitals would receive victims and the surge capacity of each hospital managed. Once a hospital had reached its maximum surge response, victims would be triaged to another hospital. Within each hospital, policies would be applied to determine, which individuals receive the most rapid medical care. The elderly, the infirm, children, and those with visible combined injuries would be those handled first [50, 51]. With respect to administration of radiation countermeasures in the case of the hospital, which was, perhaps, several miles from the detonation of a bomb, individuals would be triaged based on factors other than visible combined injuries. The "worried-well" those with significant anxiety and fear-related symptoms might be triaged differently from those, who come into the emergency rooms for evaluation and appeared to have no visible or reported prior medical condition.

A conclusion from all of these considerations is that real-time dissemination of information to care providers will be critical for management of casualties. Hospital emergency rooms will be notified as soon as possible about the nature of the explosion, whether radiation was involved, and when available information on the types of radioisotopes. Educational sessions have been carried out since 9/11, but it is also clear that after these educational sessions when a significant amount of time passes, hospital personnel and providers forget what they have been taught. Therefore, the "real time" delivery of information by the Internet and other direct communications will be critical. Most hospital personnel are skilled in disaster management, and since 9/11, radiation exposure has been added to this list of possible disaster scenarios [52].

The Radiation Injury Treatment Network (RITN) now established in the United States will be involved immediately after any recognition of a radiation disaster-fission bomb, fusion bomb, dirty bomb, and radioisotope dispersal. Triage methods will be reported to individual hospitals to assess what patients should be candidates to be evacuated to a bone marrow transplant center and which should be maintained in local communities. At the present time, there are hospital systems designated as RITN sites for evacuation of patients for bone marrow transplant, and this list is growing as the need for more bone marrow transplant beds is met.

References

1. Byhardt RW, Scott C, Sause WT, et al. Response, toxicity, failure patterns, and survival in five radiation therapy oncology group (RTOG) trials of sequential and/or concurrent chemotherapy and radiotherapy for locally advanced non-small-cell carcinoma of the lung. Int J Radiat Oncol Biol Phys. 1998;42(3):469–78. https://doi.org/10.1016/s0360-3016(98)00251-x.
2. DiCarlo AL, Ramakrishnan N, Hatchett RJ. Radiation combined injury: overview of NIAID research. Health Phys. 2010;98(6):863–7. https://doi.org/10.1097/HP.0b013e318a6ee32.
3. Jacobson LK, Johnson MB, Dedhia RD, et al. Impaired wound healing after radiation therapy: a systematic review of pathogenesis and treatment. JPRAS Open. 2017;13:92–105.
4. Bharadwaj S, Rocker J. Minor head injury: limiting patient exposure to ionizing radiation, risk stratification, and concussion management. Curr Opin Pediatr. 2016;28(1):121–31. https://doi.org/10.1097/MOP.0000000000000297.
5. Brand R, Epperly MW, Stottlemyer JM, et al. A topical mitochondria-targeted redox cycling nitroxide mitigates oxidative stress induced skin damage. J Invest Dermatol. 2017;137(3):576–86. https://doi.org/10.1016/j.jid.2016.09.033.
6. Thalji SZ, Cortina CS, Guo MS, et al. Postoperative complications form breast and axillary surgery. Surg Clin North Am. 2023;103(1):121–39.
7. Nassif TM, Brunelle CL, Gillespie TC, et al. Breast cancer-related lymphedema: a review of risk factors, radiation therapy contribution, and management strategies. Curr Breast Cancer Rep. 2020;12:305–16.
8. Senkus-Konefka E, Jassem J. Complications of breast-cancer radiotherapy. Clin Oncol (R Coll Radiol). 2006;18(3):229–35. https://doi.org/10.1016/j.clon.2005.11.004.
9. Veronesi U, Paganelli G, Viale G, et al. A randomized comparison of sentinel-node biopsy with routine axillary dissection in breast cancer. N Engl J Med. 2003;349(6):546–53. https://doi.org/10.1056/NEJMoa012782.
10. Wahl AO, Rademaker A, Kiel KD, et al. Multi-institutional review of repeat irradiation of chest wall and breast for recurrent breast cancer. Int J Radiat Oncol Biol Phys. 2008;70(2):477–84. https://doi.org/10.1016/j.ijrobp.2007.06.035.
11. Antman K, Suit H, Amato D, et al. Preliminary results of a randomized trial of adjuvant Adriamycin for sarcoma: lack of apparent difference between treatment groups. J Clin Oncol. 1984;2(6):601–8. https://doi.org/10.1200/JCO.1984.2.6.601.
12. Antman K, Amato D, Wood W, et al. Impact of patient and physician refusal of randomization of otherwise eligible patients on the results of a clinical trial. J Clin Oncol. 1985;3:1142–7.
13. Greco FA, Brereton HD, Kent H, et al. Adriamycin and enhanced radiation reaction in normal esophagus and skin. Ann Intern Med. 1976;85(3):294–8. https://doi.org/10.7326/0003-4819-85-3-294.
14. Azria D, Magne N, Zouhair A, et al. Radiation recall: a well recognized but neglected phenomenon. Cancer Treat Rev. 2005;31(7):555–70. https://doi.org/10.1016/j.ctrv.2005.07.008.

15. Kiefer J. Interaction between ultraviolet and ionizing radiation in eukaryotic cells. In: Riklis E, editor. Photobiology: the science and its applications. 1st ed. Springer; 1991. p. 61–9.
16. Manti L, D'Arco A. Cooperative biological effects between ionizing radiation and other physical and chemical agents. Mutat Res. 2010;704(1–3):115–22. https://doi.org/10.1016/j.mrrev.2010.03.005.
17. Bray FN, Simmons BJ, Wolfson AH, et al. Acute and chronic cutaneous reactions to ionizing radiation therapy. Dermatol Ther (Heidelb). 2016;6(2):185–206. https://doi.org/10.1007/s13555-016-0120-y.
18. Tran TA, Kappelhoff J, Justel T, et al. UV emitting nanoparticles enhance the effect of ionizing radiation in 3D lung cancer spheroids. Int J Radiat Biol. 2022;98(9):1484–94. https://doi.org/10.1080/09553002.2022.2027541.
19. Zhang Y, Zanos P, Jackson IL, et al. Psychological stress enhances tumor growth and diminishes radiation response in preclinical model of lung cancer. Radiother Oncol. 2020;146:126–35. https://doi.org/10.1016/j.radonc.2020.02.004.
20. DiCarlo AL, Hatchett RJ, Kaminski JM, et al. Medical countermeasures for radiation combined injury: radiation with burn, blast, trauma, and/or sepsis. Report of an NIAID workshop, March 26–27, 2007. Radiat Res. 2007;169(6):712–21. https://doi.org/10.1667/RR1295.1.
21. Gokhale AS, Epperly M, Glowacki J, et al. Small molecule GS-nitroxide and MnSOD gene therapy ameliorate ionizing irradiation-induced delay in bone wound healing in a novel murine model. In Vivo. 2010;24(4):377–85.
22. Simon DW, Vagni VM, Kochanek PM, et al. Combined neurotrauma models: experimental models combining traumatic brain injury and secondary insults. Methods Mol Biol. 2016;1462:393–411. https://doi.org/10.1007/978-1-4939-3816-2_22.
23. Jegoux F, Malard O, Goyenvalle E, et al. Radiation effects on bone healing and reconstruction: interpretation of the literature. Oral Surg Oral Med Oral Pathol Oral Radiol Endod. 2010;109(2):173–84. https://doi.org/10.1016/j.tripleo.2009.10.001.
24. Iddins CJ, DiCarlo AL, Ervin MD, et al. Cutaneous and local radiation injuries. J Radiol Prot. 2022;42(1):011001. https://doi.org/10.1088/1361-6498/ac241a.
25. Marsh D. Concepts of fracture union, delayed union, and nonunion. Clin Orthop Relat Res. 1998;355(Suppl):S22–30. https://doi.org/10.1097/00003086-199810001-00004.
26. Gomez-Barrena E, Rosset P, Lozana D, et al. Bone fracture healing: cell therapy in delayed unions and nonunions. Bone. 2015;70:93–101. https://doi.org/10.1016/j.bone.2014.07.033.
27. Ryan JL. Ionizing radiation: the good, the bad, and the ugly. J Invest Dermatol. 2012;132(3 Pt 2):985–93. https://doi.org/10.1038/jid.2011.411.
28. Phillips TL, Fu KK. Quantification of combined radiation therapy and chemotherapy effects on critical normal tissues. Cancer. 1976;37(2 Suppl):1186–200. https://doi.org/10.1002/1097-0142(197602)37:2+<1186::aid-cncr2820370830>3.0.co;2-v.
29. Kiang JG, Jiao W, Cary LH, et al. Wound trauma increases radiation-induced mortality by activation of iNOS pathway and elevation of cytokine concentrations and bacterial infection. Radiat Res. 2010;173(3):319–32. https://doi.org/10.1667/RR1892.1.
30. Michalowski AS. On radiation damage to normal tissues and its treatment: II. Anti-inflammatory drugs. Acta Oncol. 1994;33(2):139–57. https://doi.org/10.3109/02841869409098397.
31. Epperly MW, Wang H, Jones J, et al. Antioxidant-chemoprevention diet ameliorates late effects of total body irradiation and supplements radioprotection by MnSOD-plasmid liposome administration. Radiat Res. 2011;175(6):759–65. https://doi.org/10.1667/RR2398.1.
32. Li K, Epperly M, Greenberger J, et al. Longitudinal fecal microbiome study of total body irradiated mice treated with radiation mitigators identify bacterial associations with survival. Front Cell Infect Microbiol. 2021;11:715396. https://doi.org/10.3389/fcimb.2021.715396.
33. Spyropoulos BG, Misiakos EP, Fotiadis C, et al. Antioxidant properties of probiotics and their protective effects in the pathogenesis of radiation-induced enteritis and colitis. Dig Dis Sci. 2011;56(2):285–94. https://doi.org/10.1007/s10620-010-1307-1.

34. Cassatt DR, Winters TA, PrabhuDas M. Immune dysfunction from radiation exposure. Radiat Res. 2023;200(4):389–95. https://doi.org/10.1667/RADE-22-00197.1.
35. Vial T, Descotes J. Immunosuppressive drugs and cancer. Toxicology. 2003;185(3):229–40. https://doi.org/10.1016/s0300-483x(02)00612-1.
36. Hart JP, Broadwater G, Rabbani Z, et al. Cytokine profiling for prediction of symptomatic radiation-induced lung injury. Int J Radiat Oncol Biol Phys. 2005;63(5):1448–54. https://doi.org/10.1016/j.ijrobp.2005.05.032.
37. Greenberger JS, Hou W, Shields D, et al. SARS-COV-2 (COVID-19) spike protein induces oxidative stress and senescence in mouse and human lung. In Vivo. 2024;38(4):1546–56.
38. Wu YL, Christodoulou AG, Beumer JH, et al. Amelioration of fetal irradiation injury from mid-gestation total body radiation with maternal administration of the mitochondrial-targeted GS-nitroxide JP4-039. J Clin Investig. 2024. Submitted.
39. Murrain-Hill P, Coleman CN, Hick JL, et al. Medical response to a nuclear detonation: creating a playbook for state and local planners and responders. Disaster Med Public Health Prep. 2011;5 Suppl 1:S89–97. https://doi.org/10.1001/dmp.2011.13.
40. Coleman CN, Parker GW. Radiation terrorism: what society needs from the radiobiology—radiation protection and radiation oncology communities. J Radiol Prot. 2009;29(2A):A159–69. https://doi.org/10.1088/0952-4746/29/2A/S11.
41. Dainiak N, Goans RE, Iddins CJ, et al. Radiological and nuclear terrorism: the oncologic emergency response. In: Todd KH, Thomas Jr CR, editors. Oncologic emergency medicine. Springer Cham; 2016. p. 127–36.
42. Moore AV Jr. Radiological and nuclear terrorism: are you prepared? J Am Coll Radiol. 2004;1(1):54–8. https://doi.org/10.1016/S1546/S1546-1440(03)00014-0.
43. Anspaugh LR, Catlin RJ, Goldman M. The global impact of the Chernobyl reactor accident. Science. 1988;242(4885):1513–9. https://doi.org/10.1126/science.3201240.
44. Gale RP. Immediate medical consequences of nuclear accidents. Lesson from Chernobyl. JAMA. 1987;258(5):625–8.
45. Baranov A, Gale RP, Guskova A, et al. Bone marrow transplantation after the Chernobyl nuclear accident. N Engl J Med. 1989;321(4):205–12. https://doi.org/10.1056/NEJM198907273210401.
46. Hasegawa A, Ohira T, Maeda M, et al. Emergency responses and health consequences after the Fukushima accident: evacuation and relocation. Clin Oncol (R Coll Radiol). 2016;28(4):237–44. https://doi.org/10.1016/j.clon.2016.01.002.
47. Suzuki S, Suzuki S, Fukushima T, et al. Comprehensive survey results of childhood thyroid ultrasound examinations in Fukushima in the first four years after the Fukushima Daiichi Nuclear Power Plant accident. Thyroid. 2016;26(6):843–51. https://doi.org/10.1089/thy.2015.0564.
48. Clark LD, Stabin MG, Fernald MJ, et al. Changes in radiation dose with variations in human anatomy: moderately and severely obese adults. J Nucl Med. 2010;51(6):929–32. https://doi.org/10.2967/jnumed.109.073015.
49. Boccia S, Ricciardi W, Ioannidis JPA. What other countries can learn from Italy during the COVID-19 pandemic. JAMA Intern Med. 2020;180(7):927–8. https://doi.org/10.1001/jamainternmed.2020.1447.
50. Smith GL, Smith BD. Radiation treatment in older patients: a framework for clinical decision making. J Clin Oncol. 2014;32(24):2669–78. https://doi.org/10.1200/JCO.2014.55.1168.
51. Mustafa MM, Cengiz K. Real-time system for forecasting natural disasters using the social network. In: Kumar R, Sharma R, Pattnaik PK, editors. Multimedia technologies in the internet of things environment, vol. 3. Singapore: Springer; 2022. p. 107–17.

Chapter 20
Future of Radiation Oncology and the Physicians/Scientists/Radiobiologists

The History of Radiation Oncology

In the history of medicine, there have been many major changes in the approach to treating human disease, such is the case with radiation oncology [1–11]. In the specialty of surgery, many instruments that were invented in ancient times have persisted into the modern era including tools that were inserted into the bladder to remove bladder stones and specific materials that were used to produce sutures closing wounds. Resorbable sutures for surgery used materials that were designed from biological materials, and some of these have been modified over the centuries but they are still used today. Even if all cancer disappears, there will always be a need for surgeons, and subspecialty surgeons including urologists, thoracic surgeons, pediatric surgeons, neurosurgeons, orthopedic surgeons, and others.

Herbal medicines were discovered by primitive *Homo sapiens* and also have remained in the armamentarium of physicians to treat cancer well into the modern era. One example is the French lilac, which gave rise to the drug metformin that was chemically synthesized by French scientists in 1929. The history of medicine shows that the material from the French lilac was used to treat diabetes, stimulate lactation and for other medical conditions that were diagnosed by primitive humans. The Vinca alkaloid gave rise to the anticancer drug vincristine. The bark from the Yew tree was used to generate the chemotherapy drug taxol. There are many examples of medicines that have persisted for thousands of years since discovery. Multiagent chemotherapy used today includes some of these drugs [12–16].

There are many previous "standards of care," which have been discarded. One can only look at the history of medicine to see that while some of these options for care or even approaches to public health may now seem ludicrous, at the time they were logical. Building fires in the street to disperse the miasma, which was thought to have produced the plague, is one example. The use of blood-letting, and clisters (enemas) to remove harmful materials from a patient, was used routinely

J. Greenberger, *Radiation Oncology and Radiation Biology*,
https://doi.org/10.1007/978-3-031-66300-0_20

throughout Europe prior to the discovery of antibiotics. Will future generations of humans look back on the use of ionizing irradiation to treat cancer the same way? A problem, which constantly needs explanation, is why treating patients with radiation that causes cancer is the standard of care. As more patients are cured and live for decades, there are new radiation late effects being reported.

The future of the specialty of radiation oncology for the next several decades is sound. However, what about after that? Will this specialty still exist 100 years from now?

There is evidence to suggest that it will not.

With the exception of a few "benign" disease states, ionizing irradiation as a therapy is primarily used to treat cancer. The list of human cancers in which radiation oncology is the primary treatment leading to cure has been decreasing through the last 50 years. Treatments for these cancers have been replaced by a simple surgical approach for biopsy and then combination chemotherapy. Chemotherapy drugs are being augmented and, in some cases, replaced by targeted therapies including biological response modifiers and immunotherapy drugs. Medical students know this and choose the residency training now in spite of concerns (Tables 20.1 and 20.2). Several new radiation treatment devices have been introduced over the past 40 years, with different radiation beams [17–25], different targeting methods [26], and different dose rates [27–29]. Toxicity of radiotherapy has been a major focus of clinical research, particularly, late effects in cancer survivors [30].

Advances in diagnostic pathology have been revolutionary. One hundred years ago, a tumor specimen was fixed with hematoxylin and eosin stains, and slides were reviewed by pathologists, who made a diagnosis. Simple viewing of the tumor specimen under the microscope has been replaced by techniques of immunostaining in which monoclonal antibodies that are specific for certain biomarkers of a specific tumor are used to treat histopathologic slides and the immunostaining profile is

Table 20.1 Changes in utilization of Radiation Oncology in cancer patient management in USA

	Relative patient numbers by decades						
Modality	1960s	1970s	1980s	1990s	2000s	2010s	2020s
Mantle, para-aortic, pelvic, total nodal irradiation of Hodgkin's disease	+++	+++	+++	++	+	–	–
Head and neck cancer	+++	+++	+++	+++	+++	+++	+++
Gynecologic cancer: cervix, uterine, vulvovaginal	+++	+++	+++	+++	+++	+++	+++
Prostate cancer	+	++	++	++	++	++	++
Breast cancer	+	++	++	+++	+++	++	++
Treatment of metastasis, whole brain Gamma knife cyberknife, Stereotactic radiosurgery SABR, SBRT	+	+	+ +	+ ++	+ + +	+ + ++	– – +++
New modalities – Protons – FLASH	– – –	– – –	+	+	+	+ +	– +
Pediatric cancers	+++	+++	++	+	+	+	+

Table 20.2 Reasons why medical students do not choose careers in radiation oncology

Reasons	1960s	1970s	1980s	1990s	2000s	2010s	2020s
Fear of radiation	+++	+++	+++	++	+	–	–
Dislike for care of dying patients	+++	++	–	–	–	–	–
Concern over physics	+++	++	–	–	–	–	–
Limited responsibility for patient care	–	–	–	+	+	+	++
Concern for lack of available jobs	–	–	–	+	++	+++	+++
There will not be cancer since cure is imminent	–	++	+	–	–	–	–

presented to the surgeon, who carried out the biopsy, as well as to multidisciplinary tumor boards that discuss how to manage a particular tumor. In the last decade, the field of "Molecular Pathology" has exploded with the advent of techniques to identify fusion genes in individual tumor specimens, which indicate not only histopathologic type of tumor, but also the subgroup of cancers to which a specific drug can be delivered to target that fusion protein. The etiology of some cancers has changed [40–42] opening up new targets for prevention. Earlier diagnosis is common with better screening tools [43]. Given the plethora of publications on the basic science approach to diagnosing cancer, it is likely that diagnostic pathology will continue to evolve over the next 100 years, such that physicians, who have carried out the biopsy, will receive a report specifically identifying the subtype of each cancer and direct therapy to use of drug that is specific for that patient. Most recently, 30 years ago, the concept of "personalized medicine" began to evolve. This concept was interpreted to mean that a diagnosis of specific cancer and the staging of that cancer including evaluation of lymph nodes, size of original tumor, and its propensity for invasion will be modified by the individual patient's background needs. An example of this is a patient with Fanconi Anemia, which is the background condition of defective DNA repair mechanisms. That person will not be directed toward a "standard of care" approach using a specific dose of irradiation and specific combination of chemotherapy drugs, without attention to the normal tissue sensitivity of that particular patient. This is a specific example. There are also widely applied examples in which the approach to treating a cancer has been modified based on the age of the patient. The elderly do not receive the same program of aggressive chemotherapy as younger patients. Pediatric patients receive a different approach including a different spectrum of chemotherapy drugs, based on the ability of normal tissues to tolerate the treatment. All of these changes are continually being modified and adapted as more knowledge is acquired.

With respect to the specialty of radiation oncology, there is one issue that is affecting the choice of medical students, who are in decreasing numbers choosing to enter this specialty. Radiation oncologists are cancer doctors and use a single modality to treat their patients. While the approach to delivering radiation therapy has changed dramatically since the first use of an orthovoltage radiation machine, to now the availability of sophisticated linear accelerators, dose rate altering machines, and sophisticated treatment planning, it is still a single modality. Furthermore, whether the ionizing irradiation is delivered to the cancer cells by orthovoltage X-ray, implanted brachytherapy sources, or different types of particle-generating machines including protons and carbon atoms, it is still a single approach using a single modality.

Medical oncologists have a continuous change in their spectrum of drugs used to treat cancer. Medical oncologists are specialists in internal medicine, and if a particular cancer is eliminated, medical oncologists will still be able to practice medicine [12]. They have a continuing great experience in other areas including infectious diseases and knowledge of nearly all organ systems, because they manage the side effects of chemotherapy. Similarly, surgeons will always have a practical use of their training. If there is no further lung cancer, thoracic surgeons will still handle trauma, organ transplantation, and treatment of "benign" diseases that cause significant human suffering. While diagnostic radiologists can move from one specific modality to another, as an example pneumoencephalograms to diagnose tumors in the brain replaced by computerized axial tomography (CAT scanning) and magnetic resonance imaging (MRI), they will always have diagnostic capabilities to guide surgeons and provide valuable information. This may not be the case with radiation oncologists. If there is no more cancer and/or if cancers can be treated with systemic agents, what will radiation oncologists do? The answer to this question may well relate to the training program (Residency) for board certification in Radiation Oncology (Tables 20.1 and 20.2). The evolution of cancer resistance occurs over months (Fig. 20.1) compared to the evolution of species discussed in Chap. 1. However, new drugs can be developed to follow the rapid evolution of drug resistance as well as cancer recurrence, invasion, and metastasis (Fig. 20.1).

Over the last 50 years, the concept of my modality conferences or "tumor-boards" has been developed in all academic medical centers and in most community hospitals. At these conferences, radiation oncologists, surgeons, including specialty surgeons, and medical oncologists discuss each patient and develop a treatment protocol, which is modified by the current literature and recent publications. At these sessions, it has become clear that radiation oncologists have a particular focus in their training. For years, radiation oncologists have been the people at these conferences, who understand cancer biology, the natural history of all cancers, and staging systems at times better than do surgeons or medical oncologists. Part of this has been related to the training program for radiation oncology. Residents in radiation oncology spend time on pediatric cancer services, gynecologic oncology services, and work with specialty surgeons in all disciplines including urology, neurosurgery, thoracic surgery, and others. Radiation oncologists learn the mechanism of action of chemotherapy drugs and biologically targeted agents just as do medical oncologists.

Radiation oncologists learn anatomy, design treatment protocols, and in recent years now understand the toxicity of radiation and chemotherapy to specific areas within each organ. Treatment planning software now has evolved to give radiation oncologists a guideline for the dose distribution to all tissues in the clinical treatment volume (CTV), not just the area of the tumor. In fact, the treatment planning software now is very much anatomy focused, so there is separation between the

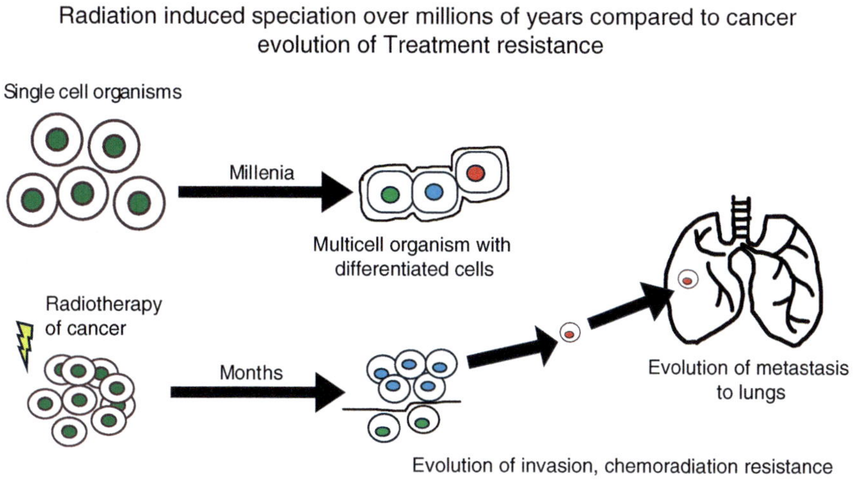

Fig. 20.1 Radiation-induced speciation: An adaptation in the evolution of species compared to the evolution of cancer metastasis. There has been much attention given to the capacity of cancer to evolve, not only to escape radiation therapy and chemotherapy, but also to change its biology. Shown in the figure is a sample of the evolution of single-cell organisms over millions of years to multicell organisms with differentiated cells capable of producing different effects, central nervous system, blood production, digestion, and elimination of waste is the example shown. This may require millions of years of natural selection of the evolving species, which evolves from single cells to multicellular organisms. In contrast, in the lower panel radiotherapy and/or chemotherapy of cancer induces natural selection and evolution of cancer subsets, where the cells have the ability to invade a background tissue, develop chemoradiation resistance, or develop the ability to metastasize to lymph nodes or through the blood to distant organs, such as the lung. The genetic changes involved in each phenomenon, both upper and lower panel, include many categories of change including gene deletion, gene adaptation, and gene replication. The fact that this happens in cancer represents a challenge not only to physicians treating the cancer, but also to understand the biology of evolution of the cancer cells. This domain has been part of the education of radiation oncologists for generations

actual tumor itself (GTV) and the treatment planning volume, which may include a margin around the tumor (PTV) [20, 21]. Radiation oncology residents learn anatomy, and in many cases, as proficiently as do diagnostic radiologists. Therefore, the training program in radiation oncology provides some degree of hope that even if there is no more cancer, there will be a great need for physicians, who are skilled in the elements of this training program. The most important thing about radiation oncology residency training is that it teaches the basics of medicine, just as does residency training programs in all surgical subspecialties and in medical oncology, namely, care for the patient. Training programs in radiation oncology include a first clinical year, formerly termed, internship. The training programs are flexible in this first clinical year, which may be an internship in internal medicine, surgery, or a so-called "Rotating" internship in which that first year can be spent in pediatrics, gynecology, general surgery, or internal medicine. Radiation oncology residents are taught to make very good use of this first year, because it teaches them principles of internal medicine that go far beyond that from medical school training. Radiation oncologists see their patients on weekly on-treatment visits and in follow-up. In some cases, the primary care physician may appreciate the help. Radiation oncologists are trained not only as medical students, but during the internship year to diagnose medical complications of radiotherapy, but also principles of general medicine. It is not uncommon for radiation oncologists seeing a patient in follow-up to diagnose deep vein thrombosis, by taking a history to diagnose the onset of diabetes, diagnose new onset of vision problems, and even some acute emergencies, such as a patient limping in for a follow-up visit, who has right lower quadrant abdominal pain, and is found after referral to the emergency department to have acute appendicitis. Radiation oncologists are physicians and will always have the ability to care for patients.

What are the factors which are likely to continue to reduce the scope of the specialty and the issues that are motivating medical students to consider residency training in specialties other than radiation oncology.

Fifty years ago, a Department of Radiation Oncology usually saw patients in categories of "curable" and "palliative" [1–4]. The spectrum of patients with curable diseases has decreased. The most prominent example is Hodgkin's disease in which large-volume radiation to the chest (mantle), abdomen (para-aortic field), and pelvis (pubic radiation field) has been replaced by combination chemotherapy. While major categories of disease have been removed from the spectrum of those that are curable by radiation therapy, others have remained a prominent focus for radiation oncologists, namely, head and neck cancer and pelvic malignancies. However, in these cases, there are dose reduction protocols in place. It has become clear that the major causes of cancer in these regions have changed. For example, tobacco smoke-related head and neck cancer has largely been replaced by human papilloma virus (HPV)-induced cancers [40, 41]. The HPV-associated head and neck cancers can be controlled with lower radiation doses, and in some protocols, these doses have been decreased markedly. Large-volume, high-dose irradiation has been replaced by targeted and focused stereotactic radiosurgery treatment for many of these curable cancers.

Radiotherapy for palliation has expanded over the last three decades. The concept of "prophylactic palliation" has gained serious consideration, because patients with cancers that are known to metastasize are followed routinely with sophisticated diagnostic radiology techniques including CAT scanning and MRI. The most prominent change has been PET scanning for following patients. When a "spot" is noted on a scan, in many cases, the patient receives stereotactic radiosurgery to eliminate this suspected site of disease, without a biopsy, and using hypofractionated approaches, which may be a single or small number of focused treatments. Stereotactic body radiotherapy (SBRT) and stereotactic ablative radiotherapy (SABR) [5] have been routinely used in most radiotherapy departments. In decades past, metastatic lesions would not be treated unless they had produced symptoms. This was the concept of palliative radiotherapy. Departments would discuss the logic of palliative radiotherapy with the question "what are you palliating?". This was a logical approach given the fact that medical students and residents were taught that a single metastatic focus usually heralded widespread metastatic disease. The revolutionary discovery that there was a phenomenon of oligometastasis and that some cancers clearly spread to only a few sites [20, 21]. Given that this molecular approach to diagnosing oligometastasis was sound, physicians now in the last decade treat single or multiple (small numbers) of metastatic disease without the need to present with symptoms associated with that lesion. Accordingly, most radiation oncology departments now have a significant number of patients, who are being treated with a new diagnostic category "localized disease" "oligometastatic disease." These patients may disappear from the schedule if the field of diagnostic pathology expands as predicted to include hundreds of tests to identify a specific tumor that can be treated with a specific drug. Targeting a metastatic lesion in the brain with a drug that will only kill the cells in that tumor would probably be preferable to a radiation therapy approach. Why would this be the case? The answer is toxicity and side effects. Just as radiotherapy replaced surgical excision as a treatment for metastases, so targeted therapies may well replace radiotherapy as a treatment for metastases. If this is the case, then there will be a decreased number of patients requiring therapeutic radiation.

While there were more applicants than the available residency slots during the years 1990–2010, the number of applicants has been decreasing (What has happened?). Cancer patients have been increasingly treated with new chemotherapy or target agents (Table 20.1). The number of medical students, who apply each year for residency slots in radiation oncology (usually 190–220 residency slots per year) and during the decades 1990, 2000, 2010, there were more applicants than available slots, but the number of applicants is now decreasing (Table 20.2). The number of slots was designed to replace the retiring physicians (5000 practicing radiation oncologists in the USA and assuming that 200 retire per year) with an equal number of new graduates, plus more based upon the estimated workforce needs [2]. The American Board of Radiation Oncology usually determines the workforce needs for the specialty. Their determination is based upon several factors including the estimated number of cancer patients in the coming years, who will be candidates for or require radiotherapy. One determination suggested that there was a decreased need for radiotherapy for breast and prostate cancer patients due to more patients choosing surgery, hormone ablation, or chemotherapy only [4]. The reasons would be outweighed by the need for more radiotherapy for patients with head and neck and lung cancer [2, 3]. The current estimate is based on a clear increased need for stereotactic radiosurgery to treat metastasis and then would increase the need for more radiation oncologists [5]. The specialty of radiation oncology was popular for medical students in past decades. It is still popular for those, who are interested in physics and mathematics, but overall fewer are interested.

Radiation oncology is a separate specialty of medicine, which evolved from the specialty of diagnostic radiology around 1965 [6, 7]. Since the specialty of radiation oncology was declared to be independent and separate with its own Board of Registration, and its own continuing medical education activities, it has always been dependent upon collaboration with surgeons and medical oncologists (internal medicine physicians, who have completed fellowships in the subspecialties of either oncology and/or hematology, both of which train physicians to safety deliver chemotherapy drugs and other new systemic cancer-targeted therapies).

The radiation oncology specialty has also evolved as a robust collaboration and dependence upon the corporate vendors, who build radiation therapy machines (linear accelerators and other supportive equipment including patient immobilization devices and computer hardware and software products that have been continually improving). There is an increasing precision of treatment planning software for radiation dose delivery to smaller volumes. During the years following 1990, radiation oncology, as a technical specialty, has exploded on the medical scene as a critical component in the multimodality management of cancer patients (Table 20.1), so why are not more medical students applying for residencies?

It is important to reflect on the history of the specialty to understand its current decreasing popularity among medical students before making any predictions about its future.

Since the 1970s, there was the voiced concern by some medical students that they did not want to plan for a career in this specialty, because of several prominent concerns (Table 20.2): (1) There would soon be no more cancer patients for them to treat, since basic research had discovered what was believed to be the cancer virus in mice, and the virus in humans was just around the corner (this concern dissipated by 1985). Early diagnosis and prevention were progressing rapidly; (2) a concern and in some cases fear of the hazard of their own cumulative radiation exposure; (3) the real advances in cancer patient management would be made by medical subspecialists in oncology and hematology with the coming of new targeted therapies and immunotherapy including genetic engineering; and (4) lack of available jobs (Table 20.2). These concerns are still voiced by medical students, but do not explain every year why fewer are choosing this specialty for their resident training. Another concern is the relative decrease in physician/scientists, or individuals, who chose to stay in academic careers including radiobiology research.

Radiation therapy was first used to treat cancer at the turn of the twentieth century. As described in a previous chapter in this book, radium sources were placed into a tumor mass, and the tumor was observed to shrink in size. This first clinical use of radiation-emitting sources also led to the first description of the side effects of irradiation for normal tissues. The first use of the Roentgen ray (X-ray machine) to treat cancer was reported in a patient in Chicago, Illinois, who received external beam radiation through a diagnostic X-ray machine (Kilovoltage emitting machine) for an enlarged spleen [18]. The spleen was observed to shrink in size and the patient had fewer symptoms and felt better. Radium source implants for treating gynecologic cancers and head and neck cancers came into use in many patients beginning in the late 1930s [8]. Of interest, the relative use of radiotherapy on those patients has not decreased (Table 20.1).

Orthovoltage radiation machines gave way to the use of Cobalt 60 teletherapy of the first Cobalt machine having been developed in Saskatchewan, Alberta, Canada. Then, around 1965, the first linear accelerators were developed [9]. By 1974, linear accelerators produced by companies such as Varian, Siemens, Thompson, Sagitaire, Elekta, and others developed sophisticated machines to deliver each of a multiple available spectrum of photon and electron energies each, which provided radiation oncologists with the ability to tailor a radiation dose to specific tissues and at specific depths, and locations within the body [10]. The Cobalt 60 machine delivered a 1.0 megavoltage energy gamma irradiation radiation beam, which had a penumbra [11], or blurred margin. The penumbra was attributable to the relatively large Cobalt source, which had to be replaced periodically, as the isotope decayed and the dose rate of production of gamma rays decreased.

The relative size of the Cobalt 60 radioisotope source in the machine produced a beam with margins that were not precise. To make the field edges more precise, the radiation beam/edge was collimated, which was carried out by attaching a device to the head of the machine at a distance from the unit-called a teletherapy machine, which did remove the penumbra effect, but which itself caused production of electrons when the gamma ray beam hit the metal in this device. The electrons due to their relatively superficial deposit in the patient caused skin irritation and in a sense obviated the advantage of the 1.0 megavoltage Cobalt gamma ray energy, which had the advantage of a superior depth dose compared to the then standard orthovoltage X-ray machines [18]. The orthovoltage X-ray machines we designed to take diagnostic X-rays over seconds of exposure not to be left open for minutes to deliver 100–200 Roentgens (rads, centigray) to a tumor masses [18]. These orthovoltage machines cause skin burns. Not surprisingly, these patients presenting in the 1970s remembered when their parents or grandparents had radiotherapy delivered by this machine and had experienced skin burns during their treatments [18], particularly, those patients, who experienced chest wall radiation skin acute moist desquamation (weeping skin lesions) and later radiation fibrosis (scarring) [18].

Once linear accelerators replaced Cobalt 60 machines, their point source and multileaf collimators eliminated the issue of skin burns. These linear accelerators had the ability to shape the radiation beam. The use of individually cut divergent-beam (sloped) blocks that were attached to the linear accelerator beam head could shape the beam. The divergent lead blocks or Sarband-heavy metal blocks [19] did not produce electrons, and patients did not experience skin burns. Once heavy metal multileaf collimators were placed inside the collimator head, these provided even more precise collimated delivery of the radiation beams [19, 43]. Furthermore, the multileaf collimator eliminated the need for heavy block trays that had to be inserted into the linear accelerator for each different treatment field. Radiation oncology residents in the 1970s observed all these changes in the equipment and enjoyed the improved outcomes for their patients.

Evolution and improvement in technologies of Radiation Oncology led to an accelerated pace in the years leading up to and following the turn to the twenty-first century. Over the same time improved chemotherapy regimens for adult and pediatric patients were becoming available and either alone or combined with reduced radiation doses cured patients [30]. High-energy photon beams and electron beams, which were the center stage of advertisements for new technology, were replaced by the availability of gamma knife radiosurgery by delivery of up to 200 pencil size diameter Cobalt 60 beams to precise areas deep in the brain in immobilized patients [20], and the linear accelerator-based stereotactic radiosurgery, which followed the technology of Cobalt 60. Stereotactic radiation therapy (SBRT) and stereotactic ablative radiation therapy (SABR) [5] became an independent subspecialty within radiation oncology. Radiation Oncology residents were trained to use this modality to deliver a lower number of high-dose fractions to very small areas in close proximity to critical tissues, while limiting toxicity. This was an exciting time for the specialty, and there were increased numbers of medical students applying to enter the field.

During the final decade of the twentieth century and first decades of the twenty-first century, new modalities arrived on the scene. Proton therapy units were provided to large medical centers and private medical facilities. The high cost of multigantry (multiple rooms) to deliver proton beams, which were generated by cyclotron in a distant location, was prohibitively expensive for many cancer treatment centers, leading to the development of single gantry proton machines. While comparative clinical trials had not yet established the superiority of proton beams, it seemed that every hospital still wanted a proton unit. The precise delivery of radiation deep in tissues through the use of the Bragg peak of physics led to proliferation of proton units [22]. Carbon ion high LET radiation therapy devices [23] became available for even more precise deep tissue deposition of radiation. Neutron beam machines, while tested in several facilities (notably Seattle, Washington) in a group using pi-meson radiotherapy at Los-Alamos, also achieved a clinical presence [24]. There was limited use of pi-mesons [25] and multiple machines were not produced nor widely used [22]. Of interest, these new machines produced for cancer therapy often involve the same kinds of radiation that have been described in prior chapters, as problematic for space travel and developing countermeasures for radiation terrorism (proton, high LET (linear energy transfer) components of GCR, and neutrons). Also, of interest is the production of unwanted forms of irradiation by inpatient delivery devices: X-ray shields near the patient skin produce electrons and high-energy photons hitting the collimator produce neutrons. Why have not more medical students with interest in physics been motivated to enter radiation oncology residencies?

The most recent technology has been the development of FLASH delivery systems [27, 28], which can provide very large doses in the range of 50–100 Gy in a fraction of a second. This technology is based on the developing biologic concepts that tumor cells cannot repair FLASH dose rates damage, while normal tissues can. The molecular mechanism of this hypothesis is yet to be tested and proven [28].

In the field of brachytherapy (implantation of radiation sources into tumors), radium was replaced by Cesium, as the preferred radioisotope for brachytherapy (Table 20.1). Furthermore, the low dose rate delivery systems developed early in the twentieth century were replaced with high dose rate after-loader technology, such that a patient could be brought to the radiation oncology department, receive high-dose brachytherapy, and then returned to a hospital bed that did not require radiation safety monitoring, since radiation sources were not in the patient [25]. Radioactive seed implantation (permanent implants with rapidly decaying isotopes) was developed for treatment of prostate cancer and other tumors. The technology continues to develop and the volume of patients requiring the treatment has remained stable (Table 20.1).

With all the technology-driven improvements in the field of radiation oncology, it is critical to evaluate the leading standard of care for cancer patients. Since radiation oncology, as a specialty, remains totally dependent on the clinical need for localized delivery of radiation therapy for patient management, the field is dependent upon collaborations with surgeons and medical oncologists. There are exceptions for the need: (1) radiotherapy for Hodgkin's disease and (2) the use of total body irradiation (TBI) to prepare patients for a donor bone marrow transplantation. The use of effective chemotherapy replaced radiotherapy to the management of Hodgkin's disease patients. Other drugs, such as busulfan and cytoxan, have replaced the use of TBI in many bone marrow transplant programs (Table 20.1). The lung toxicity of TBI that was used to reduce cancer cell numbers before marrow transplant could be replaced by chemotherapy. Many treatment facilities employed transmission blocks to reduce lung dose; however, the reduced lung dose in some cases also reduced the removal of cancer cells or leukemia cells that reside in the spinal vertebrae or rib bone marrow [31] and also reduced the removal clearance of the patient's own bone marrow to clear space for engraftment of the donor bone marrow cells [31].

Radiation Therapy Is Being Utilized in a Decreasing Number of Some, but Not All Categories of Cancer Patients

If one observes the clinical use of radiation oncology techniques to treat cancer, the history can be divided into three segments: the Orthovoltage era from 1900 to 1960, the Cobalt 60 era from 1960 to 1974, and the Linear Accelerator era from 1974 to the present.

One could add a fourth era by subdividing the linear accelerator era into the recent proton, high LET, FLASH era, or the new development era. The subdivision is interesting; however, an argument can be made that all external beam radiation therapy, whether by linear accelerator, proton, high LET carbon ion, or FLASH irradiation is a continuum of the same specialty and should not be separated. Rather there are simply improvements in technology. The dominant use of radiation therapy in the treatment of cancer over the years 1970 to the present has been accompanied by publications of a plethora of clinical protocols, randomized perspective clinical trials, and numerous new studies validating the more limited and ever decreasing dose or eliminating the use of radiation therapy in patient management. Why is this trend continuing? One reason is the increasing evidence of deleterious side effects of radiotherapy in cured patients [32, 33]. The other reason is the clear availability of an increasing number of highly effective target therapies for fusion genes and oncogenes and immunotherapy such as CAR-T cell therapy or immune checkpoint inhibitors.

The reasons for the decreased use of radiation therapy in patient management are complex and disease-specific (Table 20.1). While the number of patients referred to see a radiation oncologist may not have decreased due to the advent of SABR and SBRT treatments of metastasis (Table 20.1), the relative number of patients treated on curative protocols is decreasing in all uses of radiotherapy the exception of gynecologic cancers and head and neck cancers (Table 20.1).

Nearly every other major cancer category has observed a decrease in the use of external beam radiotherapy for "curative" intent.

There remains a significant need for radiation therapy for palliation of symptoms from recurrent cancers and for the use of stereotactic radiosurgery for patients with metastatic disease. In current radiation oncology departments, the majority of patients on treatment in many cancer treatment facilities are those in the category of curative treatment for head and neck cancer or gynecologic cancers or for stereotactic radiation for either palliation or treatment of metastatic disease.

Why Is There a Predicted Decrease in the Need for Radiation Therapy and Radiation Oncologists?

There is a complex evolution of clinical data from three sources that leads to the conclusion that radiation oncology will be used in a decreasing number of cancer patients in the future (Table 20.2). There are three major categories for this conclusion: (1) an appreciation of the side effects of radiation therapy and that higher doses do not necessarily lead to more cures or improved outcomes [29, 30]; (2) the availability of better combination chemotherapy regimen and now targeted therapies based on genetic evaluation of tumors leads to a better outcome in cancer patients than that found in previous decades; and (3) multiple techniques are now available to manage palliative control of recurrent or metastatic disease including many surgical approaches that are minimally invasive, such as photodynamic therapy, ultrasound radio-ablation without the need to worry about radiation late effects [31–35].

The Changing Landscape of Overall Cancer Patient Management

The first chemotherapy drugs were developed based on an anti-metabolism concept. Sidney Farber understood that folate metabolism of all cells including tumor cells was required for DNA repair [26]. Folate was a key component of the DNA synthetic mechanism and involved in the generation of the bases required for assembly of DNA. Dr. Farber reasoned that the concept of an anti-folate could be used to attack the increased metabolic rate of cancer. First experiments in clinical use in patients with leukemia tested aminopterin, methotrexate, as a drug to treat lymphocytic leukemia in children [12]. Excellent results led to the development of other anti-metabolism drugs including 6-mercaptopurine, as another approach to anti-metabolic effects of attacking the pyrimidines and purine components of DNA [12].

Combination chemotherapy then followed by observing the toxicities of each chemotherapy drug and allowing the body's response to one drug, which might lead to suppression of bone marrow cell counts as a side effect, to resolve, and then add a second drug, which might have had a toxicity for the nervous system or the skin, but not the bone marrow. The first combination chemotherapy regimen was the VAMP regimen developed by William C. Moloney and colleagues [13], followed shortly by the MOPP chemotherapy regimen developed by Vincent Divita, George Canellos, and others at the National Institutes of Health [14]. Combination chemotherapy became the standard of care in the 1970s and was observed to have wide ranging effects on bulky tumor masses as well as microscopic metastatic disease. The use of combination chemotherapy in lymphoma and both Hodgkin's, and non-Hodgkin's lymphoma led to the rapid decrease in use of mantle/periaortic/pelvic irradiation for lymphoma patients in the 1970s and 1980s.

Another major discovery, combination chemotherapy, the CMF (cyclophosphamide, methotrexate, F-fluorouracil) regimen, developed in Italy became the standard of care for breast cancer patients to be treated prospectively after the removal of the primary tumor and identification of metastatic lymph nodes in the axilla, mediastinum, or supraclavicular region. Another effective combination chemotherapy regimen for breast cancer patients was the Cooper regimen [15]. Both of these chemotherapy approaches heralded the development of prospective randomized clinical trials in which radiotherapy was either randomized to be decreased or eliminated.

If one looks at the number of patients on treatment in most academic and private practice radiation oncology departments in the 1970s, a majority of patients would have been those with Hodgkin's disease/lymphoma, lung cancer, head and neck cancer, and others with breast cancer, or metastatic cancer. As the number of patients in these categories decreased over the coming decades, but there was still use of radiation therapy for patients with head and neck cancer and gynecologic cancer with both breast cancer and prostate cancers [36], surgeons and urologists continued to dominate the treatment strategies until the 1980s with patient awareness demanding alternative to aggressive surgery for everyone. The reason for the increase in the use of radiotherapy at this time was based on the observed complications of attempted curative resection for head and neck cancers with positive nodes in one case, and the standard use of prostatectomy in the latter case. Patients were often not referred to radiation oncologists for the consideration of use of radiotherapy only if surgery was not possible due to comorbid disease or anesthesia risk. Only after a limited number of prospective randomized clinical trials showed an equal effectiveness of curative radiotherapy in prostate and breast cancer did more patients receive radiotherapy. Now, in the 2020s, there are more patients with breast and prostate cancer electing observation rather than treatment. This choice is based on new molecular tools to characterize the likelihood of severity or recurrence. As the evolution of techniques in cancer management evolved, there were changes in radiotherapy for head and neck cancer and prostate cancer leading to reduced toxicity.

The decreased use of radiotherapy for head and neck cancer was associated with publications of large studies showing that increasing radiation dose did not increase cancer control as well as the availability of better chemotherapy regimens, and targeted therapies, first cetuximab (epidermal growth factor receptor antagonist [16]) and others. Radiotherapy is still used for head and neck cancer in a large number of patients, but the number of treatments has decreased, patient volumes treated has decreased, and with the availability of better systemic therapy, its use is anticipated to decrease further. Head and neck cancer patients have been cured in large numbers, and their availability for study of late effects has been extended to hundreds or thousands of patients in medical centers throughout the world. The Head and Neck Cancer Survivorship Clinics [37, 38] have demonstrated an unequivocal toxicity of late radiation fibrosis in these patients associated with skin and muscle deficits, and profound changes in voice and in swallowing due to radiation fibrosis of laryngeal muscles and pharyngeal constrictor muscles. Thus, there is a clear and unavoidable spectrum of toxicities from radiotherapy for head and neck cancer and this will undoubtedly be taken into account for future clinical protocols. In addition, the decrease in head and neck cancers that are induced by cigarette and tobacco products has been replaced by concern about human papilloma virus (HPV) inducing head and neck cancers [37]. HPV cancers will continue to be controlled by reduced radiation doses [38]. There will be better vaccination and, at present, lower radiation doses have been shown to be as effective as higher doses. A short course of radiation is becoming a mainstay of clinical protocols. Patients do not like coming in for radiotherapy treatments 5 days a week for 6–7 weeks, and the fraction size of irradiation was thought to require low dose per day and spreading the treatment over 7 weeks. Now with short-course radiotherapy protocols [39] in which higher doses are delivered for fewer numbers of treatments, there are fewer patients on treatment in radiation oncology departments. This is another explanation for the decrease in the use of radiotherapy for head and neck cancer.

With no history of use of radiation therapy for prostate cancer, decades of evaluation of the PSA (prostate specific antigen) biomarker for disease have now allowed an increasing number of patients to be categorized as "low risk," or those, who have had biopsies and evaluation of low Gleason histopathologic score [42], many histopathologic score: intermediate risk, patients to elect not to have radiotherapy or prostatectomy, particularly, if over 70 years of age. Short-course radiotherapy for these patients as well as radioiodine or gadolinium seed implantation has allowed more rapid and efficient treatment of prostate cancer in fewer number of patients with intermediate or high risk. The changing landscape of referral of patients with head and neck cancer and prostate cancer for radiation oncology will undoubtedly continue to evolve.

The decreased use of radiotherapy for lung cancer is quite interesting. In a recent review of current clinical protocols, post-operative radiation for lung cancer showed no increase in survival or disease-free interval, compared to those patients, who received adjuvant chemotherapy alone. In a recent review of patients with advanced stage lung cancer that was marginally operable, pre-operative radiation showed an improvement in disease-free interval and survival only in a subgroup of patients that had N2 disease (severe metastatic disease). More clinical protocols are presenting results that show that post-operative or definitive radiation is required in fewer patients. The increasing number of targeted therapies, based on molecular diagnosis of genetic components in lung cancer, has made available many more systemic therapies, which are not only limiting metastasis, but improve local control. Surgical techniques for limited resection have also improved, and even patients with positive margins can receive adjuvant chemotherapy, and if the current publications are correct, may not need post-operative radiation.

Multiple recent publications have reported the results of clinical trials that were designed to test the hypothesis that increasing the radiation dose for some cancers including lung cancer and esophagus would cure more patients [34, 35]. Dose response relationships have shown no increase in the number of patients with disease-free survival or overall survival by increasing the radiation dose. Julian Rosenman, M.D., once was quoted as saying, "That doses of 90 Gy would be required to control bulky lung cancers [37]." At the time of this statement, there was no available IMRT or Stereotactic Radiosurgery that was widely available, so it was not possible to tailor a radiation field to not exceed a safe dose to the spinal cord and the heart. Once IMRT fields and treatment delivery techniques like VMAT were available, higher treatment doses could be safely delivered. Accordingly, radiation oncologists carried out studies increasing radiation dose.

The RTOG 0617 randomized prospective trial showed that there was no increase in cure in patients receiving 70 Gy compared to 55 Gy. The former dose was toxic to heart and lungs, such that the trial was ended early, because of toxicity. The standard of care for radiation treatment of lung cancer (when it was required) showed no improvement by giving doses over 55–60 Gy. Single treatment facilities confirmed the RTOG report [34, 35]. This principle extended to cancers in other anatomic sites in which it was thought that better treatment planning would allow higher doses and that higher doses would cure more patients [43]. Results in many of these trials are pending.

Decreased Use of Radiotherapy for Lung, Esophagus Cancer

While fewer cases of esophagus cancer are found in most medical centers compared to patients with lung cancer, the same principle holds. A better surgical approach with minimally invasive thoracoscopic or laparoscopic resection has resulted in decreased morbidity from surgical excision. Better diagnosis and detection of positive lymph nodes by PET scanning have allowed surgeons to identify positive nodes before resection. Anastomosis at most surgical centers has shown to residual disease at the anastomotic line. Therefore, post-operative adjuvant radiotherapy was tested in a multitude of clinical trials. These patients received adjuvant chemotherapy with or without irradiation. The most recent clinical trials show no significant advantage of adding irradiation to these effective chemotherapy regimens. One prominent study with esophagus cancer confirmed that, as with lung cancer, higher doses did not improve survival in the setting of pre-operative radiotherapy administration before esophagectomy [38].

Use of Radiation Therapy for Abdominal Cancers Including Pancreas Cancer, Liver Cancer, Colorectal Cancer, Bladder Cancer, and Pelvic Malignancies

Protocols are underway to evaluate the use of post-operative radiotherapy in all of these disease categories. One principle is that randomized prospective trials in which chemotherapy is supplemented with radiotherapy for example with ovarian cancer often show no effect of adding the radiotherapy [39].

Brain Tumor Radiotherapy

Protocols using pre-operative radiotherapy for glioblastoma or other CNS malignancies are currently underway.

Pediatric Radiotherapy

There is a decreasing use of radiation in all pediatric patients. In those places, where it is still used such as Wilm's tumor, pediatric lymphoma, wings sarcoma, osteogenic sarcoma, medulloblastoma and others, decreased radiation dose and fractionation are applied. This is because of the availability of better systemic chemotherapy and the clear evidence that radiation, even in the lowest dose regimens, results in significant late effects.

Radiotherapy for Palliation

This is the mainstay of clinical radiation oncology departments at the present time. Pioneering studies demonstrated that there is a phenomenon of oligometastatic disease [5, 20]. These are patients who have had a curative approach to their cancer and present with multiple, but limited metastasis. Using stereotactic radiosurgery to treat these has now become an accepted and standard of care. The better scanning techniques and follow-up of patients allow diagnosis of metastatic disease prior to development of symptoms. Therefore, delivery of SRS, SBRT, or SABR radiation to sites of clinically silent metastatic disease has become a standard. Patients can survive years or decades with a diagnosis of metastasis by the use of SRS and SABR. This is an exciting time in radiation oncology and will lead to a generation of trained radiation oncologists with expertise in this modality. However, the availability of better chemotherapy and better techniques for extending the disease-free interval and cure of patients will make it unnecessary to use proactive stereotactic radiosurgery everywhere. If patients develop symptoms, there are other ways to treat metastatic disease including surgical resection (if morbidity is low), radiofrequency ablation, and photodynamic therapy. Randomized prospective clinical trials comparing these different modalities for palliation are in progress and may lead to yet another decrease (or increase) in the use of radiation therapy for palliation.

Will there be available treatments to limit or prevent radiation late effects? Two competing phenomena are in play. The use of radiotherapy to treat metastatic disease with minimal complications is clear, but there is an increasing concern for late effects of irradiation [27, 28]. The deleterious effects of irradiation are of concern with the side effects of space radiation, environmental exposure from fallout, or radiation emitting weapons and also with the use of radiotherapy in management of cancer patients.

What do medical students know about the future of the specialty of radiation oncology that is limiting and reducing their interest in pursuing a career in this specialty? Some of the reasons that have been voiced at National Meetings that are attended by medical students are listed in Table 20.1 and Table 20.2.

Why do medical students, who also choose a career in radiation oncology not seeking to become physician/scientists? This is a separate question, which applies to nearly all medical specialties. In the current environment of academic medicine, there are two issues: (1) availability of shrinking levels of grant funding for research and (2) work/life balance. The physician scientist does, indeed, have two jobs.

References

1. Lin K, Arya N, Yu NY, et al. 9-year analysis of trends in the radiation oncology residency match. Int J Radiat Oncol Biol Phys. 2022;114(3):e494–5.
2. Srivastava A, Jalink M, de Moraes FY, et al. Tracking the workforce 2020–2030: making the case for a cancer workforce registry. JCO Glob Oncol. 2021;7:925–33. https://doi.org/10.1200/GO.21.00093.
3. Amini A, Luh JY, Bush A, et al. Radiation oncology workforce: supply and demand. J Am Coll Radiol. 2024;30:S1546–440. https://doi.org/10.1016/j.jacr.2024.01.009.
4. Tyldesley S, Delaney G, Foroudi F, et al. Estimating the need for radiotherapy for patients with prostate, breast, and lung cancers: verification of model estimates of need with radiotherapy utilization data from British Columbia. Int J Radiat Oncol Biol Phys. 2011;79(5):1507–15. https://doi.org/10.1016/j.ijrobp.2009.12.070.

5. Folkert MR, Timmerman RD. Stereotactic ablative body radiosurgery (SABR) or stereotactic body radiation therapy (SBRT). Adv Drug Deliv Rev. 2017;109:3–14. https://doi.org/10.1016/j.addr.2016.11.005.
6. Fletcher GH. Regaud lecture perspectives on the history of radiotherapy. Radiother Oncol. 1988;12(4):iii–v, 253–71.
7. Thariat J, Hannoun-Levi J-M, Myint AS, et al. Past, present, and future of radiotherapy for the benefit of patients. Nat Rev Clin Oncol. 2013;10(1):52–60. https://doi.org/10.1038/nrclinonc.2012.203.
8. Skowronek J. Current status of brachytherapy in cancer treatment—short overview. J Contemp Brachytherapy. 2017;9(6):581–9. https://doi.org/10.5114/jcb.2017.72607.
9. Thwaites DI, Tuohy JB. Back to the future: the history and development of the clinical linear accelerator. Phys Med Biol. 2006;51(13):R343–62. https://doi.org/10.1088/0031-9155/51/13/R20.
10. Hussein M, Heijen BJM, Verellen D, et al. Automation in intensity modulated radiotherapy treatment planning—a review of recent innovations. Br J Radiol. 2018;91(1092):20180270. https://doi.org/10.1259/bjr.20180270.
11. Warrington J, Adams L. Cobalt 60 teletherapy for cancer: a revived treatment modality for the 21st century. Paper presented at: IEEE Seminar on Appropriate Medical Technology for Developing Countries. 2002.
12. Goldman B. Multidrug resistance: can new drugs help chemotherapy score against cancer? J Natl Cancer Inst. 2003;95(4):255–7. https://doi.org/10.1093/jnci/95.4.255.
13. Raje N, Powles R, Kulkarni S, et al. A comparison of vincristine and doxorubicin infusional chemotherapy with methylprednisolone (VAMP) with the addition of weekly cyclophosphamide (C-VAMP) as induction treatment followed by autografting in previously untreated myeloma. Br J Haematol. 1997;97(1):153–60. https://doi.org/10.1046/j.1365-2141.1997.d01-2122.x.
14. van Eys J, Cangir A, Coody D, et al. MOPP regimen as primary chemotherapy for brain tumors in infants. N Neurooncol. 1985;3(3):237–43. https://doi.org/10.1007/BF00165184.
15. A'Hern RP, Smith JE, Ebbs SR. Chemotherapy and survival in advanced breast cancer: the inclusion of doxorubicin in Cooper type regimens. Br J Cancer. 1993;67(4):801–5. https://doi.org/10.1038/bjc.1993.146.
16. Van Cutsem E, Kohne C-H, Hitre E, et al. Cetuximab and chemotherapy as initial treatment for metastatic colorectal cancer. N Engl J Med. 2009;360(14):1408–17. https://doi.org/10.1056/NEJMoa0805019.
17. Darrar AS, Mahmoud RMM, Ezzel-Din MR, et al. Risk assessment for occupational potential exposure at cobalt teletherapy units. J Radiat Res Appl Sci. 2019;12(1):140–6.
18. Bell BI, Vercellino J, Brodin NP, et al. Orthovoltage x-rays exhibit increased efficacy compared with γ-rays in preclinical irradiation. Cancer Res. 2022;82(15):2678–91. https://doi.org/10.1158/0008-5472.CAN-22-0656.
19. Butson MJ, Cheung T, Yu PKN. Calculation of electron contamination doses produced using blocking trays for 6 MV x-rays. Radiat Meas. 2002;35(2):99–102.
20. Lunsford LD, Flickinger J, Coffey RJ. Stereotactic gamma knife radiosurgery. Initial North American experience in 207 patients. Arch Neurol. 1990;47(2):169–75. https://doi.org/10.1001/archneur.1990.00530020071018.
21. Solda F, Lodge M, Ashley S, et al. Stereotactic radiotherapy (SABR) for the treatment of primary non-small cell lung cancer; systematic review and comparison with a surgical cohort. Radiother Oncol. 2013;109(1):1–7. https://doi.org/10.1016/j.radonc.2013.09.006.
22. Lomax A. Intensity modulation methods for proton radiotherapy. Phys Med Biol. 1999;44(1):185–205. https://doi.org/10.1088/0031-9155/44/1/014.
23. Tsujii H, Kamada T. A review of update clinical results of carbon ion radiotherapy. Jpn J Clin Oncol. 2012;42(8):670–85. https://doi.org/10.1093/jjco/hys104.
24. Broerse JJ, Battermann JJ. Fast neutron radiotherapy: for equal or for better? Med Phys. 1981;8(6):751–60. https://doi.org/10.1118/1.594851.

25. Yuhas JM, Li AP, Kligerman MM. Present status of the proposed use of negative Pi mesons in radiotherapy. Adv Radiat Biol. 1979;8:51–83.
26. Hashkes PJ, Becker ML, Cabral DA, et al. Methotrexate: new uses for an old drug. J Pediatr. 2014;164(2):231–6. https://doi.org/10.1016/j.jpeds.2013.10.029.
27. Lin B, Gao F, Yang Y, et al. FLASH radiotherapy: history and future. Front Oncol. 2021;11:644400. https://doi.org/10.3389/fonc.2021.644400.
28. Bourhis J, Montay-Gruel P, Jorge PG, et al. Clinical translation of FLASH radiotherapy: why and how? Radiother Oncol. 2019;139:11–7. https://doi.org/10.1016/j.radonc.2019.04.008.
29. Malviya VK, Han I, Deppe G, et al. High-dose-rate afterloading brachytherapy, external radiation therapy, and combination chemotherapy in poor-prognosis cancer of the cervix. Gynecol Oncol. 1991;42(3):233–8. https://doi.org/10.1016/0090-8258(91)90351-5.
30. Horton TM, Sposto R, Brown P, et al. Toxicity assessments of molecularly targeted drugs incorporated into multiagent chemotherapy regimens for pediatric acute lymphocytic leukemia (ALL): review from an international consensus conference. Pediatr Blood Cancer. 2010;54(7):872–8. https://doi.org/10.1002/pbc.22414.
31. Wong JYC, Filippi AR, Dabaja BS, et al. Total body irradiation: guidelines from the International Lymphoma Radiation Oncology Group (ILROG). Int J Radiat Oncol Biol Phys. 2018;101(3):521–9. https://doi.org/10.1016/j.ijrobp.2018.04.071.
32. Ortigara GB, Bonzanini LIL, Schulz RE, et al. Late radiation effects in survivors of head and neck cancer: state of the science. Crit Rev Oncol Hematol. 2021;162:103335. https://doi.org/10.1016/j.critrevonc.2021.103335.
33. Cooper JS, Fu K, Marks J, et al. Late effects of radiation therapy in the head and neck region. Int J Radiat Oncol Biol Phys. 1995;31(5):1141–64. https://doi.org/10.1016/0360-3016(94)00421-G.
34. Bernard ME, Glaser SM, Gill BS, et al. Results of a single institution experience with dose-escalated chemoradiation for locally advanced unresectable non-small cell lung cancer. Front Oncol. 2017;7:1. https://doi.org/10.3389/fonc.2017.00001.
35. Cox JD. Are the results of RTOG 0617 mysterious? Int J Radiat Oncol Biol Phys. 2012;82(3):1042–4. https://doi.org/10.1016/j.ijrobp.2011.12.032.
36. Kupelian PA, Willoughby TR. Short-course, intensity-modulated radiotherapy for localized prostate cancer. Cancer J. 2001;7(5):421–6.
37. Rosenman JG, Halle JS, Socinski MA, et al. High-dose conformal radiotherapy for treatment of stage IIIA/IIIB non-small-cell lung cancer: technical issues and results of a phase I/II trial. Int J Radiat Oncol Biol Phys. 2002;54(2):348–56. https://doi.org/10.1016/s0360-3016(02)02958-9.
38. DeFoe SG, Pennathur A, Flickinger JC, et al. Retrospective review of patients with locally advanced esophageal cancer treated at the University of Pittsburgh. Am J Clin Oncol. 2011;34(6):587–92. https://doi.org/10.1097/COC.0b013e3181f942af.
39. Iorio GC, Martini S, Arcadipane F, et al. The role of radiotherapy in epithelial ovarian cancer: a literature overview. Med Oncol. 2019;36(7):64. https://doi.org/10.1007/s12032-019-1287-8.
40. Maxwell JH, Grandis JR, Ferris RL. HPV-associated head and neck cancer: unique features of epidemiology and clinical management. Annu Rev Med. 2016;67:91–101. https://doi.org/10.1146/annurev-med-051914-021907.
41. Chaturvedi AK. Epidemiology and clinical aspects of HPV in head and neck cancers. Head Neck Pathol. 2012;6(Suppl 1):S16–24. https://doi.org/10.1007/s12105-012-0377-0.
42. Partin AW, Yoo J, Carter HB, et al. The use of prostate specific antigen, clinical stage and Gleason score to predict pathological stage in men with localized prostate cancer. J Urol. 1993;150(1):110–4. https://doi.org/10.1016/s0022-5347(17)35410-1.
43. LoSasso T, Chui CS, Kutcher GJ, et al. The use of a multi-leaf collimator for conformal radiotherapy of carcinomas of the prostate and nasopharynx. Int J Radiat Oncol Biol Phys. 1993;25(2):161–70. https://doi.org/10.1016/0360-3016(93)90337-u.

Epilogue

While it is difficult to predict the future, particularly, at this point in 2024 with all the geopolitical challenges that face the United States and the world, there are a number of factors, which will undoubtedly affect the future of Radiation Oncology and Radiation biology.

Regarding Radiation Oncology as a medical specialty, there will be no need for therapeutic radiation once targeted therapies are available for all cancers. Systemic administration of new chemotherapies will control local disease as well as metastatic disease. Surgical biopsy will be required for diagnosis, and in some cases, local excision can be followed by systemic administration of targeted therapies. Chemotherapy drugs in use today have toxicities, but new ones will be less toxic. Late effects of chemotherapy have been established. As fewer cytotoxic drugs are used to treat cancer, and these are replaced with targeted therapies including immune stimulant drugs and agents that are specific for cancer cells, while sparing normal tissue cells, the approach to treating cancer will be entirely different. Furthermore, earlier diagnosis and better surveillance techniques will allow the use of surgical and targeted therapies to be applied earlier. For the current generation of radiation oncologists, the future will be stable, since we are just beginning to see the advent of widespread use of immune checkpoint inhibitors and targeted therapies. Translation of the research discoveries into a clinical protocol takes time and significant investment by the pharmaceutical companies that are producing new drugs will continue.

The medical specialty of Radiation Oncology will be phased out (my opinion); however, Radiation Biology will increase in its scope, importance and intensity of research.

With proliferation of nuclear weapons, breeder reactors, and eventually more nuclear power stations, there will be a need to manage the exposure of people to ionizing irradiation emitting isotopes and consequences of nuclear weapons. As more countries acquire the capacity to construct and purchase nuclear weapons, the possibility of a nation with a nuclear weapon using it increases. The development of radiation countermeasures and management of radiation exposed victims will

J. Greenberger, *Radiation Oncology and Radiation Biology*,
https://doi.org/10.1007/978-3-031-66300-0

require advances in basic radiobiology, including the discovery and development of radiation countermeasures.

It is difficult to predict the future of space radiation biology. While there remains some controversy about the dose estimation from a Mars Mission, there has been an approach to assessing the radiation biology of the estimated levels of exposure. The relative biologic effect of protons, galactic cosmic irradiation (high LET particles), and neutrons generated by GCR hitting the components of the spacecraft has been estimated. NASA and other National and International research organizations. All recognize the need for radiation countermeasures to treat astronauts for prolonged "low level" radiation exposure. There are big questions regarding the long duration space missions. The Artemis Programs of NASA have provided some data on the radiation biology that is both exciting and cautionary.

Artemis 1 produced data on yeast that have been exposed to space radiation with respect to changes in specific genes. Experiments with Salmonella bacteria maintained in an environment of space radiation have demonstrated on return to Earth infectivity levels that have changed. Experiments with Aspergillosis, also exposed to continuous space irradiation, have demonstrated changes in the biology once the organisms are returned to Earth. These experiments have produced data that is in contrast to the slow evolutionary changes in microorganisms described in Chap. 1. Is there something about the complexity of space irradiation that has led to more rapid genetic changes in microorganisms? Will such a complexity of exposure to different components of irradiation affect humans in unexpected ways? The studies with yeast, salmonella, and Aspergillosis have yielded data that is largely attributed to growth in reduced gravity conditions, but the role of radiation exposure in addition to zero gravity must be considered as also possibly relevant. Advances in understanding space irradiation will be accompanied by advances in the development of space vehicles, engines for space travel, fuel considerations for prolonged space missions, and a better understanding of the physiology of reduced gravity, artificial environments, and, above all, the need to find sources of oxygen and water, other than those that can be transported on a space vehicle, or from the result of chemical synthesis alone.

As the need for therapeutic radiation for cancer and he number of radiation oncologists decreases, the knowledge gained from understanding the late effects of radiation therapy in cancer patients will increase. Ths knowledge will be very valuable to apply to an understanding of the radiation biology of the consequences of nuclear weapons and of space travel.

This book has been a combination of two sets of information: review of the literature on many topics related to the medical specialty of Radiation Oncology, and review and predictions about advances and directions in the scientific discipline of Radiation Biology. This book contains my personal recollections from my clinical practice of Radiation Oncology over 55 years. The book also contains information from my experience, scientific publications and recollections from basic science research in my laboratories over the same 55 years at four different academic institutions: Harvard, NIH, UMASS Medical Center, and the Univereity of Pittsburgh. I have enjoyed uninterrupted NIH funding of my radiobiology and stem cell research since 1977, when I completed my Radiation Oncology residency. Having treated cancer patients for 55 years with therapeutic ionizing irradiation, I have watched the changing patterns of care and the evolution of management of cancer patients with combined modality approaches (always involving collaborations with medical oncologists and surgeons). I have also watched the evolution of radiation biology research that has incorporated discoveries in basic science including the discovery of reverse transcriptase, the advent of gene cloning, gene therapy, and a clear increase in radiation research which has been directed toward both radiation counter-terrorism, and space radiation. This book represents my personal opinions about the importance of both research publications and my observations regarding the specialty of Radiation Oncology.

Regardless of the future of the medical specialty of Radiation Oncology, I firmly believe that advances in understanding of the acute and prominently the late effects of irradiation in cancer patients will guide research in both the development of radiation countermeasures and realistic approaches to managing space irradiation for future astronauts.

Radiation Oncology as a medical specialty may disappear. One need only look at the landscape of clinical radiation oncology in 1974 that led to today. In 1974, patients with Hodgkin's Lymphoma comprised a dominant fraction of radiotherapy patients in the academic medical centers and in private practice radiation oncology settings. These patients now are primarily treated with combination chemotherapy with limited use of radiation therapy for areas of residual, recurrent, or bulk disease. In the 1970s, there was a concern that not enough radiation dose could be delivered to cancer sites, primarily, due to toxicity to the spinal cord and other sensitive structures. This conclusion led to the development of sophisticated modifications in linear accelerator designs, use of multi-leaf collimators to precisely define small target volumes, immobilization devices for patients, and new radiation beams including protons, and, most importantly, ways to deliver very high doses in a small number of treatment fractions to treat metastatic disease. Regarding radiation dose, the new technologies have facilitated the testing of the hypothesis that giving more irradiation would cure more patients. In the 1990s, with the availability of new technologies, patients with lung cancer could receive doses delivered to the cancer that were 20 to 30% higher than that, which was safely possible in the 1970s. Large published clinical outcome analyses revealed that with lung cancer as well as with many other cancers, higher doses were not more effective. In fact, these studies, some of which were terminated early, because of toxicity at the higher doses, revealed significant late effects of irradiation that had not been appreciated previously. De-escalation protocols are now prominent with respect to combined modality management of head and neck cancer, lung cancer, esophagus cancer, and many others. There is a clear desire to eliminate radiotherapy entirely from pediatric patients, as dose de-escalation protocols continue to dominate the literature. The last 15 years have seen an increase in discovery of specific gene translocations, and molecular analysis of individual tumors leading to the use of new targeted systemic therapies that are specific for individual patients. This "personalized medicine" approach to treating cancer patients has been of great benefit to the patients themselves, but also highlights the need to reduce radiation doses or to eliminate radiation. What will happen to the specialty of Radiation Oncology?

The specialty of Radiation Oncology evolved from Diagnostic Radiology and became a separate Specialty in the 1960s. There was then consensus that the use of X-ray machines to diagnose diseases and Cancer in particular would be necessary for al long time. This prediction has become fact. Diagnostic radiologists now have at their disposal new techniques including computerized axial tomography (CAT-scans), magnetic resonance imaging (MRI scans), and fusion techniques to present three-dimensional images to physicians, so they can better analyze the extent of cancer and metastatic disease. New tracer scanning techniques will replace FDG glucose targeting with positron emission tomography (PET-scan) and facilitate better diagnosis with less radiation exposure. Diagnostic Radiology has been a powerful component in the management of cancer patients as well as in all clinical diseases. Diagnostic radiologists are dynamic physicians. As one technical modality is replaced by a better one, diagnostic radiologists haved adapted an moved on, A good example is the replacement of laminography with CAT-scanning. The primitive slices of laminograms, which changed the focal point in imaging of, for example lung, has been replaced by three-dimensional CAT-scanning, but diagnostic radiologists still are involved in the process of diagnosis. Another example is the elimination of the pneumoencephalogram, in which air was injected into the cerebral spinal fluid to image the aqueducts and ventricles in the brain for CSF (cerebral spinal fluid) transport through the brain. The pneumoencephalogram was also by CAT-scanning and contrast-enhanced imaging. Central to all of these advances in Diagnostic Radiology has been the development of the ways to decrease radiation dose, such as using image intensifier screens and amplification techniques to limit radiation exposure to patients as they go through a diagnostic workup. In contrast to the expected continued need for Diagnostic radiology, Radiation Oncology, has evolved in a different direction. Radiation Oncologists have changed their mandate to deliver theraputic radiation to fewer patients and for fewer and more specific indications. Stereotactic radiosurgery, radiation ablative techniques, such as SABR, and new research in FLASH irradiation have all been designed to specifically target wither smaller volumes of tissue or exploit the different radiobiology of cancer compared to normal tissue. There is a mandate to deliver fewer radiation treatments and to reduced volumes. There is now clear evidence that higher radiation are not necessary for large tumor volumes and there are limits with small volumes as well.

The best prediction of the future of the specialty of Radiation Oncology is that concluded by medical students. Young people enter medical school with the motivation to help patients, to heal them, and to exploit the principle of "First do no harm," which happily still motivates the majority of medical students. In recent years, fewer medical students choose Radiation Oncology residencies.

The three areas of this book: Clinical Radiotherapy, Radiation Countermeasures Against a Nuclear Weapon or Nuclear Power Plant Accidents, and Space Irradiation when linked together emphasize the importance of ionizing irradiation in human existence. Ionizing irradiation is a consequence of the creation of the universe, and, specifically, the creation of life on Earth Billions of years of evolution of the different species on Earth have led to accumulation genes that both protect and limit evolution, Space irradiation and, specifically, the continuous exposure of humans outside the protective Magnetosphere around the Earth presents a challenge to the vulnerability of humans entering this foreign environment. There is increasing recognition of the importance of ionizing irradiation when preparing for the reality of future space missions.

Unfortunately, the historical events, which led to the end of World War II included the creation of a nuclear fission bomb deployment on the battlefield. A new era began with focus on understanding the hazards of ionizing irradiation. Nuclear power station accidents led to radioisotope dispersal and required the creation of an entirely new research field called "Radiation Countermeasures." With the current availability of nuclear weapons, the Earth has become a dangerous place. With understanding of the hazards of galactic cosmic irradiation, solar proton events, and generation of neutrons in a spacecraft by contact with GCR life outside the Earth may also become dangerous. Humans are particularly skilled in adaptation and improving environments. There is no doubt that we as a species will conquer and overcome all of these challenges of living with ionizing irradiation. What does radiobiology have to do with clinical radiotherapy? It is a paradox and counter-intuitive that ionizing irradiation induces cancer but has been used to treat cancer. The first treatment of patients with the Roentgen ray and implantation of radium sources at the turn of the twentieth century led to design and use of many improved machines and devices that deliver ionizing irradiation to treat cancer. A principle that links clinical radiotherapy with the other two topics of radiation countermeasures and space radiation is the continuing accumulation of knowledge regarding radiation effects on normal tissues: accelerated aging, induction of cancer, and neurocognitive deficits. Radiation Oncologists participate in curing an increasing number of cancer patients. They now must address ways to limit the late effects that radiation induces.

Ionizing irradiation is dangerous; damage caused by it must be ameliorated by the development of radiation countermeasures; and if space travel must be facilitated by careful attention to minimize ionizing irradiation effects. Medical students, who choose a career in Radiation Oncology (Radiotherapy, Radiation Medicine) will have in their training a focus on radiobiology and radiation physics. At the completion of residency, most radiation oncologists go on to a career based on patient treatment and the disciplines of radiation biology and physics are handled by other colleagues in their clinical departments. After decades of practicing radiation oncology, it is inevitable that physicians will know about radiation side effects both acute and chronic. The most important part of being a radiation oncologist is the continuing interaction in combined modality protocols with surgeons and medical oncologists. Those who choose to become physician-scientists will have basic science research and/or work in clinical protocols, on a continuing basis and will understand first hand the contning challenges. Radiation oncologists are also aware of the increase in the use of systemic drugs/agents that target cancer cells with less toxicity of chemotherapy. Immunotherapy regimens, targeted therapy, and gene correction protocols will continue to improve patient care. The knowledge about radiation side effects and the hazards of radiation, particularly, in pediatric patients and in situations in which large volumes of tissue must be treated to control cancer, have remained a challenge. One challenge is to decrease the radiation dose, volume of tissue treated, and if possible eliminate radiotherapy. Medical students are aware of the evolution of cancer patient care, and the lack of focus on Radiation Oncology may be one of the reasons why fewer medical students choose this specialty. Will Radiation Oncology continue to be a clinical discipline, and a specialty in medicine? The answer is unknown, but it is essential that medical students choosing this specialty seriously emphasize their first year of PGY1 (medical internship or surgical internship). The basics of patient care will help Radiation Oncologists prepare to be physicians, who one day may not use theraputic radiation. They will still focus on patient care and improving patient outcomes without the need for radiation therapy. At present, it is not clear whether the new technologies for radiation delivery systems will persist, evolve, and become part of the armamentarium for patient care. Modalities such as proton beam radiotherapy, FLASH radiation, radioisotope targeted cancer therapy, and multi-site simultaneous focused targeted treatment of metastasis with radiation, treating multiple sites at the same time may be used for the next decades. It may be decades before cancer is eliminated as a major cause of death. It is likely that the future will hold significant relief of the general population from the need for radiation treatment of cancer and cancer recurrence. One need only look at the history of medicine to realize that prior infectious diseases such as tuberculosis and other bacterial infections were be a major cause of death prior to the advent of antibiotic therapies. Such change in the evolution of patient disease states will undoubtedly occur with cancer. Therefore, planning a career in the management of cancer patients should also include education in general medicine, general surgery, and other disciplines to be important for physicians in the event that Clinical Radiotherapy further decreases, and may even be eliminated as a specialty. This prediction is all my opinion.

Regarding the future development of radiation countermeasures, one need only look at the history of warfare and destructive human behaviors. Prior to nuclear weapons usage in 1945, thousands of victims were killed by the so-called conventional weapons. The fire-bombing of Japan killed as many people as did the nuclear weapons deployed at Hiroshima and Nagasaki. But the concept of radiation countermeasures became a focus of basic research. One can only hope that there will never be a use of nuclear weapons, and that the current development of radiation countermeasures can be applied to other disciplines including prominently their use to protect astronauts from space radiation. As the consequences of the use of nuclear weapons also involved combined injuries, space travel will not only focus on radiation effects, but also on challenges of the potential combined injuries of weightlessness, low oxygen atmosphere, infections and isolation. Will humans be able to live outside of the Earth's environment? The answer is yes, but it will require a huge amount of work. NASA and other space agencies are focusing on the search for water on the Moon, Mars, Europa the moon of Jupiter and other star systems. Humans need water and oxygen. The chemical production of these critical molecules will be achieved and not limited by lack of ingenuity, cost, or means of production. Finding water outside the Earth's environment would be an efficient solution to need and this ghe search for water. Oxygen remains a critical element and, although, the chemistry for producing oxygen is available, the same issues of cost, availability, and production will be prominent. Research on the adaptation of humans to weightlessness has emphasized the importance of changes in human physiology and requirement for gravity, whether basic or artificial to maintain stable physiology. We will solve the issue of space radiation.

The future of both medicine and basic research is bright. The goals of curing cancer and adapting humans to live in a world with the dangers of ionizing irradiation will undoubtedly motivate young physicians and scientists to pursue careers that focus on these challenges and help humanity. I hope that this book has been helpful.

Index

J. Greenberger, *Radiation Oncology and Radiation Biology*,
https://doi.org/10.1007/978-3-031-66300-0

GPSR Compliance

The European Union's (EU) General Product Safety Regulation (GPSR) is a set of rules that requires consumer products to be safe and our obligations to ensure this.

If you have any concerns about our products, you can contact us on ProductSafety@springernature.com

In case Publisher is established outside the EU, the EU authorized representative is:

Springer Nature Customer Service Center GmbH
Europaplatz 3
69115 Heidelberg, Germany

Batch number: 10732076

Printed by Printforce, the Netherlands